AF772141

Public Health and the Pandemic in Colonial Bengal

Public Health and the Pandemic in Colonial Bengal examines the interplay between colonial governance and public health crises by focusing on the effects of the 1918–19 Spanish Influenza pandemic in Bengal.

During the time of the pandemic, Bengal was a region of stark contrasts—rich in culture and intellectual thought yet marred by deep social and economic disparities. The outbreak of Spanish Influenza coincided with a turbulent period in Bengal's history. The region was not only grappling with the effects of World War I and the challenges of colonial rule but also undergoing significant political and social changes. The pandemic added a complex layer to this already dynamic historical context. Based on archival material, newspapers, and public health records, the book unveils how colonial authorities tried to suppress the crisis and how local communities protested against colonial brutality. With a unique emphasis on the context of colonial Bengal, the author highlights the socio-economic disparities exacerbated by colonial rule.

The study contributes to the broader discourse on health crises in colonial settings, offering insights into the historical roots of public health in India. It provides essential insights into the medical, social, and economic reactions to both current and future health emergencies and will be of interest to researchers in the fields of history, including medical history, public health, sociology and medical anthropology, and political science and law.

Saumitra Basu is an independent researcher in the history of science and history of medicine. He has successfully completed three projects on the history of science as a (postdoctoral) research associate in the Indian National Science Academy (INSA), New Delhi. He is the recipient of different national and international fellowships, including Visiting Fellowship at the Oxford Institute of Ageing, Oxford, UK.

Routledge Studies in the Modern History of Asia

197. Winning Vietnam's Hearts and Minds during the Vietnam War (1954–1975)
Chosen Glories
Hai-Chung Pham

198. A History of the 1957 Federation of Malaya Constitution
Joseph M. Fernando

199. US-China Naval Co-operation Against the Soviet Union
Carter's Navy
Bruce A. EllemanPark Yu-Ha

200. Alternative Histories of Development in Japan and East Asia
Unthinking Modernization, Recreating Lifeworlds
Edited by Timothy Amos, Akiko Ishii, and Samson Lim

201. Brunei and the British in the Nineteenth Century
Of a Seer-poet, an Adventurer, and the near extinction of an Ancient Malay Sultanate
Ooi Keat Gin

202. Projecting British Ideas on Post-War Japan
Propaganda, Cultural Exchange and Overseas Information Policy, 1945–1975
Yoshiomi Saito

203. Public Health and the Pandemic in Colonial Bengal
An Analysis of the Spanish Influenza (1918–1920)
Saumitra Basu

For a full list of available titles please visit: https://www.routledge.com/Routledge-Studies-in-the-Modern-History-of-Asia/book-series/MODHISTASIA

Public Health and the Pandemic in Colonial Bengal

An Analysis of the Spanish Influenza (1918–1920)

Saumitra Basu

Routledge
Taylor & Francis Group
LONDON AND NEW YORK

First published 2026
by Routledge
4 Park Square, Milton Park, Abingdon, Oxon OX14 4RN

and by Routledge
605 Third Avenue, New York, NY 10158

Routledge is an imprint of the Taylor & Francis Group, an informa business

© 2026 Saumitra Basu

The right of Saumitra Basu to be identified as author of this work has been asserted in accordance with sections 77 and 78 of the Copyright, Designs and Patents Act 1988.

All rights reserved. No part of this book may be reprinted or reproduced or utilised in any form or by any electronic, mechanical, or other means, now known or hereafter invented, including photocopying and recording, or in any information storage or retrieval system, without permission in writing from the publishers.

Trademark notice: Product or corporate names may be trademarks or registered trademarks, and are used only for identification and explanation without intent to infringe.

British Library Cataloguing-in-Publication Data
A catalogue record for this book is available from the British Library

ISBN: 978-1-041-10752-1 (hbk)
ISBN: 978-1-041-10753-8 (pbk)
ISBN: 978-1-003-65664-7 (ebk)

DOI: 10.4324/9781003656647

Typeset in Times New Roman
by Apex CoVantage, LLC

I dedicate this monograph to the countless people who died silently without treatment during the Spanish Influenza, and I give particular respect to the doctors, nurses, and citizen volunteers who selflessly aided influenza victims

Contents

Illustrations

Figures

Tables

Abbreviations

AIDS—Acquired Immunodeficiency Syndrome
CDC—Centre for Disease Control
CRI—Central Research Institute
GDP—Gross Domestic Product
HIV—Human Immunodeficiency Virus
IMS—Indian Medical Service
IRFA—Indian Research Fund Association
NGO—Non-Governmental Organization
NPIs—Non-Proliferative Interventions
PTSD—Post-Traumatic Stress Disorder
RMPA—Registration of Medical Practitioners Act
RNA—Ribonucleic acid
WHO—World Health Organization
WWI—World War I

Preface

In the tapestry of India's rich and complex history, the study of diseases stands as a testament to the nation's enduring quest for understanding and managing the health of its diverse population. This journey, marked by scientific curiosity, traditional wisdom, and colonial influences, began long before modern medicine. India's ancient traditions and medicines, including Ayurveda and Siddha, formed the foundation of its disease research. These indigenous medical systems, developed over thousands of years, offered sophisticated understandings of health and disease, emphasizing balance and harmony in bodily systems. Texts like the Charaka Samhita and Sushruta Samhita are early examples of the comprehensive medical knowledge that existed in ancient India, addressing a range of ailments with remarkable insight.

However, a significant turning point in the study of diseases in India came with European colonists. The 16th century onwards saw an influx of European traders and later, colonizers, who brought with them new diseases, and the need for new medical understandings and practices. The British era, in particular, marked a profound shift in disease studies. The establishment of medical schools and colleges and the introduction of western medicine in the 19th century were pivotal in shaping the modern landscape of medical research and healthcare in India. Colonial rule also brought about a systematic approach to handling public health crises, such as outbreaks of cholera, malaria, and plague. This period saw the initiation of formal medical research and the establishment of institutions like the Indian Medical Service. The British administration's efforts to combat tropical diseases led to significant developments in epidemiology and public health policies, albeit often driven by the interests of colonial governance rather than purely altruistic motives. Simultaneously, there was a resurgence and reform in traditional Indian medical practices, prompted in part by the nationalistic movements of the 19th and early 20th centuries. This period witnessed an endeavour to scientifically validate and integrate traditional knowledge systems with modern medical practices, a trend that continues to this day. The study of diseases in India, thus, has been a dynamic and evolving field, shaped by a confluence of indigenous knowledge, colonial influences, and the challenges posed by India's vast and varied landscape. This rich history sets the stage for understanding the complex tapestry of health and disease in modern India, a legacy that continues to influence medical research and healthcare policies in contemporary times. In the same vein, from the perspective of the history of medicine, the study of pandemics holds immense significance, as it not only unravels the complex interplay between human societies and pathogenic organisms but also showcases the evolution of medical knowledge, public health strategies, government, and societal responses to widespread health crises.

Historically, pandemics like the Black Death in the 14th century, the Spanish Flu of 1918, and more recently, the COVID-19 pandemic, have acted as catalysts for significant medical advancements and public health reforms. They have highlighted the importance of understanding disease transmission, the development of vaccines and therapeutics, and the critical need for robust, resilient healthcare systems. Pandemics have often prompted a rethinking of broader social, economic, and political issues, including healthcare equity, global cooperation, and the balance between individual rights and public health needs. Studying these events allows us to appreciate the progress in medical science and public health while also preparing for future challenges in a world where global interconnectedness continues to rise.

During my childhood, a serious epidemic, like cholera, hit me hard. Both local and indigenous practitioners gave me treatment. It was beyond my comprehension then. Since reaching adulthood, I have considered the treatment I received and questioned the medical procedures performed by those practitioners. During India's and the world's 2020 COVID-19 crisis, nightly fears of death consumed me. The silent footsteps of death echo everywhere, accompanied by the wail of ambulances in the street. To pass my lonely night, I read John Kelly's *The Great Mortality: An Intimate History of the Black Death*. Then, I developed an insatiable desire to research historical pandemics.

The major motivation to visualize this project cropped up from this untold desire and my source of inspiration has been Prof. Jagdish N Sinha, whom I met and discussed a lot to understand the issue historically and scientifically, and the present project is a fruitful outcome. During an international workshop on History of Medicine at Philadelphia (online), one of the major themes was the impact of historical pandemic studies. The backdrop of the discussion was international perspective. Being an overseas participant and specifically from India, I pondered over the issue and, in time, it became a research concern. Instead, my current research stems from something other than a dearth of historical scholarship. Rather, it was the inadequacy of suitable historical attempt specifically in colonial Bengal which provided me with the impetus to conduct my study and the present research is a fruitful outcome of it.

The present research engages with the context of Spanish Influenza. The Spanish Influenza, a pandemic that raged across the globe in the early 20th century, left an indelible mark on human history, reshaping societies and altering the course of nations. In India, a land steeped in ancient traditions and undergoing profound transformations under British colonial rule, the pandemic unfolded with devastating consequences, unveiling a tale of tragedy, resilience, and profound social change. The present research seeks to delve into the multifaceted impacts of the Spanish Influenza in India, exploring not only its immediate effects on health and mortality but also its lasting influence on Indian society, politics, and the eventual struggle for independence.

The pandemic, ravaging India between 1918 and 1920, unfolded amidst acute food scarcities and wartime famines, exacerbating the nation's vulnerability at a pivotal historical moment. The final stages of World War I coincided with India's deep entanglement in the war effort as a part of the British Empire. The war had already strained India's resources and had kindled the flames of nationalist sentiment. The Spanish Influenza amplified these existing stresses, leading to a catastrophic impact on a population already burdened by war, famine, and colonial exploitation. History rarely witnessed a pandemic as impactful and destructive as the 1918–20 Spanish Flu. This global health crisis, which claimed millions of lives, was a catastrophe that spared no corner of the world, including the vibrant and densely populated region of Bengal in colonial India. The focus of this effort is to provide a comprehensive and detailed account of the Spanish Influenza as it ravaged Bengal, a province under British colonial rule, and to analyze its profound and lasting impacts on the region's society, politics, and culture.

The essence of the present study centres on colonial Bengal, in the eastern part of the Indian subcontinent. During the time of the pandemic, Bengal was a region of stark contrasts—rich in culture and intellectual thought, yet marred by deep social and economic disparities. The outbreak of Spanish Influenza coincided with a turbulent period in Bengal's history. The region was not only grappling with the effects of World War I and the challenges of colonial rule but also undergoing significant political and social changes. The pandemic added a complex layer to this already dynamic historical context. The present attempt begins by setting the stage, describing Bengal in the early 20th century. It delves into the geopolitical landscape, the socio-economic conditions, and the public health environment of the time, which collectively set the scene for the pandemic's arrival and its subsequent impact. This analysis scrutinizes the role of colonial policies, the state of medical infrastructure, and public health responses to understand the initial conditions influencing the pandemic's course.

The heart of the research lies in its detailed recounting of the pandemic's progression through Bengal. It draws upon a rich tapestry of sources, including colonial records, newspapers, personal diaries, and oral histories, to construct a vivid narrative of the pandemic's timeline. The analysis focuses on the demographic impact, including the staggering mortality and morbidity rates, with particular attention given to variations across different regions of Bengal and among various social and economic groups. This work's key element is exploring how the Spanish Flu impacted Bengali society and politics. The pandemic had far-reaching effects on the societal fabric, exacerbating existing class and gender inequalities and placing an immense strain on social and familial structures. The response of the colonial government to the crisis, often inadequate and marred by racial and class biases, further fueled nationalist sentiments and became a significant factor in Bengal's burgeoning independence movement.

The present research delves into the cultural and psychological impacts of the pandemic. This research examines the pandemic's collective trauma and profound societal changes' impact on Bengal's traditional beliefs, religious practices, and rich literary and artistic traditions. The concluding sections of the research reflect on the legacy of the Spanish Influenza in Bengal. It discusses how the pandemic influenced public health policies, and societal attitudes towards disease and healthcare, and contributed to a critical rethinking of colonial governance. This analysis thoroughly examines how this catastrophic event and the lessons learned shaped the course of Bengal's history, leading up to and beyond Indian independence.

Through this detailed exploration, the present effort aims not only to chronicle a tragic episode in Bengal's history but also to provide insights into how a health crisis can influence the course of history, reshape societal norms, and alter the trajectory of political movements. This work contributes to a broader understanding of the Spanish Influenza in the colonial context, offering a lens through which to view the complex interplay between disease, society, and empire.

Despite this, primary and secondary sources remain crucial; they fulfilled a vision. The archival sources were of immense help. Personal papers, diaries, letters of correspondence, minutes of meetings, newspaper articles, government reports, proceedings, microfilms, etc. not only helped the author to think in an in-depth manner but also helped to understand the perspective with varied connotations. This research built its theoretical and conceptual understanding mainly of published books, papers from national and international journals, personal interviews, and newspaper articles. To understand this research comprehensively, we divided the discussion into six chapters, including observations and conclusions. The present treatise humbly concludes with the hope that the study of historical pandemics holds immense significance from the perspective of the history of medicine, offering invaluable insights into the evolution of medical understanding, public health responses, and societal impacts of widespread disease outbreaks. By examining past pandemics, historians of medicine can trace the development of epidemiological concepts, the progress in diagnostic and therapeutic techniques, and the changing nature of doctor–patient relationships. These studies also highlight how societal, cultural, and economic factors influence the spread of disease and the effectiveness of medical responses. Crucially, understanding the successes and failures of past public health measures aids in the preparation for future health crises, emphasizing that historical pandemics are not just relics of the past but vital case studies for current and future medical strategies. This historical lens also enriches our comprehension of the social determinants of health and the ethical challenges faced in medicine, providing a more nuanced and holistic view of healthcare's role within society.

This unpublished treatise of mine is a living document of that unspoken desire.

Saumitra Basu

Acknowledgement

In June 2020, the project developed; it began in October 2021 and concluded in September 2024. This moment, a culmination of persistent effort, is truly unforgettable. I bend my head at the feet of the Almighty God whose profound grace paved the path forward. This humble work reflects the mercy emitted from the Almighty. Many contributors, individuals, and organizations significantly shaped this project's development. This work would not have been possible without the generosity of the many people in different corners of India, Bangladesh, and the United Kingdom who valued my work, offered me hours of discussion, imparted their wisdom, and welcomed me into their wider research canvas.

I cannot adequately acknowledge all those who helped during my research because there were so many. They all have extended their helping hands in unknown environs, both academic and geographic.

First, I sincerely express my heartfelt gratitude to Indian National Science Academy (INSA), New Delhi. The present research work was only made possible by the generous support of funding opportunities from the Indian National Science Academy (INSA), New Delhi. I have no words to express my heartfelt gratitude to the respectable members of the National Commission of History of Science and Research Council whose valuable suggestions and thoughtful review inspired me to complete the work successfully. I am also grateful to Mr. Madhvendra Narayan, Assistant Executive Director, History of Science for his cordial administrative assistance throughout the project period.

I also express my gratitude to Prof. Achin Chakraborty (Former Director) and Prof. Indrani Chakraborty (Present Director), Directors, Institute of Development Studies Kolkata (IDSK) for affiliating my project at their institute. The institutional administration assisted me in performing the present project successfully.

I wish to express a special gratitude and respect from the bottom of my heart to Dr. Srabani Sen and Dr. Sukta Das. Since the beginning, they gave their great wisdom in framing this project, constantly pushing my expectations of myself, of what it meant to write a history of this forgotten pandemic, and of what my sources could tell me and what I could tell for future researchers. I feel fortunate to have learned from Dr. Sen and Dr. Das.

I acknowledge my deep indebtedness to John O' Brien, Archivist, India Office Library; Edward Bishop, Wellcome Trust Library, London, UK; Mr. Elias Miah,

National Archives; and National Library of Bangladesh, Dhaka for their untiring assistance which has enabled me to complete my archival works in those esteemed institutions of London, UK and Dhaka, Bangladesh.

My special thanks to all the members of the Editorial Team of Routledge for their heartiest cooperation. I am greatly indebted to Dorothea Schaefter, Senior Editor, Asian Studies, Routledge; Stuti Goel, Squad Manager, Asian Studies/Russian & Eastern European Studies, Routledge|Taylor and Francis; Sangeetha S, Assistant Project Manager|Apex CoVantage and all other editorial assistants of Apex CoVantage team whose untiring effort make my draft manuscript into a monograph.

Such research involves many key contributors. I shall fail in my duty if I do not acknowledge the library and archival authorities of the National Archives of India (NAI), New Delhi; Mr. Kalipada Pramanik, Librarian, Town Hall Library; Abhishek Chaturvedy, Librarian, All India Institute of Hygiene and Public Health; and All the Staff of Microfilm Section and Old News Paper Section, National Library, Kolkata for their sincere and indefatigable cooperation in my library work. My work would remain incomplete without acknowledgement to Mrs. Jhumur Sengupta, Archivist, Directorate of State Archives, Kolkata, West Bengal. I am deeply grateful for her help during the post-COVID-19 project phase. I also convey my sincere thanks to Mr. Subir Chatterjee, Librarian, IRDM Faculty Centre, Narendrapur Campus for his untiring assistance starting from the COVID-19 period to the end of this project. I am immensely grateful to Dr. Satarupa Dutta Majumdar Saha, Research Associate, Indian National Science Academy (INSA), New Delhi, for her academic and editorial assistance. I am grateful to Ms. Nilanjana Patra, who has helped me immensely in finding the right materials for archival work on this subject. I am eternally grateful to her for this help. I am indebted to my students Deep Banerjee and Patatri Baidya for their constant academic and moral support, which was encouraging and provided me with generous mental support.

My family, I think the last because its contribution has been the most important. I sincerely acknowledge the role of my wife Malika Basu (Ghosh) (Associate Professor of History, Kalna College, University of Burdwan, West Bengal), and my beloved son, Soumalya, whose youthful spirit, patience, and encouragement during my work have been a constant source of inspiration. I have received incredible intellectual, emotional, and material support and patience from both of them during my challenging career as a historian of science. They significantly impact my life and work.

The absence of gratitude towards an individual renders all efforts unfulfilled, particularly in reference to Prof. K.C. Malhotra, Former Professor of Anthropometry and Human Genetics Unit at the Indian Statistical Institute in Kolkata, whose academic guidance, moral support, critical feedback, recommendations, and essential assistance from the initial stages have been instrumental in facilitating the proper continuation and timely completion of this research work.

Saumitra Basu

Introduction

The study of public health in colonial India, especially in Bengal, emerged as a significant focus for scholars across various disciplines, including history, anthropology, sociology, and history of science and medicine. This interest stemmed from the intricate relationships between colonial governance, social structures, and health practices during that era. Colonial Bengal, a vital region of British India, faced many epidemics such as cholera, plague, and malaria, which not only costed several lives but also underscored the difficulties in managing public health within a colonial framework. Historians and anthropologists were particularly interested in how colonial policies influenced local health systems, as the British imperial agenda transformed health infrastructure in both urban and rural areas. Colonial authorities interpreted the implementation of western medicine and public health initiatives in Bengal through a colonial lens, using western scientific approaches to reinforce colonial dominance and diminish traditional medical practices (Prakash, 1999, pp. 11–12, 136–137, 143–144).

Historians and historical sociologists have shown a keen interest in how the colonial state perceived the health of its subjects as a mechanism of control, influencing both public health and social hierarchies. Implementing sanitation measures, vaccination initiatives, and quarantine protocols not only aimed at improving public health but also reinforced the authority of colonial governance. The state's involvement in health regulation fostered a pronounced class divide, with Europeans frequently receiving superior medical care compared to the indigenous population (Harrison, 1994, pp. 36–60, 117–139, 202–211). The tensions between modern western medicine and traditional health practices have attracted medical and public health researchers to colonial Bengal, making it a significant area for examining the evolution of medical knowledge and practices within an imperial context. Scholars such as David Arnold in *Colonizing the Body* (1993, pp. 14, 114–115, 240–241, 291–292) have investigated how colonial policies not only shaped public health measures but also established racial and social hierarchies in healthcare. In her work *History of Public Health: Colonial Bengal, 1921–1947* (2008, pp. 50, 157, 343–348), Kabita Ray explores the relationship between colonial policies and public health efforts in rural Bengal, emphasizing the influence of western medical practices on local populations during the final years of British governance. The history of science and medicine during this era sheds light on the global dissemination of diseases,

DOI: 10.4324/9781003656647-1

the emergence of epidemiology, and the influence of scientific institutions within the colonial framework. Colonial Bengal presents a complex and nuanced case for researchers interested in the interplay of power, health, and society throughout the colonial period. In this perspective, the works of Sumit Sarkar *Modern India: 1885–1947* (1989, pp. 20–21) and Ray's contributions to public health history further clarify how colonial power dynamics used health as a means of governance.

The present study examines the Spanish Influenza[1] as a case study of public health in colonial Bengal, as it represented a crucial moment in both global and local health responses. The swiftly spreading 1918 pandemic catastrophically affected India, particularly Bengal, where the mortality rate was alarmingly high; historians may not have adequately documented its impact. Within the framework of colonial Bengal, the Spanish Influenza underscored the vulnerability of the public health system under colonial administration, as the colonial government struggled to effectively address such a widespread and deadly health emergency. The pandemic revealed the shortcomings of colonial governance in handling public health crises, highlighting not only the deficiencies of the medical infrastructure but also the colonial state's neglect of the indigenous population's needs regarding timely intervention and sufficient medical care.

Examining the Spanish Influenza as a case study enables to highlight the widening gap between colonial authorities and the indigenous population. The pandemic acted as a framework for scholars to investigate the enforcement of western medical practices and to reveal how colonial administrators, despite their dependence on modern medicine, struggled to effectively manage the outbreak. Colonial interests frequently shaped the execution of public health initiatives in colonial Bengal during the Spanish Influenza, often harming the local population. This incident not only represented a pivotal moment in colonial Bengal's public health history but also emphasized the fundamental shortcomings of the colonial government's public health management, making it a significant point of interest for scholars examining the broader consequences of colonialism on health and governance.

Why Colonial Bengal Was Mournfully Underexamined?

Colonial Bengal, despite being one of the most severely affected regions during the Spanish Flu pandemic, remains remarkably understudied in both official colonial records and subsequent historical analyses. This lack of documentation stems from a complex web of political, administrative, and ideological factors intrinsic to the nature of colonial governance in British India. At the heart of this neglect was the imperial state's utilitarian approach to public health, where the value of life was assessed not in human terms but based on economic productivity and administrative necessity. Although Bengal was a populous and economically significant region in earlier colonial periods, by 1918, it was increasingly marginalized in the eyes of the colonial bureaucracy, especially compared to presidencies deemed more "strategically vital", such as Bombay and Madras.

The Spanish Flu reached Bengal at a critical time for the British Empire. The First World War had exhausted colonial resources, and much of the heavily

Anglicized and militarized Indian Medical Service (IMS) was deployed either to the war front or to protect British military and civilian personnel in India. The IMS was never intended to comprehensively serve the Indian population; its primary focus was the health and safety of British soldiers and officials. In Bengal, this resulted in an alarming lack of medical infrastructure, especially in the rural areas where the majority of the population resided. When influenza spread with devastating speed and lethality, there were few doctors, no operational surveillance system, and virtually no logistical support to document the spread or the number of deaths. Furthermore, most deaths occurred outside the reach of state institutions, in homes, villages, along roadsides, and near riverbanks, where bodies often went uncremated due to the magnitude of mortality. As a consequence, most of these deaths went unrecorded. Another very surprising fact in this context is that in the rural areas of colonial Bengal, the data on influenza deaths were kept by the uneducated village watchmen (*chowkidar*). Their job was to register births or deaths. If the cause of death was unknown, it was written that the person died of fever. The colonial death registration system was rudimentary at best and limited primarily to urban municipalities. It also suffered from chronic undercounting, especially among marginalized populations such as women, lower castes, Muslims, and rural masses (Arnold, 1993, pp. 221–224). These systemic administrative deficiencies contributed to a severe underestimation of mortality and morbidity rates in colonial Bengal.

A major reason for the lack of adequate documentation was the colonial state's active disinterest in recognizing the magnitude of the pandemic's impact. Acknowledging the deaths of hundreds of thousands of Indian subjects due to unpreparedness and governmental neglect would have exposed the moral and structural flaws of imperial rule. British authorities had little political or diplomatic incentive to thoroughly investigate or publish detailed reports from a region like Bengal, which had already been politically unstable following the 1905–11 Partition controversy and the rise of nationalist unrest. The state prioritized maintaining order over safeguarding lives and collecting data. Furthermore, vernacular Bengali sources—newspapers, magazines, and personal diaries—that addressed the pandemic with emotional intensity and graphic descriptions were neither preserved nor valued by colonial archivists. These indigenous sources, often written in Bengali, Urdu, or regional dialects, were considered unofficial and therefore excluded from the state's documentation apparatus. As a result, the lived experiences of suffering, death, and despair in Bengal during the pandemic remained localized, oral, or lost over time.

Furthermore, Bengal's social structure, characterized by dense slums, communal burial practices, and close-knit rural communities, intensified the pandemic's effects, making them even more overwhelming and, at the same time, difficult to track statistically. For example, Calcutta experienced massive excess mortality in its overcrowded districts, but the city's medical system quickly collapsed under the pressure, leading to improvised mass burials and the unceremonious disposal of bodies. Public health officials failed to keep pace with the crisis, and no systematic epidemiological surveys were conducted after the pandemic to assess the regional impact. In conclusion, the scant documentation of the Spanish Flu in colonial Bengal is not simply the result of accidental omission; it is the product of a deeply entrenched colonial logic that devalued native lives, prioritized imperial needs over humanitarian ones, and willfully ignored crises that did not directly threaten the colonial apparatus (Chandra, 1996, p. 90). The devastating toll the pandemic took on Bengal—estimated in the hundreds of thousands, if not more—was rendered invisible in official archives, leaving generations of historians with only fragments of memory, anecdotes, and unofficial records to piece together one of the deadliest episodes in the subcontinent's modern history. This historical erasure reveals much about the politics of imperial record-keeping and the silent suffering of millions whose deaths were never recorded in the annals of empire.

The present study underscores the catastrophic, somberly under-examined consequences of the 1918–20 Spanish Flu in colonial Bengal. Pandemics profoundly affect human life, revealing both disease and societal structures. Pivotal in our collective history, these junctures mark periods of struggle, resilience, and transformation. During this crisis, it's vital to reflect on the past, learn from past lessons, and prepare for the future (Athukorala & Athukorala, 2022, pp. 5–11). Global health crises expose the interconnectedness of our modern world by highlighting societal strengths, healthcare system vulnerabilities, and governance weaknesses. Pandemics, acting as catalysts, force a re-evaluation of priorities and values, and they confront us with the fragility of human life and the resilience of the human spirit (Gordon, 2021, pp. 35–37).

Historical pandemics provide valuable insights into medical practices, public health policies, and societal responses to health crises when studied. We can see the evolution of diagnostic methods, treatments, drugs, and vaccines from the Black Death to COVID-19.[2] These events also provided a timeline of medical advancements, with their triumphs and failures, shaping current medical practices. Crucially, understanding historical pandemics illuminates epidemiology,[3] revealing insights into disease transmission, control measures, and the effects of public health[4] interventions. For managing current health issues and preparing for future outbreaks, this knowledge is essential (Humphreys, 2018, pp. 220, 223, 225). By studying past pandemics' epidemiological data, we can identify patterns and trends vital for predicting and mitigating disease spread. Social and economic structures, behaviours, and geopolitical landscapes are all influenced by pandemics. Analysis of these effects reveals crucial health disparities based on socio-economic status, race, and geography for health equity and healthcare inclusion (Tambolkar et al., 2022, pp. 1642–1645).

Revealing diverse cultural attitudes towards health and illness, historical pandemics illuminate the ethical and cultural dimensions of healthcare. In addition, they spur innovation in medical science, interdisciplinary approaches, and technological advancements. Significant breakthroughs often arise from the urgent need for pandemic solutions, underscoring the importance of collaborative and innovative healthcare thinking (Frankema & Tworek, 2020, pp. 333–334). Regarding the present discourse, the 1918 influenza pandemic in India, along with other early 20th-century pandemics, offers valuable insights into the interplay of disease, society, and colonialism. Within the Indian context, examination of these pandemics offers a crucial understanding of the era's public health difficulties and societal reactions, influenced by colonialism (Ojo, 2020, p. 1026). British colonial rule's impact on public health infrastructure influenced disease spread and management. In diverse populated regions with varied socio-economic realities, such as India, pandemics illuminate the challenges in implementing public health measures. Crucially, traditional medicine and local health practices address the limited access to western medical care. Frequently, the fight for independence and self-determination intertwines with these crises (Mukherjee, 2010, p. xx). Early 20th-century Indian health crises, when studied, provide valuable insights into resilience, adaptation, and sensitive healthcare. Studying these crises reveals the social, political, and cultural dynamics of a critical era in Indian history. Historical pandemics can be understood both as pathological realities and as socially constructed events. A history of medicine perspective on past pandemics improves current and future healthcare practices, policies, and responses. Comprehensively, this perspective shows how medical knowledge, societal structures, and ethical considerations have influenced health crises (Kumar, 2013, pp. 25, 27, 29, 33).

Etymology of the Words "Influenza" and "Pandemic"

The word *pandemic* derives from the Latin word *pandemus*, which itself comes from the Greek word "pan demos", the first meaning all, every, and the second meaning the people (Honigsbaum, 2009b, p. 34). This refers to a simultaneous, widespread epidemic of contagious disease across a nation or continent(s). First documented at the beginning of the 1500s, the Italian word influenza described an illness thought to be caused by celestial alignments. People believed astrological influences caused outbreaks of disease, so they called any outbreak "Italian Flu". A catarrhal epidemic, dubbed "influenza di catarro" by Italians, ravaged Europe in 1743, eventually shortening to "influenza" in English (Breedlove, 2006, p. 179).

The Concept of "Pandemic"

Kessler (2020, p. 17) defines a pandemic as an epidemic spreading across multiple countries or continents, affecting many people. A pandemic is a widespread outbreak of a contagious disease affecting people across regional and national borders. Across multiple countries or continents, the rapid and widespread transmission of an infectious agent, like a virus or bacteria, signifies a pandemic. Pandemics potentially cause widespread illness, overwhelmed healthcare systems, and significant social and economic disruptions. Frequently, the term links diseases with sustained human-to-human transmission and serious public health threats (McMillen, 2024, pp. 1–5). For effective pandemic management and control, coordination among healthcare professionals, governments, and the public at the local, national, and international levels is essential. Governments and healthcare professionals implement public health interventions, travel restrictions, and vaccination campaigns. However, Burnet (1953, p. 155) notes that the term "pandemic" has different connotations.

The first one considers pandemics as an episodic chapter in human civilization, characterized by the emergence and spread of infectious diseases across populations (Arnold, 2022, p. 46). From the Black Death[5] to the Spanish Flu, these global outbreaks have challenged healthcare systems, tested societal structures, and prompted innovation. The recurring theme is collective response, as communities and nations face the dual challenges of containing infectious agents and mitigating socio-economic fallout. Each pandemic, like the HIV/AIDS[6] crisis and COVID-19, has spurred advancements in medical science, public health strategies, and international cooperation. Understanding the historical context of pandemics highlights the importance of global solidarity in addressing shared threats to human well-being (Harrison, 2016, pp. 129–135).

One can view the second one from the point of a pandemic's impact. Pandemics impact social, demographic, and political spheres, reshaping interpersonal dynamics, highlighting inequalities, and altering population structures. They highlight vulnerabilities, test governance systems, and shape policy priorities. Studying these effects from multiple perspectives helps build resilient societies and understand complex interactions, enhancing our understanding of future challenges and promoting international collaboration. Understanding these impacts is crucial for addressing future challenges (Mander, 2020, p. 25).

The third approach considers pandemic as a public health crisis that requires a coordinated global response from governments. Governments face surges in cases, healthcare infrastructure, urgent need for diagnostics, antiviral therapies,[7] and vaccines. Interventions include social distancing, quarantine, travel restrictions, and testing (Mills, 1986, pp. 11, 19–25). The pandemic highlights the importance of government policies in promoting public health adherence, emphasizing the need for agile, evidence-based policymaking. Governments must balance safeguarding public health by minimizing socio-economic disruptions, deploying robust strategies, and fostering collective responsibility (Ministry of Health, 1920, pp. iv–xxiii).

The fourth perspective of a pandemic reveals a multifaceted interplay of people's perceptions, narratives, scientific understanding, and societal and governance theories, influenced by cultural beliefs, socio-economic status, and information access (Peckham, 2016, p. 3). The pandemic has exposed the strengths and weaknesses of governance models and societal structures, prompting a re-evaluation of priorities and strategies. It emphasizes the importance of transparent communication, trust in scientific expertise, and agile governance. Navigating a global health crisis requires a multidisciplinary and collaborative approach (Polu, 2010, p. 50).

The fifth perspective, which is an alternative and innovative method for comprehending pandemics, involves examining the intricate connections between environmental and ecological factors. This viewpoint highlights how human activities, such as environmental degradation, contribute to the rise of infectious diseases. Activities like deforestation, urban expansion, and intensive farming have heightened interactions between humans and wildlife, which facilitate the transmission of zoonotic pathogens. Climate change worsens disease patterns by modifying ecosystems, altering the distribution of vectors, and affecting biodiversity. Recognizing pandemics as ecological events emphasizes the critical necessity for sustainable development, enhanced environmental policies, and international collaboration to protect ecosystems. This perspective reinforces the importance of environmental stewardship in reducing the likelihood of future outbreaks, fostering a healthier equilibrium between human advancement and the health of our planet (Daszak et al., 2001, pp. 103–108).

So, considering the earlier approaches, it is present author's endeavour to highlight the perspectives of pandemic studies from history of medicine point of view. The history of medicine offers a valuable perspective on pandemic studies, tracing the evolution of medical knowledge and responses to infectious diseases (Kenneth, 1993, pp. 20–30). Past pandemics, like the Black Death or COVID-19, provide insights into medical understanding, diagnostic capabilities, and treatment modalities. These studies also unveil successful patterns, lessons, and strategies in various contexts. They underscore the interconnectedness of global health and the need for international collaboration. Pandemic studies within the context of the history of medicine serve as a vital resource for shaping contemporary medical practices, informing future public health strategies, and advancing our collective ability to confront emerging health threats (Ramanna, 2003, pp. 86–90).

Spanish Influenza—The Real Story Behind the Nomenclature

The Spanish Flu's devastating impact and rapid spread killed millions in 1918. However, the name "Spanish" can be misleading. An influenza virus epidemic was first identified in Spain because of censorship during the First World War.[8] Spain's neutrality during wartime meant they lacked strict press restrictions, allowing for open reporting on the viral disease. This led people to believe that the influenza virus was specific to Spain, that is why the pandemic came to be known as the "Spanish Flu". Although the disease was associated with Spain because of its neutrality in World War I, the flu did not originate in this country. The first documented cases emerged in the United States and elsewhere, but wartime censorship restrictions limited the disclosure of information about the illness in many nations. Spain, not subject to censorship, and reported on the flu, leading to the erroneous perception that the epidemic started there. In reality, the name "Spanish" reflects more the freedom of the press than an actual geographical connection (Hoyle & Wickramasinghe, 1977, p. 402).

In 1918, Spanish intelligence reported a new epidemic disease in Madrid, causing 100000 people to contract the flu. The virus hit hard, infecting politicians and King Alfonso XIII. Almost 40% of people living in enclosed spaces contracted the virus, disrupting telegraph services and curtailing track driver businesses. The Spanish Flu overburdened hospitals, and Britain received it. British media blamed Spain's windy spring for the flu wave, arguing that the dusty winds carried microbes that Britain's humid climate couldn't survive. This incident underscored the importance of transparency and accuracy in information during global crises (Langford, 2005, pp. 473, 482–490).

Concept of Pandemic in Ancient Indian Medical Texts

Ancient Indian medical texts, Ayurveda,[9] offer a nuanced understanding of pandemics, even without using the term. Ayurveda, recognized as one of the oldest holistic healing systems globally, focuses on the collective effects of diseases on communities and underscores the interrelation between individual and community health. The foundational Ayurvedic texts, such as the Charaka[10] Samhita and Sushruta Samhita, elaborate on how diseases can be transmitted via air (Vayu) and water (Jala), thereby stressing the importance of personal hygiene and environmental purity. Ayurveda also recognizes the role of seasonal factors and planetary influences in the onset and spread of diseases. Concepts such as *Janapadoddhvamsa* allude to the devastation caused by epidemics at the community level (Acharya, 2000, p. 30).

Ayurvedic Concept of Janapadoddhvamsa

Charaka Samhita Vimana Sthana Chapter-3 Janapadoddhvamsa means destruction or demolition of communities. Ayurvedic authors such as Sushruta[11] and Charaka recorded communicable diseases as Aupasargika Roga and Janapadoddhvamsa (Acharya, 2000, p. 55).

Janapadoddhvamsakara Bhava (most dangerous Bhava) *Impairment of Vayu* (air), *Udaka* (water), *Desha* (land), and *Kala* (season) are more lethal in their increasing order. Seasonal impairment is the most dangerous.

The wise man should know that water is more important than air, land is more important than water, and Kala is yet more important than Desha by virtue of their degree of indispensability (Tripathi, 2007b, p. 31).

General Treatment of *Janapadoddhvamsa*

Yesham Na Mrityusaamanayam Saamnayam Na Ch Karmnaam |
Karm Panchvidham Teshaam Beshjam Parmuchyate ||
Rasayanaam Vividhch Upyogha Shashyte |
Shashyte Dehvritisch Bheshaje purvamudhytrite || ^

One does not suffer from these diseases even if all four vitiated factors are at work if people are assured with proper medicaments which are already collected and processed. Proper administration of Panchakarma[12] and *Rasayana* therapies is recommended for the effective management of *Janapadoddhvamsa* (communicable diseases). The herbs used for the medicine preparation should be collected prior to the onset of diseases in that particular area.

Along with this, *Satyabhuta* (truthfulness), *Bhoote Daya* (compassion for living beings), *Dana* (charity), *Bali* (sacrifice), *Devatarchana* (prayer to the gods), *Sadvritta Anuvritti* (good deeds), protection of the self by *Mantra*, etc. are very effective. These practices—devotion to God, service to those observing celibacy, discussions of religious scriptures, befriending great sages, and associating with self-controlled, religious, sattvic, and learned individuals—are also very effective. These therapies, which when adopted during the spread of communicable diseases (*Janapadoddhvamsa*), can save the lives of individuals provided the epidemics can save the lives of individuals provided the death of the individuals is not predetermined (Tripathi, 2007b, p. 26).

Causes for the vitiation of Janapadoddhvamsa factors

> "*Tasyamoolam Adharmah Tanmoolam Vaa Asat Karma Purvakrit Karma Tyoryoni Pragyapradha*" ^

The primary cause of the corruption of all elements is Adharma (unrighteousness), which arises from *Pragyapradha* (intellectual error). When leaders of nations, cities, and other entities govern their populations irresponsibly, failing to adhere to the virtuous path, they guide their followers towards wrongdoing. The citizens, communities, and merchants also stray from their responsibilities and further propagate these sinful behaviours. Such actions result in the erosion of virtue. As righteousness diminishes, even the divine beings abandon the inhabitants of these regions. This abandonment adversely affects the climate of those areas, leading to irregular rainfall, drought, or excessive precipitation; improper winds; extreme heat; and rising temperatures. Water sources may dry up, and medicinal properties may diminish. The community ultimately suffers from the consequences of consuming contaminated food and water, resulting in widespread illness (Tripathi, 2007a, p. 43).

Adharma—The Cause of War and Destruction

Individuals who experience overwhelming greed, anger, and attachment, while showing contempt for the vulnerable, may engage in violent conflicts with one another, either assaulting their adversaries or becoming victims of such assaults. *Aatamswajanpar Upaghatayeti*—It even leads to harm inflicted by one's own close relatives. Sinful acts lead to affliction by demons, variety of other creatures, and curse of sages.

Shusruta Samhita Nidana Sthana Chapter-5

Acharaya Shusruta (The Father of Surgery) has explained *Aupasargik Rogas*^. *Anupasargika* diseases are communicable diseases that spread through direct contact or contaminated objects of the patient.

> "*Parsangaat gaatrasansparsshaat Nishvaasaat Sah Bhojnaat* | *Sahsayya Aasana Ch Api Vastramaalya Anulepnaat* ||."^

Physical contact, expired air, eating with others by sharing plates, sharing bed, clothes, and cosmetics spread the communicable diseases from one person to another person. According to Acharya Dalhana, Prasangaat means "frequently, if these activities are performed".

The ancient medical texts also discuss the symptoms and signs of pandemics. They describe how pandemics often manifested with high fever, severe respiratory symptoms, and spread among the population. The texts emphasized the need for immediate recognition and diagnosis of these diseases to prevent their transmission and manage their impact on individuals and society. The texts highlight preventive measures to contain the spread of pandemics. These measures included maintaining personal hygiene, observing dietary restrictions, practicing social distancing, and disinfection of living spaces. The texts also emphasized the importance of strengthening the immune system through the use of herbal remedies, dietary modifications, and lifestyle practices to prevent and combat pandemics (Tripathi, 2007d, p. 19). Acharya Charaka and Acharya Sushruta outline three unique approaches for addressing disease-inducing conditions and for preventing the elements that lead to the development of diseases. This is the initial measure to avert pathogenesis. Ayurvedic literature states that manifesting disease requires involvement and vitiation of the body's channels as part of pathogenesis. The treatment includes *Samprati Vighatana*, which refers to the breakdown of pathogenesis. *Rasayana therapy* is anticipated to be advantageous in the management of Janapadoddhvamsa, which encompasses infectious and communicable diseases. To avert *Janapadoddhvamsa*, it is recommended to employ *Rasayana therapy* for rejuvenation and vitality, along with Panchakarma procedures for detoxification and body purification, adherence to Sadvrit Palan as a code of right conduct, and Aachara Rasyana for behavioural therapy (Tripathi, 2007c, p. 31).

The texts also emphasize prizing mental and emotional well-being in the recovery process. The concept of pandemics in ancient Indian medical texts shows the sophisticated understanding of disease management and prevention in early Indian civilization. These texts recognized the interconnectedness of human health with the environment and the need for a comprehensive approach to combat pandemics. While the medical practices and remedies mentioned in these texts may differ from modern medicine, they provide valuable insights into the historical perspectives on pandemics and the efforts made to mitigate their impact.

Overall, including the concept of pandemics in ancient Indian medical texts highlights the rich medical heritage of India and serves as a reminder of the continuous evolution of scientific knowledge in understanding and managing infectious diseases. The ancient Indian physicians acknowledged the importance of quarantine measures (Disease Eradication—*Roga Nivritti*) and also outlined guidelines for preventing the spread of contagious diseases. Ayurvedic principles emphasize the significance of enhancing personal immunity (Ojas) to combat infections. Using medicinal herbs, dietary practices, and lifestyle recommendations aimed at enhancing overall well-being also aligns with a holistic approach to pandemic prevention.

In summary, while the ancient Indian medical texts might not use the specific term "pandemic", ancient Indian medical texts offer a comprehensive understanding of contagious diseases, emphasizing preventive measures, hygiene, and individual and community health, reflecting timeless wisdom and contemporary global health perspectives.

Trans-Atlantic Diffusion of a Terrible Menace

Trans-Atlantic diffusion refers to the movement, exchange, or transfer of ideas, practices, goods, diseases, or other elements across the Atlantic Ocean. It is often used to describe historical interactions between Europe and the Americas during periods of exploration, colonization, trade, and cultural exchange (Thornton, 1998, pp. 43–71). In the Spanish Influenza, it refers to the rapid transmission of the influenza virus from one side of the Atlantic Ocean to the other. In 1918, the spring wave of influenza began in Kansas City and spread to the eastern seaboard, France, and China. By May 1918, the virus reached neutral Spain to gain the popular but inaccurate soubriquet "Spanish Flu". The virus reached Scandinavia, Britain, and Germany in June, and spread along the railway network in Bombay. New South Wales, Victoria, and New Zealand were also infected by June. Russia, Latin America, and sub-Saharan Africa escaped infection. The infection waned in July and August because of seasonal factors, and overall mortality rates were low (Kuperberg, 2008, pp. 48–59).

The trans-Atlantic diffusion of the Spanish Influenza in 1918 stands as a significant chapter in the history of pandemics, marking a critical moment in the global spread of infectious diseases. The rapid transmission and devastating impact of the virus across continents were indisputable. Combining factors such as World War I, the movement of military personnel and civilians, and the interconnectedness of nations facilitated the swift diffusion of the virus. Ports, transportation hubs, and the movement of troops acted as major conduits for the influenza, leading to widespread outbreaks in Europe, North America, South America, and beyond (Mills et al., 2004, pp. 904–905). World War I influenced the spread of the Spanish Influenza across the Atlantic because of the movement of troops, refugees, and goods, as well as the efficient transmission of the virus because of its mutating nature. During the Spanish Influenza, the virus spread across continents because of interconnectedness, international trade, and the movement of troops which allowed the influenza to transcend geographical boundaries.

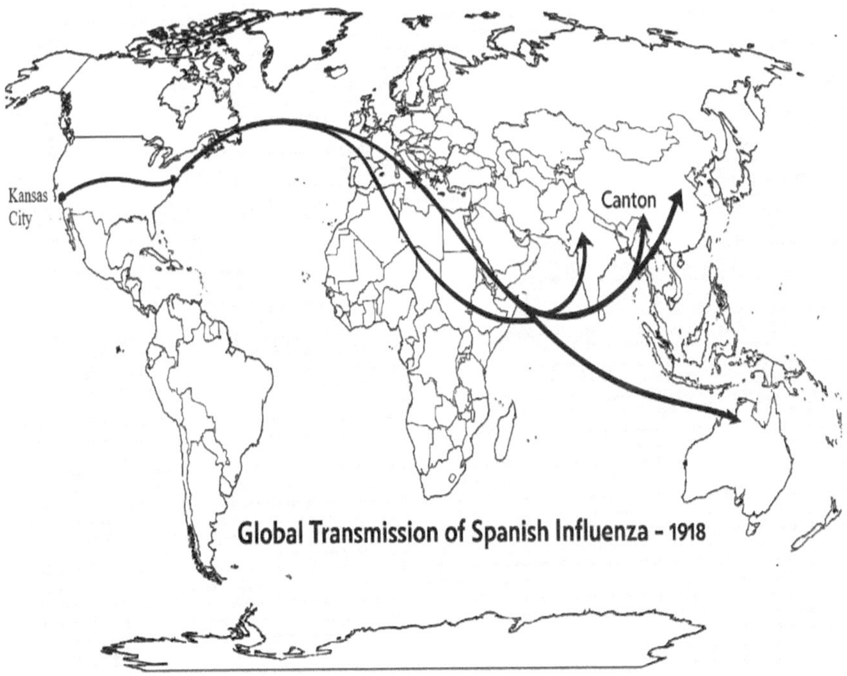

Figure 0.1 Trans-Atlantic Diffusion of Spanish Influenza (Prepared by Author)

Europe experienced a swift outbreak, while lack of communication hindered a unified global response, causing profound effects on different continents (Roser, 2020, p. 15). Europe, amid war-related hardships, experienced a devastating toll on its population. The virus spread, overwhelming healthcare systems and causing unprecedented mortality rates. In North America, the influenza made its presence felt, with major cities experiencing significant outbreaks. The virus affected communities, both urban and rural, with alarming speed, leaving a trail of illness and death. South America, Africa, Asia, and Oceania also witnessed the consequences of the trans-Atlantic diffusion, with varying degrees of severity.

The Spanish Influenza spread across the Atlantic, highlighting the vulnerability of populations to global health threats and the interconnectedness of the world. The pandemic highlighted the challenges of coordinated global responses during crises, especially in conflict-ridden times. The lack of a coordinated international response during World War I exacerbated the impact of the Spanish Influenza, as nations prioritized military efforts over public health measures. Wartime censorship limited information dissemination, hindering early detection and response efforts. The scarcity of accurate information further impeded the implementation of effective public health measures (Tsoucalas et al., 2016, pp. 23–25). The Spanish Influenza had profound social, economic, and political ramifications, with high mortality rates straining communities and families worldwide. The pandemic disrupted sectors like agriculture, industry, and trade, affecting the labour force. The economic repercussions of the pandemic contributed to post-war reconstruction challenges. The trans-Atlantic spread of the disease raised questions about naming the pandemic, as Spain reported, leading to the perception that the outbreak originated there. This historical episode underscored the importance of accurate and transparent information dissemination during pandemics to prevent misunderstanding and stigmatization (Saunders et al., 2016, p. 66). The 1918 trans-Atlantic diffusion of the Spanish Influenza marked a seminal moment in pandemic history, highlighting global populations' vulnerability to infectious diseases. The 1918 Spanish Influenza pandemic highlighted global vulnerability to infectious diseases, highlighting the importance of global cooperation, transparent communication, and coordinated responses in addressing challenges posed by interconnected worlds. The pandemic had profound consequences on health, economies, and social structures.

Specifically in India, the spread pattern of the Spanish Flu pandemic between 1918 and 1919 followed a distinctive trajectory influenced by transportation networks, troop movements, climatic conditions, and urban density (Mihika et al., 2020, p. 167). The virus initially entered India through western ports, likely brought by Indian soldiers returning from World War I, especially via Bombay (present-day Mumbai), which served as the main gateway for maritime traffic. From Bombay, the pandemic spread rapidly eastward and northward, affecting major cities such as Poona (Pune), Madras (Chennai), and Delhi. Railway lines, which were extensive under colonial rule, played a crucial role in facilitating the inland spread of the virus, allowing the infection to reach even remote districts within weeks. The timing also coincided with the end of the monsoon, a season that weakened the general health of the population, making them more vulnerable to respiratory illnesses. As noted by Davis (2001, pp. 207–210), the virus disseminated in successive waves and displayed regional disparities in intensity and mortality, influenced by climatic variations, nutritional deficiencies, and differing public health measures.

In colonial Bengal, the influenza outbreak was particularly catastrophic, exacerbated by high population density, inadequate sanitation, and existing deficiencies in public health. The virus likely entered the region through Calcutta (now Kolkata), a significant administrative and commercial hub linked by sea and rail to the rest of India. From Calcutta, it disseminated northward and into rural areas via congested railway lines, rivers, and postal networks. In contrast to the western provinces, where the epidemic surged quickly and then receded, Bengal faced multiple waves of infection with extended mortality, especially in rural districts where medical assistance was nearly absent. The effects were particularly harsh on the impoverished, women, and children, who had limited access to healthcare and were often malnourished. The lack of an effective colonial response further worsened the crisis, as public health services were ill-prepared and overwhelmed. Mukherjee (2011, p. 195) observes that the scarcity of qualified medical personnel, particularly in rural Bengal, combined with insufficient governmental action, resulted in rampant disease spread and unaccounted fatalities. This situation was exacerbated by the colonial government's unwillingness to allocate resources away from the war effort, culminating in a humanitarian disaster that is still inadequately documented in official historical accounts.

Voice of the Deadliest Influenza Pandemic in Different Provinces of India

The Spanish Influenza of 1918 affected India's provinces, including Punjab, Bengal, and Bombay, with the rapid spread of the virus and ill-equipped healthcare systems. Major cities like Lahore and Amritsar experienced high mortality rates, while Bengal, Calcutta faced significant challenges. Bombay, because of its trade and populated areas, faced challenges in controlling the spread. The pandemic's impact underscored the need for better public health infrastructure and preparedness for future health crises, emphasizing the importance of historical lessons in shaping contemporary public health strategies (Hill, 2011, p. 24). The following report will highlight the horror of death by Sanitary Commissioner Norman White, the sanitary commissioner of India during India's pandemic nightmare, in his Preliminary Report on the Influenza Pandemic of 1918 in India. Here, the author tries to portray the silent horror of death by mentioning the following paragraph from Norman White's report:

> *The overwhelming number of patients in the hospitals prevented the swift removal of the deceased to make room for the dying; The postal and telegraph systems were in complete disarray; although train services persisted, at major stations, the bodies of the deceased and the gravely ill were being taken off the trains. Corpses inundated the cremation sites and burial grounds, while an even larger number awaited removal. The already strained medical services,*

> *heavily affected by the epidemic, could only address a minuscule portion of the illnesses that required care. Almost every household was mourning a loss, and an atmosphere of fear and chaos prevailed everywhere.*
>
> *(White, 1918, p. 9)*

The 1918 Spanish Influenza in India caused significant devastation and upheaval, from populated urban centres to remote corners of villages. The crisis emphasized the need for better public health infrastructure and preparedness for future crises, underscoring the importance of historical lessons in shaping contemporary public health strategies. Here, an attempt has been made to give a brief account of the Spanish Influenza infection in various provinces of India.

Western India

Influenza was well-known in Bombay city because it served as the first point of entry in India before the disease spread (it was called *nayi sardi bukhar* means *new cold fever),* through troop movements (Liston, 1918, p. 8). In 1918, the medical community in Bombay faced challenges because of the flu pandemic, which began spreading in late June (Liston, 1918, p. 8). Between June 1918 and March 1919, Bombay City and the Bombay Presidency experienced a devastating event, losing over 6% of its population (Mills, 1986, pp. 25, 28, 33, 37). The Dangs in Gujarat lost over 15% of their indigenous tribe population, comprising Bhils[13] while in Portuguese-ruled Goa, the virus spread, in the Salsette district (Times of India, 1918, p. 10).

Drought, flu, and famine affected the Deccan plateau's rural areas, with districts like Sholapur, Ahmednagar, Nasik, and Satara experiencing significant mortality. In Bombay, various organizations, including the Hindu Medical Association, Social Service League, community-based hospitals, St. George's Nursing Association, Young Men's Mahomedan Association, Bombay Humanitarian League, Telugu Free Library, and others, provided assistance (Ramanna, 2003, pp. 87, 92–96). They distributed food and medicines and often ran travelling dispensaries. In Poona, V.R. Shinde spearheaded the relief initiatives of the Depressed Classes Mission, supported by the Poona Volunteer Corps and Arogya Mandal (Report of the Director of Public Instruction in the Bombay Presidency, 1918–19, p. 10). The Spanish Influenza in Western India in 1918–19 marked a significant chapter in the region's history, with merchant associations and the Gujarat Sabha playing crucial roles in relief efforts (Sanitary Commissioner's Report, 1918–19, p. 17).

Northern India

The Punjab province in northern India served as a crucial recruitment area for the British Indian army during World War I. Additionally, postal services emerged as a significant means of transmission in Punjab, with the public associating the spread of infection with letters and parcels (Report on the Sanitary Administration of the Punjab, 1919, p. 13). The initial sources of the infection were postal workers in Bombay and Karachi, with the Railway Postal Service facilitating the flu's arrival in Punjab (Herriot, 1920, pp. 8–9). The 1918 influenza pandemic had a profound impact on Punjab, Delhi, Gurgaon, and Rohtak, resulting in a population loss exceeding 10%. Rural regions were more severely affected than urban areas, with mortality rates decreasing further west, while Rawalpindi experienced higher death rates and Simla recorded the lowest at approximately 2% (Punjab Sanitary Board Report, 1918, p. 31). Districts such as Lahore and Amritsar faced significant challenges, prompting voluntary relief initiatives and assistance from medical students, as reported by census officials (Census of India, 1921b, p. 82). In several areas of northern India, particularly outside of Punjab, the destruction faced in 1918 was significantly more intense. The princely states of Rajputana were particularly affected, with an estimated loss of over 10% of their population (Census of India, 1921e, p. 60). The influenza outbreak impacted western Jaisalmer and Marwar, resulting in a mortality rate of one-fifth of the population. Jammu and Kashmir faced two subsequent waves, which affected all demographics (Adams, 1899, pp. 218–229). The United Provinces (currently Uttar Pradesh) also endured a significant drought that year, which only slightly alleviated in its easternmost regions, with approximately 50–70% of the population contracting the flu (Census of India, 1921c, p. 13). The pandemic had a detrimental effect on the districts of Agra, Hamirpur, Meerut, Bijnor, Jhansi, Bulandshahr, Unnao, Lucknow, Farrukhabad, Banda, and Muzaffarnagar, leading to a population decline of 10–20% (White, 1919, p. 19). Mortality rates in urban areas such as Agra, Lucknow, Varanasi, Kanpur, Allahabad, and their cantonment regions rose significantly, while the United Provinces faced a distinct challenge (Arnold, 2019, pp. 181, 189–195).

Central India

During the pandemic, Central India, a region with high death rates, experienced severe distress, including present-day states like Madhya Pradesh, Chhattisgarh, Odisha, Telangana, Maharashtra, and northern Karnataka, and was under the British-ruled Central Provinces and Berar or the Nizam-ruled[14] Hyderabad state or the many princely states that made up the Central India Agency. Indigenous people inhabited rural and remote territories in this region, including Gond, Bhil, Baiga, and Kolam, who often suffer during times of stress (Census of India, 1921d, p. 4). The province suffered significant losses, with around 10% of its population of 14 million people losing their lives during the 1918 pandemic (Tumbe, 2020, pp. 152–155). The districts that were most severely impacted comprised Damoh, Sagar, Betul, Mandla, Hoshangabad, Seoni, Yavatmal, Akola, Amravati, and Chanda, in addition to the Hyderabad State (Census of India, 1921a, p. 6). The flu's virulent nature allowed for rapid transmission, even in human contact, causing deaths in remote areas of India. Table 0.1 will highlight the occurring influenza deaths in different provinces of India.

South and East India

The pandemic devastated west, central, and north India, with improved conditions in south India and eastern parts. Travancore, modern-day Kerala, had minimal

Table 0.1 Influenza Deaths in Different Provinces of British India—1918

Province	*Population (Census 1911)*	*Total Estimated Influenza Deaths*	*Influenza Death Rate per Thousand*
Central Provinces and Berar	13916308	790820	56.8
Delhi	416656	23175	55.6
Bombay	19587383	900000	45.9
Punjab	19337146	816317	42.2
North-West Frontier Province	2041077	82000	40.0
United Provinces	46820506	1072671	22.9
Coorg	174976	3382	19.0
Madras	40005735	509667	12.7
Assam	6051507	69113	11.4
Bihar and Orissa	34489846	359482	10.3
Burma	9855853	60000	6.0
Bengal	45329247	213098	4.7
British India	**238026240**	**4899725**	**20.6**

Source: A Preliminary Report on the Influenza Pandemic in India by the Sanitary Commissioner With the Government of India, Simla: Government Monotype Press, 1919

influenza impact. Madras Presidency, with over 40 million people, experienced the most severe flu impact in Deccan districts. Madras faced "twin epidemics" of influenza and grain riots in 1918 (Arnold, 1979, pp. 111, 117–129). The war effort led to increased rice prices and widespread distress, causing looting of grain shops and warehouses. The government focused on food supply to avoid a pandemic crisis. The sanitary commissioner of Mysore released a list of cures and treatments for influwenza, including rest, food, warm coverings, and thymol solution[15] (Sekher, 2007, pp. 194–211). Tumkur and Shimoga were the worst-affected districts, and in the Kolar Gold Fields mining belt, 960 out of 13600 influenza-infected people died, reflecting a 7% case fatality ratio (The Economist, 1919, p. 624). Influenza affected eastern India, Bihar, and Orissa, reducing population growth rates from 1911 to 1921. Death toll decreased as people moved east to Bengal and Assam, with arrivals reported via tea estates. Various tea estates reported the disease in early December through Marwari shopkeepers returning from Calcutta, coolies from Nagpur, and via the bastis and bazaars outside the tea plantations (Bhattacharya, 2012a, p. 89). Calcutta and Madras underwent considerable upheaval due to the Spanish Influenza in eastern India between 1918 and 1919, marking a pivotal moment in the region's historical narrative (Minutes of the Syndicate for the Year 1919, p. 66). The pandemic exposed healthcare system vulnerabilities, economic effects, and societal changes, emphasizing preparedness, resilience, and international collaboration in addressing infectious diseases like the Spanish Influenza (Annual Report of the Sanitary Commissioner, 1918, 1920, pp. 33–35).

India faced significant challenges during the Spanish Influenza pandemic of 1918–19 because of its dense population, crowded urban areas, inadequate sanitation, and limited healthcare infrastructure. The lack of awareness and education about the virus further exacerbated the situation. India's involvement in World War

I also contributed to the severity of the pandemic. The deployment of military personnel, displaced individuals, and supplies throughout the conflict contributed to the worldwide dissemination of the virus. Economic strain, widespread poverty, malnutrition, and inadequate healthcare access further weakened the population's resilience, making them more susceptible to the virus's severe effects. The combination of these factors created a perfect storm, causing India's significant suffering during the pandemic.

Brief Outline About the History of Influenza

Throughout history, the occurrence and impact of influenza have been recorded, although its origins remain uncertain. K. F. Kiple associates its emergence with the advent of agriculture and the establishment of human settlements following the Paleolithic era (Kiple, 1993, pp. 1–8). Influenza, an infectious disease, first appeared in Italy in 1504, influenced by stars. In 1510, a severe lung disease spread across Europe from Africa (Quinn, 2008, pp. 111–135). Honigsbaum suggests that the outbreak of 1580, which spread from the Mediterranean to the Baltic Sea, could be regarded as the first genuine influenza pandemic. The 17th century witnessed multiple outbreaks, with reports indicating that influenza was widespread across Europe in 1610, resulting in significant illness but relatively low death rates. Additionally, in April 1658, Dr. Willis noted a severe influenza outbreak (Honigsbaum, 2009a, p. 1939). Dr. Willis documented the influenza outbreak of 1675, during which Thomas Sydenham noted the impact on entire families, leaving few unaffected. The 18th century saw improvements in the documentation of pandemics, accompanied by enhanced scientific insights. In 1743, the term "influenza" was officially used to describe an epidemic that was occurring in Italy at that time (Quinn, 2008, pp. 111–135). The word "influenza" was initially introduced in Britain in 1729, with the first recorded influenza epidemic taking place in Paris in 1803. The 19th century experienced its first pandemic in Paris, succeeded by another outbreak in 1847–48, which resulted in 5000 fatalities in London and rapidly disseminated throughout Britain within a span of six weeks (Johnson, 2006, pp. 180–205). Numerous individuals succumbed to pneumonia, bronchitis, and asthma (Creighton, 1891, p. 568). The influenza pandemic of 1889–91, which began in southern China, made its way to Europe through Russia and the United States due to large-scale migration. It subsequently spread to Japan, Latin America, and other parts of Asia. Dr. Parsons arrived in Scotland in 1889 and conducted four visits between 1889 and 1894, during which time 100000 individuals in Britain succumbed to the illness. Notably, there were no significant outbreaks of influenza reported after 1894 until the 1918 pandemic, which is the primary subject of this analysis (Scientific American, 1977, p. 21).

Pathological Perspectives of Influenza Pandemic

Past theories suggest various causes for the virus, but pathological perspectives offer insights into its unique nature and unprecedented severity of the outbreak.

The true cause is a virus. An influenza virion (virus particle), the size of which is so tiny that "an ordinary pinhead can accommodate a billion and to photograph them an electron microscope has to magnify their image at least 200,000 times" (Winternitz et al., 1920, pp. 13–14). The virion, spherical, can become elongated. Two types of glycoproteins, haemagglutinin and neuraminidase, are involved in the virus's spread. Haemagglutinin binds to the host's red blood cells, establishing infection. Neuraminidase cleaves sialic acid residues, promoting the release of progeny viruses, which spread the infection to uninfected cells, causing the host to succumb to the disease (Beveridge, 1978, p. 39).

The influenza virus exhibits adaptability, comprising eight individual RNA[16] strands that each carry distinct genetic information. This allows for infinite reproductive possibilities and recombination of genetic information, making disease combating difficult. The virus changes its structure at regular intervals, known as antigenic drift, allowing antibodies to recognize the virus from the last infection. However, when the virus undergoes an antigenic shift, the structure changes, making it difficult for previous outbreaks to recognize, leading to epidemics and pandemics. This adaptation allows the virus to grow and grow, making disease control challenging. The influenza virus, type A, can transform into various subtypes, causing epidemics and global pandemics. Surface protein configurations identify these subtypes, with 15 forms of haemagglutinin and 9 forms of neuraminidase identified. Only three haemagglutinin and two neuraminidase subtypes connect to human infection. These are H1, H2, and H3 and N1 and N2 (Johnson, 2006, pp. 105–109). The H1N1 influenza A virus is accountable for the 1918 pandemic.

The 1918 H1N1 influenza A virus[17] caused the pandemic, affecting young, healthy adults, leading to high mortality rates. Pathological studies revealed severe lung damage, necrotizing bronchitis, and bronchiolitis, in the lower respiratory tract, causing profound destruction of bronchial and alveolar epithelium. The aggressive attack of the 1918 influenza on the respiratory system and secondary bacterial infections, such as pneumonia, caused significant morbidity and mortality. The virus induced a cytokine storm, leading to systemic hyper-inflammation and severe lung pathology, making healthy young adults susceptible to complications. The immune response triggered by the virus became a double-edged sword, attempting to control the infection and causing collateral damage to the host's own tissues (Johnson, 2006, p. 116). The 1918 influenza virus had systemic effects, affecting vital organs and causing cardiovascular complications. Autopsies revealed myocarditis and multi-organ failure. Advancements in virology and immunology have allowed for a detailed genetic characterization of the virus, providing insights into its virulent nature. In 1918, the Spanish Influenza, also known as the Spanish Flu, was the world's worst pandemic of influenza until then. The spread of the virus was because of the H1N1 influenza A virus, a microscopic pathogen that infiltrates the respiratory system and infects epithelial cells. The germ theory, fundamental to contemporary microbiology, asserts that the entry of microorganisms into the body is responsible for numerous diseases. The virus spreads through respiratory droplets produced by infected individuals during coughing or sneezing, which are inhaled by susceptible individuals. Once inhaled, the virus gains entry into the respiratory tract, the upper and lower airways. The virus exploits host cells to replicate, leading to a cascade of pathological events. The influenza virus has a predilection for the respiratory epithelium and attaches to sialic acid receptors on the surface of host cells, starting the infection. This adherence triggers the virus's entry into the host cell, where it hijacks cellular machinery to replicate and produce new viral particles.

The influenza virus, which causes respiratory symptoms like cough, fever, and difficulty breathing, can undergo rapid genetic changes through antigenic drift and shift, evading pre-existing immunity. This evasion contributes to the periodicity and severity of influenza pandemics. Germ theory highlights the importance of understanding viral dynamics in disease transmission and evolution. Secondary bacterial infections, such as Streptococcus pneumonia and Staphylococcus aureus, complicated the cases of Spanish Influenza, contributing to high mortality rates during the 1918–19 pandemic (Morens et al., 2008, pp. 962, 967–968).

Germ theory offers insights into the host's immune response to the influenza virus, highlighting the balance between the immune defense and the pathological consequences of an overactive response. It provides a comprehensive framework to explain the pathology of the Spanish Influenza of 1918–19, explaining viral transmission, cellular invasion, host immune response, and secondary bacterial infections. This understanding has not only enriched our knowledge of historical pandemics but also contributed to contemporary strategies for preventing and managing influenza outbreaks.

Retrospective Literatures on Influenza Pandemic

Systematic studies on pandemic date back to the post-independence era. The nature of development of the subject is not always similar in the two places, both in India and the West. Here, mention will however have to be made of those literary works that provide background material for the present research. For a better and comprehensive understanding, the author has divided the consulted literatures into two groups—the Indian and the western. First, the light will throw on the Indian literatures and then on the western literatures. However, the illustrious journey reveals that scholastic research on pandemic Spanish Influenza is a scant phenomenon in India, and in Bengal, is almost non-existent.

The study of historical pandemics in India has been a complex endeavour, reflecting the rich tapestry of the country's history and its dynamic sociocultural landscape. Encompassing a diverse array of sources, such as ancient writings, medieval narratives, and medical documents. During the Mughal and British colonial periods, systematic documentation emerged, with colonial administrators and medical officers recording outbreaks and implementing public health measures like quarantine.[18] Post-independence, the focus shifted to epidemiological studies, healthcare infrastructure, and vaccine development. Contemporary scholars use archival research, interdisciplinary approaches, and advanced scientific methods to understand the nation's resilience, adaptive strategies, and evolution of public health practices

(Yeole et al., 2020, pp. 167–168). Systematic studies on historical pandemics in India reveal that, with the changing sociopolitical and public health circumstances, late 18th, 19th, and early 20th centuries witnessed billowy wave in health, medicine, and administration. The 1918–19 Spanish Influenza pandemic in India was a significant event, with most studies focusing on the US and Europe, only few historians and economists have studied this devastating pandemic on the Indian subcontinent. Researchers documented some systematic attempts to study the 1918–19 influenza pandemic in India.

K.C. Bose's (1920, p. 169) paper titled *Influenza in and Around the City of Calcutta* provides a comprehensive and detailed analysis of the occurrence and impact of influenza in Calcutta during a specific time period. The paper provides a comprehensive analysis of the epidemiology, spread, and response to influenza in Calcutta, India. It uses hospital records, medical reports, and local newspapers to provide a detailed view of the disease's impact on urban and rural areas. The historical context of the time and socio-economic conditions enhance the reader's understanding of the challenges faced in combating the outbreak.

Mills (1986, pp. 7–27) in his paper *The 1918–1919 Influenza Pandemic—The Indian Experience* provided a detailed analysis of the impact of the 1918–19 influenza pandemic on India. The author described the spread of the disease in different regions of India and its impact on public health, economy, and social life.

The paper "*Coping with the Influenza Pandemic: 'The Bombay experience'*" by Mridula Ramana in, Howard Phillips and David Killingray (2003, pp. 86–92) edited *The Spanish Influenza Epidemic of 1918–19: New Perspectives*, provided a detailed account on the 1918–19 influenza pandemic in Bombay, India, reveals the city's colonial administration's measures, tensions with Indian nationalists, and the challenges to existing power structures.

The paper *The Evolution of Pandemic Influenza: Evidence from India, 1918–19* by Siddharth Chandra and Eva Kassens-Noor (2014, pp. 2–5) explored the evolution of the 1918–19 influenza pandemic in India. The authors studied the spread of the disease in India, examining public health policies, colonial policies, and traditional healing practices' impact on the pandemic's course.

Chhun (2015, pp. 56–96) in her unpublished doctoral dissertation *Death and disorder: The 1918–1919 influenza pandemic in British India* examined the influenza pandemic's devastating effects on British India, focusing on Bombay, and analyzed the colonial government's responses, revealing their limitations and failures.

Arnold (2015, pp. 111–129) in his chapter titled *Disease, Rumor, and Panic in India's Plague and Influenza Epidemics, 1896–1919* published by Robert Peckham in his edited volume *Empires of Panic: Epidemics and Colonial Anxieties* stated that the seriousness of a crisis and the level of panic it incites are not necessarily proportional. Arnold's Chapter 5 explores the contrasting epidemiology of bubonic plague and influenza pandemics, arguing that the latter caused a more sudden and severe mortality crisis in India than the plague does. The chapter examines the cultural construction of the diseases, governmental and public health responses, timing of epidemics, and the international situation surrounding them to understand why the influenza pandemic was the "dog that did not bark".

Arnold (2019, pp. 181, 183–195) in his article *Death and the Modern Empire: The 1918–19 Influenza Epidemic in India* provided an interesting analysis of the devastating impact of the influenza epidemic on India during the early 20th century. The author analyzed the epidemic as a multifaceted public health crisis, highlighting the intricate interplay between colonial power, local responses, and global health governance.

Tumbe (2020, pp. 127–246) in his book *The age of pandemics (1817–1920): How they shaped India and the World* offered a comprehensive overview of the history of pandemics. The author examines the origins and spread of past pandemics like cholera, bubonic plague, influenza, and COVID-19, analyzing political, economic, and social factors, and their impact on societies, emphasizing global interconnectedness.

Arnold (2020, pp. 569–575) in his article *Pandemic India: Coronavirus and the Uses of History* highlighted the onset of the COVID-19 pandemic and has produced two different narratives in India. The author discusses two narratives: "historical" and "insurgent". The former compares colonial pandemics like the 1896 plague and 1918–19 influenza, highlighting past events like victimization and state authority. The latter questions the validity of historical analogies and postcolonial Indian politics. The author cautions against using colonial history to critique contemporary events.

The Mystery of the Missing Pandemic by Dwaipayan Banerjee (2023, pp. 57, 59–65) is a thought-provoking and intriguing exploration of an often-overlooked aspect of history. Banerjee explores the lack of evidence about the Spanish Influenza pandemic's impact on India, highlighting factors like limited documentation, naming conventions, and social conditions. He presents various hypotheses and theories without definitive conclusions, allowing readers to explore the historical puzzle and engage in their own exploration.

The edited volume *Pandemics and Literature: Regional and Global Perspectives,* by Kamlesh Mohan and Saurav Kumar Rai (2025) provides a detailed analysis of epidemics and pandemics, examining their historical context, effects on individuals, social upheaval, and reactions. It explores themes like evolving perceptions, public reactions, gendered dimensions, and rumours. It is a valuable resource for students and researchers in cultural studies, medical anthropology, public health, pandemic history, sociology of medicine, and South Asian studies.

Besides the earlier Indian literatures, the author also considered studies by foreign scholars on various aspects of the influenza pandemic. These are thorough examination of the influenza virus, detailing its origins, mutations, and the scientific challenges faced during the pandemic (Barry, 2005, pp. 89–195); scientific, historical, and societal dimensions of influenza (Brown, 2018, pp. 151–164); insightful analysis of how communities and individuals have responded to major disease outbreaks, offering a multifaceted view of the complex interplay between infectious diseases and human society (Hays, 2009, pp. 179–213); importance of studying pandemics and the role of historical analysis in understanding their impact (Honigsbaum, 2009a, pp. 35–150); valuable contribution to the understanding of the global impact of the 1918 influenza pandemic and offering a more nuanced understanding of the pandemic's impact on different regions and populations (Johnson & Mueller, 2002, pp. 105–107); comprehensive examination of the profound consequences of the 1918–19 influenza pandemic on the British Empire and also tries to explore the global reach of the pandemic and its specific impact on various regions within the empire (Killingray, 2003, pp. 30–37); a captivating exploration of the 1918 influenza pandemic, blending historical narrative with scientific investigation (Kolata, 1999, pp. 35–55); highlighted significant pandemics recorded in human history, and the pandemic-related crises have caused enormous negative impacts on health, economies, and even national security in the world (Qiu et al., 2016, pp. 3–7, 9); a major and wide-ranging study of the great epidemic scourges of humanity—plague, leprosy, smallpox, syphilis, cholera, and yellow fever/malaria—over the last six centuries (Watts, 1997, pp. 1–200); emphasized an interesting and enlightening exploration of a historical event and the devastating impact of the 1918 influenza pandemic, shedding light on its far-reaching consequences and the collective amnesia that followed (Crosby, 2012, pp. 17–37); tried to explore an informative exploration of one of the most devastating global health crises in history. The author also navigates the complexities of the 1918 influenza pandemic, providing readers with a clear and engaging account of the virus's origins, rapid spread, and profound impact on societies worldwide (Kupperberg, 2009, p. 23).

The researcher consulted various sources, including books, reports, and journals, to study the influenza pandemic's consequences in India and abroad, in Bombay, where the Spanish Flu arrived first and spread. No one can deny the fact that the Bombay Presidency did not tell the entire story. In addition, several Indian newspapers both in English and also in local vernaculars, like, *the Amrita Bazar Patrika, The Bengalee, Hindoo Patriot, The Indian Daily News, The Statesman, The Englishman, Times of India*, etc. reported the incidences of the death tolls, colonial bureaucracy, and common people's response about this unimaginable public health crisis. The author also addresses the inadequacy of systematic coverage of Bengal's devastating situation, despite not being an exhaustive list of publications. This inadequacy instils the present author to think over the issue, and the present mission is a fruitful outcome. This is, however, in no way an exhaustive list of publications and any omission, therefore, is unintentional.

Aim and Objectives

Retrospective studies on the Spanish Influenza provide insights into the pandemic's historical and epidemiological aspects. Studies highlight the unprecedented scale and challenges faced by healthcare systems worldwide. In India, the study reveals unique socio-economic conditions and public health infrastructure. International studies provide a comprehensive understanding of transmission patterns, morbidity, and mortality rates. The Spanish Influenza in India has provided valuable insights into the pandemic's historical impact, but there are gaps in understanding sociocultural and regional variations. Existing research often generalizes experiences without exploring diverse factors. We have limited comprehensive analysis of long-term socio-economic repercussions. Bridging these gaps would enhance our comprehension of the pandemic's impact and contribute to contemporary public health challenges. The primary focus of the present study revolves around uncovering the region-specific nuances of the outbreak. By honing in on colonial Bengal, the author aims to contribute to a more nuanced understanding of how historical and contextual factors influenced the trajectory of the Spanish Influenza in colonial Bengal, offering insights that can inform contemporary public health strategies and preparedness.

The study explores the Spanish Influenza pandemic in India, focusing on colonial Bengal. It examines the impact of colonial medical institutions, practitioners, and policies on influenza containment and management. The study also examines indigenous healing practices and common peoples' responses, providing a holistic understanding of healthcare dynamics during the pandemic. The historical perspective allows for an analysis of the adaptability and limitations of medical interventions, contributing to a broader understanding of the Spanish Influenza's impact on public health in colonial Bengal.

In such a panorama, the feelings instil the present author to think over the matter that the fundamental aim of this project is to explore a comprehensive medico-historical understanding of the 1918–19 influenza pandemic, its management, and how the wider "society" impacts upon medicine in colonial Bengal. The present study tries to explore (i) how the influenza pandemic took entry in India? (ii) how the influenza pandemic began and spread in different districts of colonial Bengal? (iii) how the colonial governance handled this challenge? (iv) what role did the indigenous practitioners perform during this pandemic? (v) what was common peoples' attitude about the pandemic and the colonial governance? (vi) how native press reported and monitored in handling this pandemic? (vii) what lessons and long-term consequences we have experienced from this devastating pandemic?

On the whole, the present study explores the relationship between disease medicine and society, focusing on sociocultural and economic factors that influenced healthcare during the pandemic, emphasizing the adaptability and limitations of medical interventions in colonial Bengal during a critical historical period.

Situating the Discourse: A Foucauldian Theoretical Approach

The present discourse utilizes Michel Foucault's theories of bio-power and bio-politics as its primary theoretical framework to critically analyze the Spanish Influenza pandemic (1918–20) in colonial Bengal. These theories, integral to Foucault's extensive examination of power and governance, offer a profound perspective for understanding the complex interplay between disease management and colonial authority (Foucault, 1978, pp. 135–159; Rabinow & Rose, 2006, pp. 195–217). Foucault's concept of bio-power signifies a form of power that emerged in modernity, emphasizing the regulation, optimization, and control of life itself. This type of power manifests through public health policies, surveillance systems, medical institutions, and statistical tools that monitor and influence populations. In colonial Bengal, bio-power was implemented by the British administration's efforts to manage the pandemic, often masked as humanitarian concern, yet fundamentally motivated by economic interests and imperial dominance (Arnold, 1993, pp. 139–164; Harrison, 1994, pp. 101–126). Health interventions, including the distribution of medical resources and the management of mortality rates, were applied inconsistently, frequently favouring urban elites and colonial officials while disregarding the rural impoverished (Chandavarkar, 1992, pp. 95–120).

Foucault's notion of bio-politics is intricately linked to the political strategies and technologies employed to manage populations, particularly in relation to health, hygiene, and demographic oversight (Foucault, 2003, pp. 239–263; Esposito, 2008, pp. 37–59). The colonial government's reaction to the Spanish Flu was fundamentally bio-political, driven by the need to sustain order and productivity amid a significant mortality crisis (Bhattacharya, 2012b, pp. 19–45). The utilization of census data, the classification of illnesses, and the execution of restricted health measures were not merely public health initiatives, they were governance instruments aimed at maintaining colonial stability rather than promoting the welfare of the indigenous population (Bashford, 2004, pp. 75–102; Vaughan, 1991, pp. 45–68). Foucault's theoretical framework is particularly effective for examining this historical pandemic, as it facilitates a more profound critique of the dynamics of power during crises. It illustrates how disease serves as a battleground for reinforcing and challenging political and racial hierarchies. Furthermore, it redirects attention from the biomedical dimensions of the pandemic to the sociopolitical mechanisms that dictated survival and mortality, as well as the conditions surrounding them (Lakoff & Collier, 2008, pp. 3–25). By applying Foucault's perspectives, this thesis contests Eurocentric narratives and positions colonial Bengal as a vital area of study, demonstrating how the pandemic functioned as both a public health crisis and an expression of colonial bio-political authority.

Therefore, Michel Foucault's theories of bio-power and bio-politics act as an illuminating lens for re-evaluating the Spanish Influenza pandemic in colonial Bengal. Rather than being a mere medical occurrence, the pandemic served as a pivotal moment that allowed colonial authorities to reinforce and solidify their dominion over life itself. By examining the mechanisms of power exercised through health policies, surveillance, and the varied treatment of different populations, this theoretical perspective uncovers the colonial rationale behind public health measures—or the absence of such measures. It highlights that the responses to the pandemic were not applied uniformly, but were significantly influenced by pre-existing hierarchies of race, class, and imperial interests (Anderson, 2006, pp. 67–92). Foucault's viewpoint facilitates a profound re-evaluation of historical pandemics, viewing them not solely as biological events but as political phenomena with lasting implications. In the context of Bengal, this perspective necessitates an acknowledgement of the intertwined nature of disease management and the overarching agenda of colonial rule. It underscores the transformation of bodies into focal points for political action, illustrating how entire communities were subjected to state policies that prioritized imperial stability over human welfare. Consequently, this theoretical framework not only enriches our historical comprehension of the 1918–20 pandemic but also fosters a critical awareness of the ongoing intersections of power, health, and inequality in contemporary global health challenges (Adams, 2016, pp. 11–35). Through this Foucauldian lens, the Spanish Influenza in colonial Bengal[19] emerges not merely as a numerical tragedy but as a significant episode in the narrative of bio-political governance and colonial oppression.

Methodology

Data and information were collected from primary and secondary sources at various Kolkata institutions and also from sources outside India (London, UK and Bangladesh). Archival documents had been collected from the Directorate of State Archives, Kolkata, West Bengal; All India Institute of Hygiene and Public Health; School of Tropical Medicine, Kolkata; West Bengal Secretariat Library; Writer's Building; Town Hall Library; National Library, Kolkata; National Archives of India; and also from the India Office Library; Wellcome Trust Library; University College of London; and the National Archives of London, UK. I have also used the digitized reports available online at the National Medical Library of Scotland website and the United States National Library of Medicine. Online journals available through JSTOR, SAGE, OXFORD, TAYLOR & FRANCIS, and CAMBRIDGE ONLINE were of great help for this investigation.

Plan of the Report

The present report contains seven chapters, including observations and conclusion.

Introduction encompasses the whole plethora of the present research. The introduction discusses the impact of the influenza on India, focusing on colonial Bengal. It highlights the importance of understanding sociopolitical and demographic factors influencing the pandemic's spread and its implications in colonial Bengal, connecting the study to broader historical contexts.

Chapter 1 outlines the staggering impact of the influenza pandemic on both urban Calcutta and its surrounding rural areas. This chapter analyzes the 1918–19 influenza outbreak's unprecedented mortality rates, focusing on socio-economic conditions, healthcare infrastructure, and population density in Calcutta. It also discusses the public health response and challenges faced by local communities.

Chapter 2 illuminates the extensive impact of the 1918–19 influenza pandemic beyond Calcutta, focusing on various districts within colonial Bengal (Bangladesh). This section explores the challenges faced by rural communities and smaller towns during the pandemic, analyzing demographic, economic, and healthcare variations across colonial Bengal, highlighting unique features and responses.

Chapter 3 tries to explore the 1918–19 influenza pandemic and famine in colonial Bengal, examining the interconnected dynamics and socio-economic factors that exacerbated famine conditions. It provides a nuanced understanding of the complex web of vulnerabilities that marked this historical period.

Chapter 4 investigates the 1918–19 influenza pandemic's impact on public health, medical responses, and colonial governance in Bengal. It delves into the dynamics of disease control, medical interventions, and the politics of imperialism, revealing complex relationships shaping health policies.

Chapter 5 examines the long-term socio-economic, demographic, and health effects of the 1918–19 influenza outbreak in colonial Bengal, offering valuable epidemiological lessons for contemporary public health strategies and contributing to a broader understanding of enduring effects.

Chapter 6 summarizes the discussion and concludes, offering a glimpse into future research to comprehend the pandemic's implications. The report ends with Bibliography and primary sources in the Annexure.

The present study titled, *Public Health and the Pandemic in Colonial Bengal: An Analysis of the Spanish Influenza (1918–1920)* offers a nuanced perspective on the historical, social, and economic implications of a global pandemic in a region with its unique dynamics. By delving into archival materials, medical records, and contemporary accounts, researchers can unravel the intricate tapestry of the pandemic's impact on Bengal's communities. This includes assessing the disparities in the toll on various demographic groups, analyzing the role of pre-existing health conditions, and understanding the socio-economic consequences such as disruptions in trade, agriculture, and labour markets. The historical research on the Spanish Influenza in Bengal also contributes to our understanding of the epidemiological features of the virus within a localized setting. We can explore in-depth variations in transmission patterns, susceptibility factors, and the effectiveness of public health interventions. This knowledge is pivotal for contemporary epidemiologists and virologists, aiding them in developing more targeted and region-specific strategies for controlling infectious diseases. A detailed examination of Bengal's response to the Spanish Influenza provides invaluable insights into the effectiveness of public health measures implemented during the crisis. This includes studying the role of government interventions, quarantine[18] measures, healthcare infrastructure, and community-based initiatives. Understanding what worked and what didn't in Bengal can inform the development of robust and adaptable public health strategies for managing pandemics today. The Spanish Influenza in Bengal's development trajectory has had long-term consequences on the region's health systems. Researchers can connect historical pandemics to the evolution of public health systems, assessing resilience and guiding policymakers in creating sustainable infrastructures. The study also sheds light on cultural and social dimensions of the pandemic, revealing how communities coped with grief, societal changes, and the role of cultural practices in health behaviours. This knowledge is crucial for developing sensitive and community-driven public health approaches, ensuring interventions resonate with the local population. This knowledge is valuable for contemporary public health endeavours, helping to navigate and mitigate challenges posed by current and future pandemics.

In short, study on the Spanish Influenza in colonial Bengal cause a comprehensive understanding of the pandemic's impact on the region. It explores socio-economic, epidemiological, and cultural dimensions of the crisis, emphasizing the need for understanding how communities, healthcare systems, and governance structures responded. This study offers valuable lessons for contemporary researchers and policymakers, emphasizing the importance of historical insights in managing and mitigating pandemics in the ever-evolving global health landscape.

Notes

1 Spanish Influenza—The "Spanish Flu" or the Great Spanish Influenza was the deadliest pandemic in human history. People believed the disease originated in Spain. However,

the actual story was that Spain was one of the few major European countries that remained neutral during the First World War. Unlike the Allied and Central powers, where the freedom of the press was low as compared to the Spanish press where the freedom of the press was high. Spanish media first reported the pandemic; therefore, it became known as "Spanish Influenza".

2 COVID-19—COVID-19, caused by the novel coronavirus SARS-CoV-2, emerged in late 2019 and spread worldwide, leading to a global pandemic. It spreads through respiratory droplets, with symptoms ranging from mild respiratory issues to severe pneumonia, especially affecting older adults and those with underlying health conditions. Governments implemented various measures, such as lockdowns, social distancing, and mask mandates to curb the spread. Governments started vaccination campaigns to control the virus's impact. Ongoing research continues to deepen our understanding of the virus and its variants, emphasizing the importance of public health measures and vaccination in managing the ongoing situation.

3 Epidemiology—Epidemiology is the study of the distribution and determinants of diseases in populations. It involves analyzing patterns, causes, and effects of health and illness, aiming to improve public health outcomes. Epidemiologists collect and interpret data to understand the frequency and spread of diseases, identify risk factors, and inform preventive strategies. This field plays a crucial role in outbreak investigations, disease surveillance, and the development of evidence-based interventions. By studying the patterns of diseases, epidemiology contributes to the advancement of healthcare policies and practices, ultimately enhancing overall community well-being.

4 Public health—Public health is a multidisciplinary field focused on safeguarding and improving the health of communities and populations. It encompasses the organized efforts of society to prevent disease, promote health, and prolong life through various interventions, such as health education, policy development, and disease prevention initiatives. Public health professionals work to address health disparities, create health policies, and implement strategies that enhance overall well-being on a societal level. This field emphasizes preventive measures and the promotion of healthy behaviours to achieve optimal health outcomes for the entire population.

5 Black Death—The Black Death, occurring in the 14th century, was one of the deadliest pandemics in human history. The bacterium Yersinia pestis caused it, and fleas infesting rats transmitted it. Originating in Central Asia, the plague spread along trade routes, reaching Europe in 1347. Characterized by severe flu-like symptoms and swollen lymph nodes, the disease led to unprecedented mortality rates, wiping out about 25 to 50% of Europe's population. The Black Death had profound social, economic, and cultural effects, reshaping medieval societies and influencing subsequent historical developments.

6 HIV/AIDS—HIV/AIDS, caused by the human immunodeficiency virus (HIV), is a global pandemic affecting millions of people. First identified in the early 1980s, the virus spreads through unprotected sexual intercourse, contaminated blood transfusions, and the sharing of needles. HIV weakens the immune system over time, making individuals susceptible to opportunistic infections and cancers. Antiretroviral therapy (ART) has improved the prognosis for those with HIV, transforming it into a manageable chronic condition. However, challenges such as stigma, discrimination, and access to treatment persist. Global efforts focus on prevention, education, and expanding access to healthcare to mitigate the impact of HIV/AIDS on individuals and communities worldwide.

7 Antiviral therapies—Antiviral therapies are medications designed to treat viral infections by inhibiting the replication of viruses within the host's cells. Unlike antibiotics, which target bacteria, antivirals aim to disrupt specific stages of the viral life cycle. These drugs are crucial in managing various viral infections, including influenza, HIV, hepatitis, and herpes. Antiviral medications work by blocking viral enzymes, preventing the virus from entering cells, or interfering with its ability to replicate. Their effectiveness varies, and continuous research is underway to develop new antiviral drugs and improve existing ones. Antiviral therapies play a vital role in both preventing the spread of viral diseases and treating individuals infected with viruses.

8 The First World War acquired the nickname "the Great War" (1914–1918) in the history of humankind. The Allied and Central Powers fought the war. The Allied powers included Great Britain and the Commonwealth countries, the USA, Italy, France, and the Russian Empire, whereas the Central powers comprised the German Empire and its colonies, the Austro-Hungarian Empire, the Tsardom of Bulgaria, and the Ottoman Empire.

9 Ayurveda—Ayurveda is a traditional system of medicine with roots in ancient India, dating back thousands of years. The word "Ayurveda" translates to "knowledge of life" in Sanskrit. This holistic healing system focuses on achieving balance and harmony within the body, mind, and spirit to promote overall well-being. Ayurveda emphasizes individualized treatments based on a person's unique constitution, or "dosha", which comprises three elements: Vata, Pitta, and Kapha. Herbal remedies, dietary guidelines, yoga, and lifestyle practices are integral components of Ayurvedic treatments. While Ayurveda has gained global interest, it coexists with modern medicine, offering alternative and complementary approaches to health and healing.

10 Charaka—Charaka, often referred to as the "Father of Ayurveda", was an ancient Indian physician and sage who contributed to the development of Ayurvedic medicine. Scholars believe Charaka lived around 300 BCE, and his teachings and insights comprise the foundational Ayurvedic text, the "Charaka Samhita". This comprehensive work encompasses principles of diagnosis, treatment, and prevention of diseases, emphasizing the holistic approach of Ayurveda. Charaka's contributions have played a pivotal role in shaping the theoretical and practical aspects of traditional Indian medicine, and his work continues to influence Ayurvedic practices today.

11 Sushruta—People often regard Sushruta, an ancient Indian physician and surgeon, as one of the founding figures in surgery. He is also associated with the development of Ayurvedic medicine. Scholars believe he lived around 600 BCE, and his teachings comprise the "Sushruta Samhita", an ancient Sanskrit text. Scholars recognize this compilation as one of the earliest details of surgical techniques, medical procedures, and principles of anatomy. Sushruta's contributions to medicine include innovative surgical practices, such as plastic surgery procedures and descriptions of various surgical instruments. His work has affected the evolution of surgical knowledge.

12 Panchakarma—It is a classical Ayurvedic therapy that aims to restore body balance by eliminating accumulated toxins. It comprises five therapeutic procedures: Vamana, Virechana, Basti, Nasya, and Raktamokshana. These treatments are personalized based on an individual's constitution and health condition. Panchakarma revitalizes the mind and strengthens immunity, making it a core component of preventive and curative Ayurveda.

13 Bhils—The Bhil tribe, living in the central and western regions of India, is one of the largest indigenous communities in the country. Known for their rich cultural heritage, the Bhils have a distinct language and traditionally practice agriculture, cultivating crops such as millet and maize. They are skilled in various crafts, including pottery and weaving. The Bhil community has a strong connection to nature, often reflected in their folklore and rituals. People have worked overtime to preserve and celebrate their unique traditions.

14 Nizam rules—The Nizam rules refer to the period of governance by the Nizams, the monarchs of the princely state of Hyderabad, which existed from the late 18th century until integrating Hyderabad into the Indian Union in 1948. The larger Indian subcontinent knew the Nizams' distinctive and autonomous rule. During this time, Hyderabad was one of the largest and wealthiest princely states, marked by a unique blend of Hindu and Muslim cultures. The Nizams played a crucial role in regional politics and administration, maintaining a level of autonomy until the state's merger with India. The end of the Nizam rule marked a significant chapter in Indian history as Hyderabad became part of the newly formed Republic of India.

15 Thymol solution—Thymol solution is a liquid formulation derived from thymol; a natural compound found in thyme oil. Thymol's antiseptic and antimicrobial properties make it common in various medical and cleaning applications. People use thymol

solutions to disinfect and treat wounds and minor skin infections. Their antibacterial properties lead to their use in mouthwashes and oral care products. Thymol solutions have shown effectiveness against a range of bacteria and fungi, contributing to their use in both medical and household settings for maintaining hygiene and promoting health.

16 RNA—RNA, or ribonucleic acid, is a vital molecule found in cells that plays a key role in various biological processes. Like DNA, nucleotides compose RNA, but it differs in structure and function. There are three main types of RNA: messenger RNA (mRNA), transfer RNA (tRNA), and ribosomal RNA (rRNA). mRNA carries genetic information from DNA to the ribosomes, where protein synthesis occurs. tRNA helps translate the genetic code into proteins by bringing amino acids to the ribosomes. rRNA forms an integral part of the ribosomes, the cellular machinery responsible for protein synthesis. RNA is essential in the process of gene expression, allowing cells to convert genetic information into functional proteins and perform crucial functions in the cell's life cycle.

17 H1N1 Influenza A Virus—H1N1 influenza, a subtype of influenza A virus, is a contagious virus that causes upper and sometimes lower respiratory tract infections in the host. The name "H1N1" refers to the unique properties that tell the immune system to recognize the virus and allow it to bind and multiply. "H" (hemagglutinin) and "N" (neuraminidase) are two proteins found in the coat or envelope.

18 Quarantine—The concept of quarantine has ancient roots, and one of the earliest known instances dates back to the 14th century in Dubrovnik, now in Croatia. Public health officials use quarantine to isolate and restrict the movement of individuals or communities exposed to contagious diseases, thus preventing the spread of illness. It aims to separate and monitor those infected, even if they are not displaying symptoms, during the incubation period of the disease. Historically, outbreaks of infectious diseases like influenza, tuberculosis, and COVID-19 prompted the use of quarantine measures. It is a crucial tool in preventing the transmission of infectious agents, protecting public health, and mitigating the impact of epidemics or pandemics.

19 Colonial Bengal—Colonial Bengal, under British rule, comprised a vast territorial jurisdiction that included present-day Bangladesh and the Indian states of West Bengal. Initially, part of the Bengal Presidency, one of the three administrative divisions established by the British East India Company, Bengal played a pivotal role in the administration of British India. In 1911, the British government partitioned Bengal for administrative convenience, creating a reduced Bengal Presidency and the new province of Eastern Bengal and Assam. However, widespread protests against the partition led to its annulment in 1912. Bengal remained a crucial centre for colonial administration, commerce, and cultural exchange until India gained independence in 1947, leading to the eventual partition of Bengal along religious lines.

References

Books

Acharya, Y. T. (2000). *Charaka Samhita* by Agnivesha revised by Charaka and Dridabala, Commentary of Chakrapanidutta. Vimanasthana; Janapadodhwamsa Vimanam (1st ed., Chapter 3, Verse 6). Chowkhamba Surbharati.

Adams, A. (1899). *The western Rajputana states: A medico-topographical and general account of Marwar, Sirohi, and Jaisalmir*. Junior Army & Navy Stores.

Adams, V. (2016). *Metrics: What counts in global health*. Duke University Press.

Anderson, W. (2006). *Colonial pathologies: American tropical medicine, race, and hygiene in the Philippines*. Duke University Press.

Annual Report of the Sanitary Commissioner with the Government of India for 1918–1920 (pp. 5–6).

Arnold, D. (1993). *Colonizing the body: State medicine and epidemic disease in nineteenth-century India*. University of California Press.

Arnold, D. (2015). Disease, rumor, and panic in India's plague and influenza epidemics, 1896–1919. In R. Peckham (Ed.), *Empires of panic: Epidemics and colonial anxieties* (pp. 111–129). Hong Kong University Press.
Arnold, D. (2022). *Pandemic India: From Cholera to Covid-19*. C. Hurst & Company.
Athukorala, P., & Athukorala, C. (2022). *The 1918–20 influenza pandemic: A retrospective in the time of COVID-19*. Cambridge University Press.
Bala, R. (1918). *The spread of influenza epidemic in the Punjab (1918–1919)*. Punjab Sanitary Board Report.
Barry, M. J. (2005). *The great influenza- the story of the deadliest pandemic in history*. Penguin Books.
Bashford, A. (2004). *Imperial hygiene: A critical history of colonialism, nationalism and public health*. Palgrave Macmillan.
Beveridge, W. I. B. (1978). *Influenza: The last great plague: An unfinished story of discovery*. Prodist.
Bhattacharya, N. (2012a). *Contagion and enclaves: Tropical medicine in colonial India*. Liverpool University Press.
Bhattacharya, S. (2012b). *Expunging variola: The control and eradication of smallpox in India, 1947–1977*. Orient Blackswan.
Brown, J. (2018). *Influenza: The hundred-year hunt to cure the deadliest disease in history*. Touchstone.
Burnet, F. M. (1953). *Natural history of infectious diseases* (2nd ed.). Cambridge University Press.
Census of India. (1921a). *Vol. XI, Central Provinces and Berar, Part I—Report* (Nagpur, 1923) (p. 4).
Census of India. (1921b). *Vol. XV, Punjab, and Delhi, part I–Report* (p. 60).
Census of India. (1921c). *Vol. XVI, United Provinces of Agra and Oudh, part I–Report* (Allahabad, 1923) (p. 13).
Census of India. (1921d). *Vol. XXI, Hyderabad–Report* (Hyderabad, 1923) (p. 6).
Census of India. (1921e). *Vol. XXIV, Rajputana, and Ajmer–Merwara, part I–Report* (Calcutta, 1923) (p. 16).
Chandavarkar, R. (1992). Plague panic and epidemic politics in India, 1896–1914. In P. Chatterjee & G. Pandey (Eds.), *Subaltern studies VII: Writings on South Asian history and society* (pp. 62–132). Oxford University Press.
Chhun, M. (2015). *Death and disorder: The 1918–1919 influenza pandemic in British India* [Unpublished PhD Dissertation, History Department, University of Colorado].
Creighton, C. (1891). *A history of epidemics in Britain*. Cambridge University Press.
Crosby, W. A. (2012). *America's forgotten pandemic: The influenza of 1918*. Cambridge University Press.
Davis, M. (2001). *Late Victorian holocausts: El Niño famines and the making of the third world*. Verso Books.
Esposito, R. (2008). *Bios: Biopolitics and philosophy* (T. Campbell, Trans.). University of Minnesota Press.
Foucault, M. (1978). *The history of sexuality, volume 1: An introduction* (R. Hurley, Trans.). Pantheon Books.
Foucault, M. (2003). *Society must be defended: Lectures at the Collège de France, 1975–1976* (D. Macey, Trans.). Picador.
Gordon, P. (2021). *Complete guide on great influenza, historical analysis of pandemics and precious teachings on how to deal with actual and future epidemics*. Giancarlo Toscano.
Harrison, M. (1994). *Public health in British India: Anglo-Indian preventive medicine, 1859–1914*. Cambridge University Press.
Harrison, M. (2016). Pandemics. In M. Jackson (Ed.). *The Routledge history of disease* (pp. 129–146). Routledge.
Hays, J. N. (2009). *The burdens of disease–epidemics and human response in western history*. Rutger University Press.

Herriot, P. T. (1920). *The influenza pandemic, 1918, as observed in the Punjab, India* [MD thesis, University of Edinburgh].
Honigsbaum, M. (2009a). *Living with Enza: The forgotten story of Britain and the great flu pandemic of 1918*. Springer.
Johnson, N. (2006). *Britain and the 1918–19 influenza pandemic: A dark epilogue*. Routledge.
Kenneth, F. K. (1993). *The Cambridge world history of human disease*. Cambridge University Press.
Kessler, M. (2020). *Strengthening health systems during a pandemic: The role of development finance*. Centre for Global Health US Centers for Disease Control and Prevention.
Kiple, K. F. (Ed.). (1993). *The Cambridge world history of human disease*. Cambridge University Press.
Kolata, G. (1999). *Flu-The story of the great influenza pandemic of 1918 and the search for the virus that caused it*. Simon & Schuster.
Kumar, D. (2013). Probing history of medicine and public health in India: A study of encounters at multiple sites. In D. Kumar & R. S. Basu (Eds.), *Medical encounters in British India* (pp. 23–39). Oxford University Press.
Kuperberg, P. (2008). *Great historic disasters: The influenza pandemic of 1918–19*. Chelsea House.
Kupperberg, P. (2009). *The influenza pandemic of 1918–1919*. Infobase Publishing.
Lakoff, A., & Collier, S. J. (Eds.). (2008). *Biosecurity interventions: Global health and security in question*. Columbia University Press.
Mander, H. (2020). *Locking down the poor: The pandemic and India's moral centre*. Speaking Tiger.
McMillen, C. W. (2024). *Pandemics: A very short introduction* (2nd ed.). Oxford University Press.
Ministry of Health. (1920). *Report on the pandemic of influenza, 1918–19*. His Majesty's Stationery Office.
Minutes of the Syndicate. (1919). *University of Calcutta*, 3rd March (p. 356); Also, for 22nd April (p. 66).
Mukherjee, M. (2010). *India in the shadows of empire: A legal and political history*. Oxford University Press.
Peckham, R. (2016). *Epidemics in modern Asia*. Cambridge University Press.
Polu, S. L. (2010). *Infectious disease in India, 1892–1940: Policy-making and the perception of risk*. Palgrave Macmillan.
Prakash, G. (1999). *Another reason: Science and the imagination of modern India*. Princeton University Press.
Quinn, T. (2008). *Flu: A social history of influenza*. New Holland Publishers.
Ramanna, M. (2003). Coping with the influenza pandemic: The Bombay experience. In H. Phillips & D. Killingray (Eds.), *The Spanish influenza pandemic of 1918–19: New perspectives* (pp. 86–98). Routledge.
Ray, K. (2008). *History of public health: Colonial Bengal, 1921–1947*. K.P. Bagchi & Co.
Report of the director of public instruction in the Bombay presidency. (1918–19). Govt. Printing.
Report on the sanitary administration of the Punjab and proceedings of the sanitary board for the year 1918. (1919). Govt. Printing.
Rice, G. W. (2005). *Black November: The 1918 influenza pandemic in New Zealand*. Christchurch. (Originally cited in *Scientific American*, 1977, p. 22).
Roser, M. (2020). *The Spanish flu: The global impact of the largest influenza pandemic in history*. https://ourworldindata.org/spanish-flu-largest-influenza-pandemic-in-history.
Sarkar, S. (1989). *Modern India: 1885–1947*. Macmillan.
Sekher, T. V. (2007). Public health administration in princely Mysore: Tackling the influenza pandemic of 1918. In W. Ernst & B. Pati (Eds.), *India's princely states: People, princes, and colonialism* (p. 198). Primus Books.

The excess mortality estimates are in the range of 7–8 per cent and correcting for under-registration, it would exceed 10 per cent. The Inspector of Schools in Berar estimated a minimum of 10 percent of the population to have died from influenza in his circle. Report on the State and Progress of Education in the Central Provinces and Berar for the year 1918–19 (Nagpur, 1919) (p. 9).
The Economist. (1919, April 12). *Mysore gold mining company limited* (p. 624).
Thornton, J. (1998). *Africa and Africans in the making of the Atlantic world, 1400–1800*. Cambridge University Press.
Times of India. (1918, October 15). *Influenza in Goa* (p. 10).
Tripathi, B. (2007a). *Charak Samhita with Charak Chandrika Hindi commentary: Sutra Sthan* (Vol. 5, verse 99, p. 139). Chaukhamba Surbharti Prakashan.
Tripathi, B. (2007b). *Charak Samhita with Charak Chandrika Hindi commentary: Sutra Sthan* (Vol. 5, verse 94, p. 137). Chaukhamba Surbharti Prakashan.
Tripathi, B. (2007c). *Charak Samhita with Charak Chandrika Hindi commentary: Sutra Sthan* (Vol. 8, verse 25, p. 10). Chaukhamba Surbharti Prakashan.
Tripathi, B. (2007d). *Charak Samhita with Charak Chandrika Hindi commentary: Sutra Sthan* (Vol. 8, verse 19, p. 199). Chaukhamba Surbharti Prakashan.
Tumbe, C. (2020). *The age of pandemics 1817–1929: How they shaped India and the world*. Harper Collins.
Vaughan, M. (1991). *Curing their ills: Colonial power and African illness*. Stanford University Press.
Watts, J. S. (1997). *Epidemics and history: Disease, power, and imperialism*. Yale University Press.
White, N. (1919). *A preliminary report on the influenza pandemic of 1918 in India*. Government of India Press.
Winternitz, M. C., Wason, I. M., & McNamara, F. P. (1920). *The pathology of influenza*. Yale University Press.

Articles

Arnold, D. (1979). Looting, grain riots and government policy in South India 1918. *Past & Present*, *84*(1), 111–145.
Arnold, D. (2019). Death and the modern empire: The 1918–19 influenza epidemic in India. *Transactions of the Royal Historical Society*, (29), 181–200.
Arnold, D. (2020). Pandemic India: Coronavirus and the uses of history. *Journal of Asian Studies*, *79*(3), 569–577.
Banerjee, D. (2023). The mystery of the missing pandemic. *History of the Present*, *13*(1), 57–70.
Bose, K. C. (1920). Influenza in and around the city of Calcutta. *Indian Medical Gazette*, *55*, 169.
Breedlove, B. (2006). Title of subordinate document. *Etymologia: Influenza. Emerging Infectious Diseases*, *12*(1), 179. Retrieved April 4, 2023, from https://doi.org/10.3201/eid1201.et1201
Chandra, S. (1996). The demographic impact of the 1918–19 influenza pandemic in India. *Population Studies*, *50*(1), 89–102. https://doi.org/10.1080/0032472031000149506.
Chandra, S., & Kassens-Noor, E. (2014). The evolution of pandemic influenza: Evidence from India 1918–19. *Bio Medical Central Infectious Diseases*, (510), 1–10.
Daszak, P., Cunningham, A. A., & Hyatt, A. D. (2001). Anthropogenic environmental change and the emergence of infectious diseases in wildlife. *Acta Tropica*, *78*(2), 103–116.
Frankema, E., & Tworek, H. (2020). Pandemics that changed the world: Historical reflections on COVID−19. *Journal of Global History*, *15*(3), 333–335.
Hill, K. (2011). Influenza in India 1918: Excess mortality reassessed. *Genus*, *67*(2), 24.
Honigsbaum, M. (2009b). Historical keyword pandemic. *The Lancet*, *373*, 1939.

Hoyle, F., & Wickramasinghe, C. (1977). Does epidemic disease come from space? *New Scientist*, *76*(1078), 402–404.
Humphreys, M. (2018). The influenza of 1918: Evolutionary perspectives in a historical context. *Evolution, Medicine, and Public Health*, *1*, 219–229.
Johnson, N. P. A. S., & Mueller, J. (2002). Updating the accounts: Global mortality of the 1918–1920 "Spanish" influenza pandemic. *Bulletin of the History of Medicine*, *76*(1), 105–115.
Killingray, D. (2003). A new imperial disease: The influenza pandemic of 1918–9 and its impact on the British empire. *Caribbean Quarterly*, *49*(4), 30–49.
Langford, C. (2005). Did the 1918–19 influenza pandemic originate in China? *Population and Development Review*, *31*(3), 473–505.
Liston, G. (1918, October 11). Influenza epidemics: History and experience. *Times of India*, p. 8.
Mihika, Y., Shaikh, S., & Phatak, M. (2020). The history of pandemics and epidemics in India. *International Journal of Advance Research, Ideas, and Innovations in Technology*, *6*(5), 167–170.
Mills, E. C., Robins, J. M., & Lipsitch, M. (2004). Transmissibility of 1918 Pandemic Influenza. *Nature*, *432*(7019), 904–906.
Mills, I. D. (1986). The 1918–1919 influenza pandemic: The Indian experience. *Indian Economic and Social History Review*, *23*(1), 1–40.
Morens, D. M., Taubenberger, J. K., & Fauci, A. S. (2008). Predominant role of bacterial pneumonia as a cause of death in pandemic influenza: Implications for pandemic influenza preparedness. *Journal of Infectious Diseases*, *198*(7), 962–970.
Mukherjee, S. (2011). The 'Spanish flu' in India, 1918–19: Mortality, politics and memory. *Indian Economic and Social History Review*, *48*(2), 191–220. https://doi.org/10.1177/001946461104800204
Ojo, O. B. (2020). Socio-economic impacts of 1918–19 influenza epidemic in Punjab. *Journal of Asian and African Studies*, *55*(7), 1023–1032.
Qiu, W., Rutherford, S., Mao, A., & Chu, C. (2016–17). The pandemic and its impact. *Health, Culture, and Society*, *9–10*, 3–11.
Rabinow, P., & Rose, N. (2006). Biopower today. *Bio Societies*, *1*(2), 195–217. https://doi.org/10.1017/S1745855206040014
Saunders, H., Patrick, R., & Krewski, D. (2016). Reviewing the history of pandemic influenza: Understanding patterns of emergence and transmission. *Pathogens*, *5*(4), 66.
Tambolkar, S., Pustake, M., Giri, P., & Tambolkar, I. (2022). Comparison of public health measures taken during Spanish flu and COVID-19 pandemics: A narrative review. *Journal of Family Medicine and Primary Care*, *11*(5), 1642–1647.
Tsoucalas, G., Kousoulis, A., & Sgantzos, M. (2016). The 1918 Spanish flu pandemic, the origins of the H1N1-virus strain, a glance in history. *European Journal of Clinical and Biomedical Sciences*, *2*(4), 23–28.
Yeole, M., Shaikh, S., & Phatak, M. (2020). The history of pandemics and epidemics in India. *International Journal of Advance Research, Ideas, and Innovations in Technology*, *6*(5), 167–170.

1 Calcutta Under Siege

Spanish Influenza in Calcutta and Beyond

The year 1918 is indelibly etched in history due to the influenza pandemic, a worldwide health emergency that significantly affected communities globally. In 1918, Calcutta encountered a catastrophic influenza pandemic because of its densely populated streets and neighbourhoods. The city turned into a battlefield against a hidden enemy with a staggering death toll. The pandemic ripped apart the social structure, dividing families, and affecting everyone irrespective of wealth or age. The pandemic overwhelmed hospitals and strained medical resources, while temporary clinics sprang up, silencing Calcutta's lively cultural centre (Tumbe, 2020, p. 127). The 1918–19 influenza pandemic in Calcutta disrupted the farming cycle, penetrating villages, resulting in crop failures and family losses. The story emphasizes resilience, grief, and community reactions to an unprecedented crisis (Sen, 1920, pp. 89–90).

Footsteps of the Deadliest Pandemic in the City of Calcutta

The jurisdiction of the 1918 Calcutta Municipal Corporation is essential for comprehending the dissemination of the Spanish Flu in Calcutta and its effects on different wards. The 1918 Calcutta Municipal Corporation divided Calcutta into 25 wards, specifically,

I-Shampooker, II-Coomertooly, III-Burtollah, IV-Sookea's Street, V-Jorabagan, VI-Jorasanko, VII-Bara Bazar, VIII-Colootollah, IX-Moochipara, X-Bowbazar, XI-Poddopukur, XII-Waterloo Street, XIII-Fenwick Bazar, XIV-Taltollah, XV-Collingah, XVI-Park Street, XVII-Baman Bustee, XVIII-Hastings, XIX-Entally, XX-Beniapukur, XXI-Ballygunge and Tollygunge, XXII-Bhowanipur, XXIII-Alipur, XXIV-Kidderpur and Ekbalpur, XXV-Watgunge and Garden Reach (Minutes of the Proceedings of the Special Meeting of the Calcutta Corporation, July 1918).

The 1918 surge of panicked Rajputana[1] immigrants challenged public health. Smallpox, plague, and the Spanish Flu (recurring in October) caused increased mortality (Minutes of the Proceedings of the Special Meeting of the Calcutta Corporation, June 1918, p. 62).

The Spanish Influenza epidemic in Calcutta from 1918 to 1919 was a serious assault that affected the city and its inhabitants. The illness spread swiftly because

DOI: 10.4324/9781003656647-2

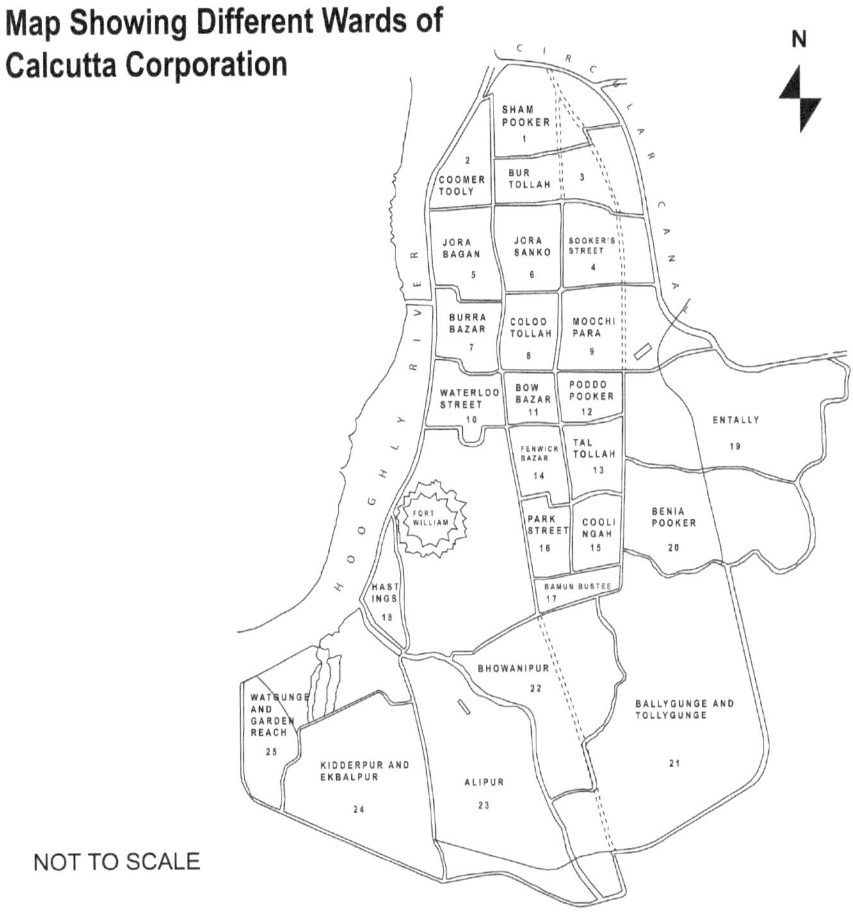

Figure 1.1 Different Wards of Calcutta Corporation in 1918 (Prepared by Author)

of the city's high population density and congested living conditions, influencing individuals across all ages and social strata. The absence of immunity to the unfamiliar strain facilitated its quick spread. Calcutta's healthcare system was unprepared, resulting in overcrowded hospitals and individuals lying in the streets. The number of fatalities was enormous, prompting mass graves and cremations. Losing lives had a significant effect on families and communities, leaving a lasting mark on the city's social structure (Minutes of the Proceedings of the Special Meeting of the Calcutta Corporation, September 1918). The 1918–19 Spanish Influenza epidemic in Calcutta affected the city's economy, resulting in business closures and the cancellation of public events. This underscored the necessity for strong public health interventions, such as early detection and medical help to curb pandemic propagation and reduce high death rates (Minutes of the Proceedings of the Calcutta Corporation, September 1918).

Box 2.1 The New Fever: Report by Health Officer of Calcutta

On the 12th of this month, the health officer of Calcutta to the General Committee of the Calcutta Corporation submitted a report regarding the ongoing fever epidemic. This morning, a special meeting of the Board of Health convened to deliberate on the precautionary measures. The preliminary statement that follows reflects the board's perspective; however, it is important to note that it is based on incomplete information and may need to be revised in the future.

People reported a few isolated cases of a short-duration, influenza-like fever 2–3 weeks ago. In the past week, the disease has spread rapidly and extensively, now manifesting as an epidemic throughout the city. Fortunately, it appears to be relatively mild, with no fatalities reported thus far. We expect the overall death rate to eventually rise, especially among older adults and weakened, who might succumb to a severe fever posing minor threat to healthier individuals. The swift spread of the illness underscores its highly contagious nature. The incubation period is notably brief, ranging from 2 to 6 days. The widespread susceptibility to the disease and its short incubation period caused the sudden and nearly simultaneous onset of symptoms in many individuals, following a few isolated cases. Regrettably, a previous infection does not confer immunity, and relapses are common. The disease appears to spread primarily through contact. Infections can occur through respiratory secretions, meaning that direct physical contact is not necessary. An infected individual who coughs, sneezes, or talks, especially in crowded or poorly ventilated spaces, can easily transmit the illness to those nearby. The risks associated with shared drinking cups, utensils, and personal items, such as handkerchiefs and towels, are clear, while the prevalent habit of spitting in public places in Calcutta will undoubtedly contribute to the spread of the disease.

H.M. Crake, Health Officer to the Calcutta Corporation
(Minutes of the Proceedings of the Special Meeting
of the Calcutta Corporation, October 1918)

The initial phase of influenza infection in Calcutta needs to emphasize its severity and characteristics, as well as the widespread outbreak in various wards, to ensure a full comprehension. The following discussion will address this issue succinctly.

Onset, Course, and Spreading Pattern of the Disease in Different Wards of Calcutta

In June 1918, the influenza pandemic began with dispersed cases, but the distribution remained unclear. By the close of June, several brief "Fever" clusters akin to Dengue[2] emerged in Wards XIX and V. The Kidderpore dispensary was exposed to

Spanish Flu in June. The disease escalated to epidemic proportions in July, but did not spread until July 13. The peak attendance for fever and influenza cases occurred on July 11. The death count from influenza climbed from 16 to 107 during the week ending July 20, reaching a peak of 179 in the week ending July 27, 1918. The average mortality rate for the entire city was 35.0 per mile, with 20 of the 25 wards surpassing 30 per mile. They instituted a revised standard to compile a "Black List" of wards with elevated death rates. The city's vital statistics were clear, with the most affected regions being Kidderpore and nearby areas (Preliminary Report on the Epidemic in India by the Sanitary Commissioner with the Govt. of India, File No. S. 2D–8, Proceedings Nos. B27–29).

The purdah system[3] in Kidderpore and Bara Bazar[4] areas resulted in high mortality rates among females because of the large coolie population living in unsanitary conditions and refusal of advice, leading to rapid infection spread.

Table 1.1 Deaths from "Spanish Flu" for Weeks in the City of Calcutta from July 1 to August 10, 1918

Wards	*Population*	*Deaths*	*Rate per 1000 Population*
I	53036	41	0.77
II	33073	27	0.81
III	54610	30	0.54
IV	48112	24	0.49
V	52114	25	0.47
VI	59541	38	0.63
District I	**300486**	**185**	**0.61**
VII	30495	18	0.59
VIII	57094	11	0.19
IX	63362	25	0.39
X	25014	9	0.35
XI	29966	13	0.43
XII	6284	3	0.47
District II	**212215**	**79**	**0.37**
XIII	28436	4	0.14
XIV	32112	7	0.21
XV	11385	2	0.17
XVI	5294	–	–
XVII	3125	1	0.32
XIX	45072	19	0.42
XX	37881	15	0.39
District III	**163305**	**48**	**0.48**
XVIII	5550	1	0.18
XXI	39952	24	0.60
XXII	54569	32	0.58
XXIII	19749	7	0.35
XXIV	21869	23	1.0
XXV	43806	17	0.38
District IV	**185495**	**104**	**0.56**

Source: (Proceedings of the Govt. of Bengal, Municipal Department, Sanitation Branch, File No. S.2D–8 (5))

Sex Differences in Death Rates

From September 1 to December 31, 1918, the colonial authorities documented 3673 deaths related to influenza in Calcutta. Males reported death rates of 30.6 per mile, whereas females had rates of 44.1 per mile. Contextual analysis shows that Kidderpore (XXIV) experienced the highest mortality rate compared to other inland wards such as Ballygunge (XXI), Beniapukur (XX), Jorabagan (V), Hastings (XVIII), and Entally (XIX). Although densely populated, the other wards lacked coastal access, thus resulting in relatively lower disease transmission. This is quite clear that Kidderpore being connected with waterways was prone to infection being carried by sailors, which intensified because of it being a densely populated area. Table 1.2 shows that the city faced the highest female mortality rate because of the purdah system, poor living conditions, and patriarchal influence. Both Hindus and Muslims faced elevated community-specific death rates because of influenza, underscoring the pandemic's substantial effect on public health (Proceedings of the Government of Bengal in the Municipal Department Sanitation, for the Month of October 1918, Prevention of the Outbreak and Spread of Influenza in Bengal, File No. S. 2D-1(1)).

The Spanish Flu outbreak posed difficulties because of ignorance and superstition among the general populace. Areas with a Christian majority experienced lower death rates because of greater health awareness. The death rate among males was 30 and the cost was 6 per mile. Figure 1.2 graphically represents Table 1.2 to enhance readers' comprehension.

Figures 1.3 and 1.4 visually illustrate Tables 1.3 and 1.4 to enhance understanding for the reader. Death rates have risen considerably across all age groups, with

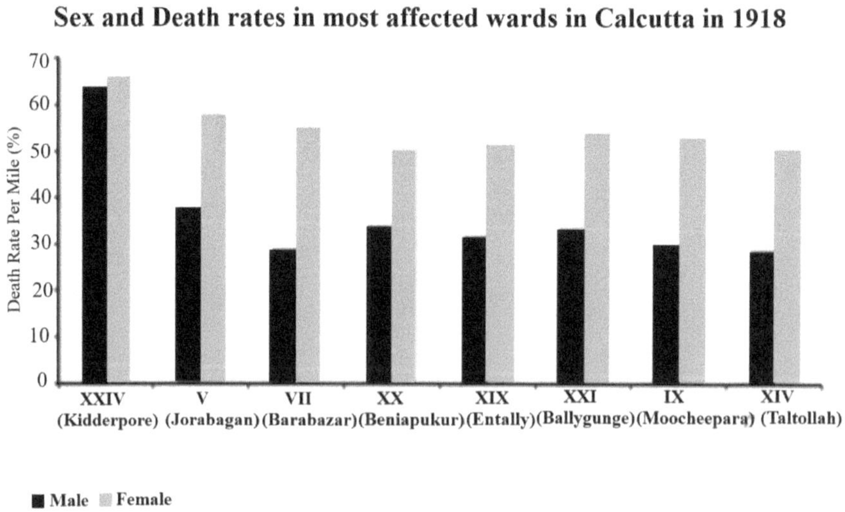

Figure 1.2 Graph Showing Sex and Death Rates in Most Affected Wards in Calcutta City in 1918

Table 1.2 Sex and Death Rates in Most Affected Wards in Calcutta City in 1918

Ward	*Male Death Rate (per Mile)*	*Female Death Rate (per Mile)*
XXIV (Kidderpore)	63.6	65.7
V (Jorabagan)	37.7	57.9
VII (Bara Bazar)	28.9	55.0
XX (Beniapukur)	34.0	50.3
XIX (Entally)	31.7	51.4
XXI (Ballygunge)	33.5	53.6
IX (Moocheepara)	29.7	52.8
XIV (Taltollah)	28.6	50.6

Source: (Proceedings of the Govt. of Bengal, Municipal Department, Sanitation Branch, File No. S.2D–8 (5))

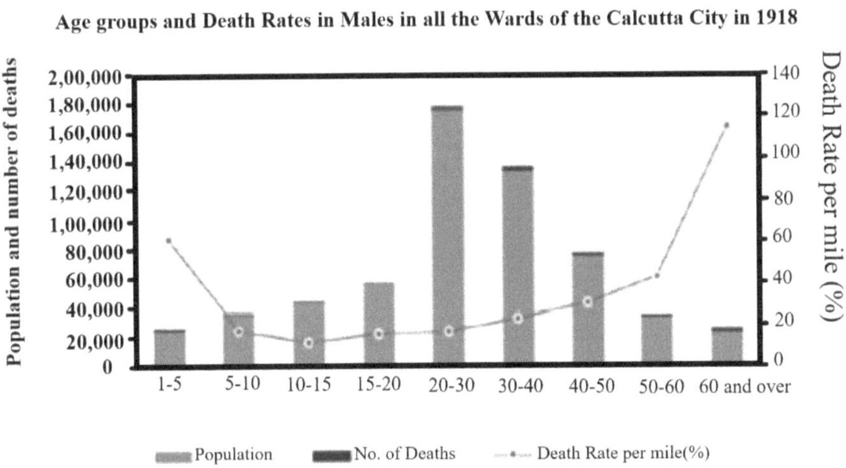

Figure 1.3 Graph Showing Age Groups and Death Rates of the Males in All the Wards in Calcutta City in 1918

the highest rates seen in children aged 5–10 years, followed closely by those aged 5–20 years and 30–50 years. Among older adults aged 60 and above, the mortality rate was the highest. The ageing immune system's immune senescence, limited access to medical treatment, pre-existing chronic conditions, and improper social isolation hindered older adults' (aged 60 and above) ability to effectively combat the virus, resulting in their high Spanish Influenza mortality rate. The death rate among females across all age groups was 44.1 per mile. The city's high mortality rate among females, particularly those of childbearing age, is primarily because of issues such as poverty, overcrowding, unsanitary conditions, child marriage, untrained midwives, and the purdah system. The infant mortality rate for the city stood at 357.8 per thousand registered births. This represents the highest rate recorded in 1902. Ward No. V exhibited the highest rates of infant mortality

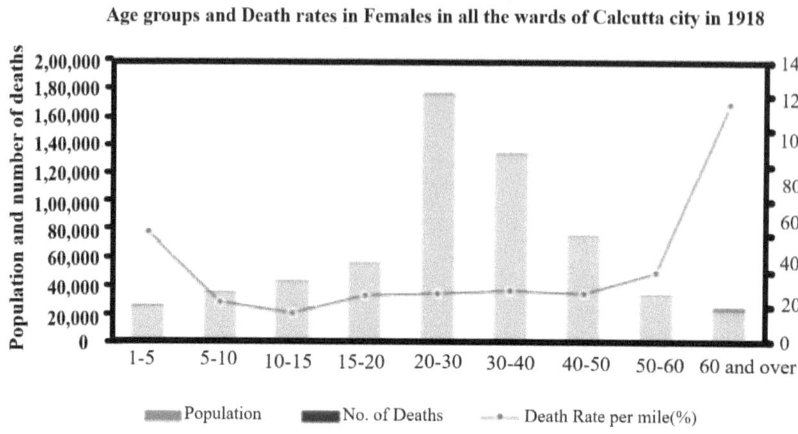

Figure 1.4 Graph Showing Age Groups and Death Rates of the Females in All the Wards in Calcutta City in 1918

Table 1.3 Age Groups and Death Rates of the Males in All the Wards in Calcutta City in 1918

Age Group	*Population*	*No. of Deaths*	*Death Rate per Mile*
1–5	24617	1507	61.2
5–10	35400	622	17.5
10–15	43478	508	11.7
15–20	56316	888	15.7
20–30	174951	2951	16.9
30–40	133664	3067	22.9
40–50	75109	2248	29.9
50–60	33879	1454	42.9
60 and over	22602	2595	114.8

Source: Annual Report of the Health Department, Section–I, Meteorology and Vital Statistics, 1918

Table 1.4 Age Groups and Death Rates of the Females in All the Wards in Calcutta City in 1918

Age Group	*Population*	*No. of Deaths*	*The Death Rate per Mile*
1–5	23191	1446	62.3
5–10	31909	709	22.2
10–15	24285	387	15.9
15–20	26325	703	26.7
20–30	59983	1654	27.5
30–40	45085	1337	29.6
40–50	31789	877	27.5
50–60	20065	794	39.5
60 and over	18719	2528	135.0

Source: Annual Report of the Health Department, Section–I, Meteorology and Vital Statistics, 1918

(Jorabagan 581), followed by the other wards namely VII (Bara Bazar 473), XIV (Taltollah 285), XXIV (Kidderpore 351), IX (Moocheepara 345), and XIII (Fenwick Bazar 325). The Spanish Flu epidemic in Jorabagan and Bara Bazar resulted in elevated infant mortality rates because of cramped buildings and narrow alleys, worsened by the Spanish Flu.

The Spanish Flu,[5] a severe epidemic leading to widespread infections and fatalities, mainly because of respiratory illnesses and fever, started in October 1918 and peaked in January 1919 (Minutes of the Proceedings of the Special Meeting of the Calcutta Corporation, November 1918). First-class residential areas with fewer women and children experienced death rates of 15.3 and 26.5 per thousand, respectively. Ward XIII had the lowest rate at 25.2 per thousand. All wards with a death rate exceeding 42.2 per thousand maintained a general rate of 42.2 per thousand and reflected the primary causes of mortality.

Figure 1.5 visually illustrates Table 1.5 to provide a clearer understanding of the causes of mortality situation. The city saw a notable rise in mortality rates across all wards, with respiratory ailments and fevers significantly increasing. In Wards XVI and XVII first-class residential areas, deaths because of respiratory diseases increased from 6914 in 1918 to 8236 in 1919, while deaths from fevers grew from 2085 to 2392 in 1919. The recurrence of the Spanish Flu contributed to a decline in community vitality and resilience, resulting in a high death rate from all existing diseases in the area (Table 1.6). The mortality rate in Kidderpore was 36.7 per thousand for males, which resulted in 22339 fatalities, while for females, it stood at 53.7 per thousand, showing an almost 50% higher rate. The significant coolie population and inadequate living conditions contributed to the elevated death rates. In Bara Bazar, female mortality was over twice that of males (Table 1.7). The second wave of the influenza epidemic began in October 1918 and peaked in December,

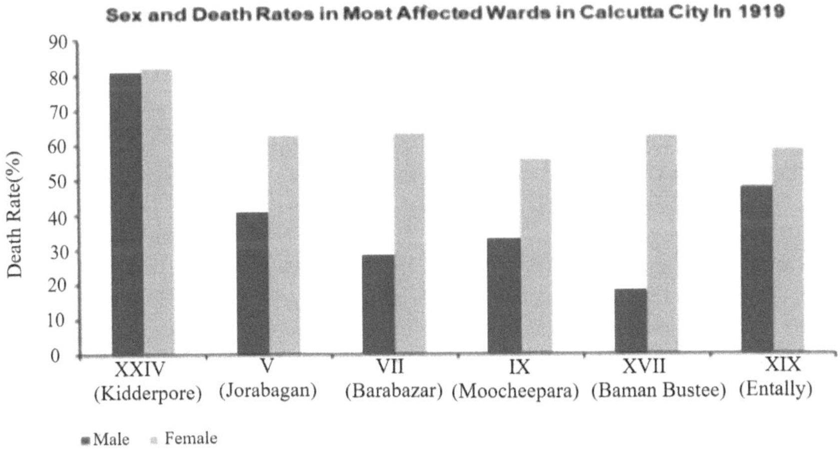

Figure 1.5 Graph Showing Death Rate (per Mile) in Most Affected Wards in Calcutta City in 1919

Table 1.5 Death Rate (per Mile) in Most Affected Wards in Calcutta City in 1919

Ward and Area	*Year 1919*	*Principal Causes of Death—Influenza and Respiratory Disease*
Kidderpore (XXIV)	81.1	Influenza, respiratory disease, and malaria
Entally (XIX)	51.3	Influenza, cholera, and smallpox
Jorabagan (V)	47.4	Influenza, respiratory disease, and diarrhoea
Ballygunge (XXI)	46.9	Influenza, respiratory disease, diarrhoea, and malaria
Hastings (XVIII)	44.5	Influenza, respiratory disease, and cholera
Beniapukur (XX)	44.4	Influenza and respiratory disease

Source: Minutes of the Proceedings of the Calcutta Corporation, January 1919

Table 1.6 Principal Burning Ghats in Calcutta City

Burning Ghats	*Calcutta Dead*	*Outside Dead*	*Total*
Nimtolla	13013	1199	14212
Kasi Mitter	5877	1305	7182
Shahnagore	4612	998	5610
Total	23502	3502	27004

Table 1.7 Burials in Calcutta by Cemetery, Religion, and Origin of the Deceased

Burial Grounds	*Calcutta Dead*	*Outside Dead*	*Total*
Topsia (Hindu)	2951	326	3277
Muraripukur (Hindu)	1048	840	1888
Gobra (Mohamedan)	4742	53	4795
Ekbalpore (Mohamedan)	1856	26	1882
Lower Circular Road Cemetery (Christian)	1115	22	1137
Other Christian Cemeteries	92	5	97
Other Mohamedan Burial Ground	580	33	613
Total	12384	1305	13689

Source: Report of the Health Officer of Calcutta Corporation for the Year 1919—H M Crake (Chief Registrar of Births and Deaths and Suptd. of Vaccination, Calcutta, Calcutta Corporation Press, 1920)

showing a gradual increase until January 1919. The severity lessened each month, concluding after June, but not fully resolved by the year's end. The third wave in 1920 was sporadic and mild (Minutes of the Proceedings of the Special Meeting of the Calcutta Corporation, December 1918).

During the pandemic, hospital accommodation became a major concern because of the high number of influenza patients in Rural Bengal. Because of space constraints, they built temporary sheds at Cambell and Sambhu Nath Pandit hospitals. Campbell and Shambu Nath Pandit Hospitals provided two sheds with 20 beds each. With the second ward at Shambhu Nath Pandit Hospital full, authorities opened two temporary hospitals—one at the Kalighat Rest House and another in a rented house on Mominpur Road. However, these hospitals were unhygienic and lacked proper medical professionals, leading to a choked environment and inability to move dead bodies. Corpses filled the burning ghats and crematoriums. Misunderstandings, ill-advised interventions, and bureaucratic policies caused widespread scepticism of the Indian Medical Service among the common people, creating widespread alarm and distress (Minutes of the Proceedings of the Calcutta Corporation, November 1918).

Disposal of Dead

In 1918, 37839 deaths were registered, with most due to influenza. 3179 bodies were disposed of outside Calcutta, while 35896 were disposed of through cremation or burial. Additionally, 4809 bodies were brought from outside, resulting in a total of 40705 bodies disposed of within the city. Of these, 27016 were cremated and 13689 were disposed of by burial.

Starting February 18, 1919, a portion of the Bhatchala Hindu Burial Ground was opened due to the closure of the Jingerpole Burial Ground by the South Suburban Municipality. Plans for additional area and construction of boundary walls, pathways, pucca quarters, office, rest house, and mortuary were sanctioned and ongoing. Block Nos. 14 and 15 of the Hindu Burial Ground at Topsia were raised, and a mail shed was constructed. Work was also undertaken to extend the Hindu Burial Ground at Murari Pukur, and at the Gori Goriban cemetery, lowlands were raised, compound walls repaired, and pucca foundations provided for fencing. The Tiljala cemetery constructed a shed for malies and coolies, and improvements have been made at the Shahnagore Burning Ghat. The north of the paved approach has been moved to a garden, and electric lights have been provided. A second sub-registrar has been appointed, and a whole-time police guard has been hired at Kasi Mitter Burning Ghat. A new contract was made for the supply of cremation articles for three years at Nimtolla Burning Ghat from September 1, 1919.

European Civilians During the Spanish Flu Pandemic of 1918–19 Calcutta

The plight of European civilians in Calcutta during the Spanish Influenza pandemic of 1918–19 underscored notable inequalities in healthcare availability, living situations, and preventive measures compared to the larger Calcutta community. While the influenza virus affected all social classes, European residents—particularly those in wealthy areas like Park Street—experienced relatively lower death rates and less severe outbreaks. Enhanced living conditions, superior healthcare, and preventive measures account for this distinction. The virus itself was remarkably aggressive, exhibiting symptoms such as abrupt high fever, severe headaches, body aches, and significant respiratory distress that often escalated to fatal pneumonia. Despite the virus's strength, European occupants had better resources to mitigate its impact. Park Street, a primary residential zone for Europeans in colonial Calcutta, included various factors that led to reduced infection rates. Homes in this area were spacious, well-ventilated, and met higher sanitation standards, which aided in decreasing overcrowding and the chance of virus spread. European families enjoyed greater access to medical practitioners trained in western medicine, who provided symptomatic treatments such as quinine, aspirin, and oxygen therapy for severe respiratory problems. Wealthier individuals could also afford immune-boosting diets abundant in fresh fruits, vegetables, and proteins, enhancing their resistance to illness. Preventive actions were more thoroughly enforced in regions primarily occupied by Europeans. British residents often practiced self-isolation, minimized social engagements, and routinely disinfected their homes using carbolic acid and other sanitizers. Colonial officials prioritized the distribution of medical resources, hospital facilities, and staff to European neighbourhoods, ensuring prompt treatment for this helpful group (Arnold, 1993, pp. 61–65).

The more advanced urban infrastructure of the Park Street area, compared to other crowded and impoverished districts of Calcutta Corporation, clarifies its comparatively low mortality rates. Unlike the cramped slums and bustees, where many working-class individuals lived, Park Street benefited from organized drainage systems, cleaner surroundings, and better air circulation, which helped to reduce the rapid spread of the virus. The crowded circumstances in other city regions created a setting that favoured the swift and lethal dissemination of the virus. This disparity emphasizes how class privilege, with environmental factors and unequal healthcare access, influenced the diverse effects of the Spanish Influenza in colonial Calcutta.

Alarming Death Toll in Rural Bengal

The Spanish influenza pandemic of 1918–1919 had a catastrophic impact on rural Bengal, leading to extensive suffering and loss of life. The virus spread swiftly through agrarian communities that were already grappling with overcrowded living conditions, insufficient sanitation, and inadequate nutrition. Limited healthcare resources and a lack of public awareness worsened the situation. Inaccessibility to medical facilities primarily caused the high mortality rate. This pandemic disrupted traditional practices, caused economic instability, and profoundly affected family dynamics. The prolonged recovery period left communities struggling to restore their lives and livelihoods (White, 1919, p. 8). The experience of Spanish Influenza in Bengal during this time underscored the vulnerability of marginalized populations, highlighting the urgent need for fair access to healthcare and preparedness, as well as the colonial government's indifference towards rural fatalities.

Statement referred to in the answer by the Hon'ble Mr. O'Malley to the questions asked by the Legislative Council Member Hon'ble Babu Brojendra Kishore Roy Chowdhury at the Council Meeting of January 21, 1919 is as follows:

The response provided by Hon'ble Mr. O'Malley to Hon'ble Mr. One can interpret Brajendra Kishore Rai Chaudhuri's inquiry at the Bengal Council on Tuesday regarding the influenza situation in the mofussil as an admission of the Government's shortcomings. Mr. Rai Chaudhuri's inquiry included the following points:

(a) Is the Government able to specify, on a district-by-district basis, the estimated number of influenza-related deaths over the past two months?
(b) Is it true that the mortality rate has been higher in rural areas compared to urban areas, relative to the number of infections?
(c) (i) What measures has the Government implemented, and (ii) what measures have the District Boards implemented to provide medical help in rural regions affected by influenza?

In response, Mr. O'Malley, representing the Government, stated:

(a) The Government regrets it cannot provide the requested information because of the inadequacy of the reporting agency in accurately diagnosing the various causes of mortality.
(b) There is insufficient data available to facilitate such a comparison.

[Source: Proceedings of the Govt. of Bengal, January 1919, Municipal Dept. Sanitation Branch, File No: S Q-5 and S Q -2].

The letter emphasizes the colonial government's attitude towards rural fatalities, underscoring the necessity to analyze the various Presidency divisions of Bengal in 1918–19. The division is:

Presidency Division of Colonial Bengal

Presidency Division—24 Parganas, Calcutta, Nadia, Murshidabad, Jessore, Khulna
Burdwan Division—Burdwan, Birbhum, Bankura, Midnapore, Hooghly, Howrah
Rajshahi Division—Rajshahi, Dinajpur, Jalpaiguri, Darjeeling, Rangpur, Bogra, Pabna, Malda
Dacca Division—Dacca, Mymensingh, Faridpur, Bakar Ganj
Chittagong Division—Chittagong, Noakhali, Tippera
The map of colonial Bengal's jurisdiction, depicted in Figure 1.6, clearly illustrates the various divisions, facilitating a better understanding of the context for the reader.

Burdwan

The Civil Surgeon identified the first cases of a disease in the district in July, originating from Calcutta. Major towns and villages with railway connections to Calcutta, such as Memari, Burdwan, and Asansol, experienced initial outbreaks. The infection was primarily transmitted through oral and nasal secretions, with no evidence suggesting contaminated clothing or similar items can facilitate its spread. The disease persisted during humid conditions in July, but decreased in August due to excessive rainfall. In mid-September, the disease reached isolated villages, aided

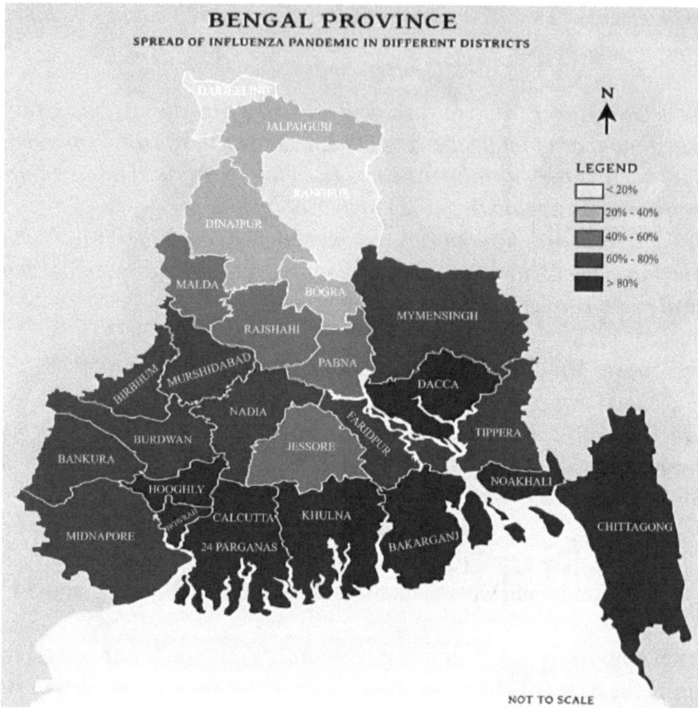

Figure 1.6 Map of Colonial Bengal (Drawn by Author)

by Puja holidays. Colder weather reduced the disease's incidence, but the subsequent epidemic affected only a few individuals who contracted the disease in July.

Asansol Mining Settlement: *Influenza outbreak in Settlement began in July, subsided in October, and re-emerged in December, affecting rural areas more than Asansol and Raniganj municipalities, causing more lethal effects among impoverished classes.*

Burdwan Municipality: *The severe disease outbreak occurred in July, August, November, and December, affecting the town except European districts and Indian gentlemen's residences. Economic strain led to reduced vitality, resulting in higher disease rates among lower-income populations.*

Dainhat Municipality: *In October and November, the local dispensary saw a surge in patients, particularly among the economically disadvantaged, due to an influx of cases.*

Asansol Municipality: *Influenza, first reported in July, initially appeared mild and subsided by August. However, it re-emerged in a highly virulent form in September, escalating in severity until December, affecting all regions, including the Railway Settlements.*

Kalna Municipality: *The influenza outbreak, first originating in Calcutta in July, was mild and severe, causing fatalities. The most critical cases were among older* *adults and those weakened by chronic malaria. In November, a resurgence affected areas previously unscathed, targeting remote villages and causing severe cases.*

Raniganj Municipality: *The epidemic began in September and intensified in October, November, and December, affecting densely populated impoverished areas and European quarters. Previous illness-weakened individuals were more susceptible to severe cases.*

Katwa Municipality: Someone imported the initial case from Calcutta, leading to the spread of infection to nearby homes and areas. *The second wave, which emerged in late October, was more virulent. The neighbourhoods of Tantipara and Baganpara, characterized by poor ventilation and overcrowding, were hard hit.*

Birbhum

The outbreak of broncho-pneumonia began in mid-July and spread across various areas, with symptoms persisting for two weeks. The infection originated from Calcutta and was transmitted through contact with an existing case. The disease was more severe in thana areas with significant railway stations, with eight experiencing severe effects. A second wave emerged in October, causing more severe symptoms, fatal outcomes, and a broader geographical impact. The disease spread from urban centres to nearby villages, affecting three-quarters of the district's total area, while regions distant from key trading locations experienced the least effects.

Bankura

Railway lines in Calcutta spread malaria from urban to rural areas, causing two outbreaks in August and October. The first was mild and recovery-oriented, while the second was severe and fatal due to respiratory complications. High malaria prevalence areas were most affected, with villages avoiding the disease due to lack of personal contact and communication.

Vishnupur Municipality: *The disease, initially sporadically appearing in Calcutta and surrounding villages, spreads through person-to-person contact, with outdoor labourers being the last group affected, and those in densely populated areas and cramped housing experiencing the most severe effects.*

Sonamukhi Municipality: *The disease, introduced by individuals from other locations, intensified in densely populated areas and persisted until November. Pneumonia complications were common, particularly among impoverished families and lower socio-economic groups. The infection spread from urban centres and river contamination by deceased bodies likely contributed to its transmission to riverside communities.*

Midnapore

The disease first emerged in the Midnapore District in early July, affecting Maisadal and the town. The heat and limited rainfall led to widespread belief that the illness was due to the unusual heat. The outbreak persisted for over a month before diminishing, with most individuals recovering and a low mortality rate. A second outbreak occurred in October, primarily affecting the Ghatal region, and spreading to Mohanpur, Egra, and Binpur areas. The cold season escalated the epidemic, resulting in an increased death rate, particularly among pneumonia-complicated cases. The disease spread primarily along railway lines and transportation routes, with personal contagion contributing to the spread. The disease was most intense in densely populated rural regions, suffering more severely than in urban areas.

***Ramjibanpur Municipality** reported no instances of influenza.*

***In Tamluk Municipality,** the initial influenza epidemic severely impacted the town's core, with high atmospheric temperatures potentially contributing. Despite aquatic occupations, the highly contagious disease spread through close human contact.*

***In Ghatal Municipality,** a few fatal cases of malaria were introduced, causing widespread illness in infected households. Poorly lit and poorly ventilated spaces were most affected, while hygienic individuals avoided infection. The disease spread from the town to surrounding villages, often preceding influenza infections, with those taking preventive measures unharmed.*

***In Khirpai Municipality,** the outbreak began at the onset of the cold season and persisted intensely for approximately two months, predominantly affecting lower-income individuals.*

***In Hooghly,** the epidemic was notably more severe in rural regions compared to urban areas.*

***In Arambagh Subdivision,** the disease was first detected in July in Khanakul and intensified by September, causing many fatalities. The infection was traced back to imports from Calcutta, affecting nearby villages. The spread was not uniform across villages, with some areas showing immunity. Transmission occurred primarily through personal interactions. Higher regions, away from rivers, experienced severe outbreaks, while areas near rivers were less affected. Pursurah thana had a lower mortality rate, but the district suffered losses across the board. As colder weather arrived, the death toll rose, particularly among those already afflicted with malaria.*

***In Serampore Municipality,** the disease has affected all parts of the town, with some bustees experiencing more severe effects. The proportion of virulent cases is small compared to the total number of infections, highlighting the impact of the disease on various areas.*

***In Arambagh Municipality,** the disease, first arising in July in southwestern villages, has affected all wards in the municipality, particularly those from impoverished and middle-class backgrounds.*

***In Baidyabati Municipality,** the disease spread throughout the municipal region, disproportionately affecting lower-income groups, peaking in November and December.*

***Many individuals in the Bhadreswar Municipality were simultaneously affected.** A mild outbreak occurred in mid-July, followed by a more severe one in early November. The first outbreak was sudden and widespread, while the second had a higher mortality rate. Mill quarters were most severely affected. The disease* *initially manifested in early July and escalated in severity over two to three weeks before subsiding. Angus Jute Co. reported only a few cases in December.*

The initial epidemic spread from Calcutta and affected nearly every household in the Rishra-Konnagar Municipality. *The disease was highly contagious and severe in the southern part of the town, particularly in the mill bustee. The second outbreak at Wellington Mill had lower cases but higher mortality rates. Europeans exhibited lower susceptibility due to their cautious lifestyle. The second epidemic at Indian Jute Co., Ltd. emerged in December with a milder form.*

Hooghly-Chinsurah Municipality: External sources introduced the disease. *The disease, spread through air transmission, exhibited fluctuating patterns, with higher incidences among the impoverished compared to the affluent.*

Bansberia Municipality: Outside sources introduced the disease. *In December, a severe weather event occurred, causing a drop in temperature and disproportionately affecting the poor, particularly females.*

Uttarpara Municipality: *A mild outbreak of a disease occurred in July, imported by Calcutta, followed by a more virulent epidemic in October. The spread was facilitated by environmental contamination, lack of precautionary measures, and cold weather. The most severely affected individuals were those living in overcrowded, damp, and poorly ventilated homes. Railway communication with towns also contributed to the disease's spread. The municipality was first attacked in the south.*

Howrah

In October, a second epidemic emerged in a town, affecting multiple villages simultaneously. The disease was notably infectious, with sputum and nasopharyngeal secretions as the primary agents. Key factors included exposure to cold and diminished vitality. The epidemic reached its peak from September to November. The second outbreak was less contagious than the first, with approximately 50% of individuals affected. Factors contributing to the second outbreak included exposure to cold, poor sanitary conditions, and excessive alcohol consumption. The virus spread through the air and contact with infected individuals. Hindus were three times more affected than Muhammadans. The New Central Jute Mills had a highly contagious epidemic, exacerbated by unsanitary living conditions. Caregivers of infected patients frequently contracted the illness through respiratory secretions and exhalation. The disease initially surfaced in June and July and re-emerged in the winter months, affecting both well-maintained residences and unsanitary slums.

Bally Municipality: Someone brought the disease from Calcutta, and initial suspicion arose in July. *A second outbreak emerged in mid-October, primarily in densely populated, low-lying areas, characterized by unhealthy conditions and rapid spread through people and air.*

24 Parganas

The first epidemic in Calcutta occurred in June and July, affecting mill workers, and postal and telegraph employees, and causing a few fatal cases of pneumonia. The second epidemic, less widespread, saw a higher incidence of broncho-pneumonia cases resulting in fatalities. The infection spread quickly through human interaction, originating in Calcutta. Kidderpore was the first area to be affected, moving northward through Kalighat and Bhowanipore. The second epidemic affected St. Vincent's Home, primarily affecting Indians and Eurasians. The contagious nature of the disease remains uncertain, as it was only fatal due to complications. The second wave emerged in November, initially affecting poorer cultivators in the abads of Diamond Harbour and Canning Town. The disease did not extend to nearby villages but occurred in isolated centres.

Baruipur Municipality: *The illness has been widespread throughout the municipality since September.*

Rajpur Municipality: *The disease peaked in August, with a high mortality rate in densely populated areas, while milder symptoms or avoidance were observed in less crowded environments.*

Various means of transportation, including road, rail, and steamer, introduced the disease to Budge Budge Municipality. *The Budge Budge Jute Mills reported that the disease was introduced by outside sources, spreading through direct contact and overcrowding. Factors such as unsanitary living conditions, poor ventilation, and poverty contributed to its transmission. The severity of the disease fluctuated with climate changes, with densely populated areas being most affected. However, the Caledonian Jute Mills reported minimal impact on their operations, with only 15 cases reported among 4000 workers.*

Garden Reach Municipality: Direct contact transmitted the disease. *A non-virulent illness primarily affected low-income labourers in overcrowded, poorly ventilated conditions in July and August, followed by a second wave in November and December, with normal mortality rates.*

South Suburban Municipality: *The Health Officer identifies the current epidemic as "Catarrhal Fever" rather than influenza, stating it began in October and subsided by November.*

Tollygunge Municipality: *The disease, first observed in July, initially appeared mildly in Tollygunge but spread throughout the municipality, causing a few deaths. The severity was more severe in Tollygunge and Arrackpur, but Russa, Mollahat, Dhakuria, and Kasba experienced less severe effects. The infection was primarily transmitted through respiratory secretions.*

Calcutta directly imported the disease into Cossipore-Chitpur Municipality. *The municipality of Jeliapara in Calcutta experienced mild disease effects, with only two deaths among 20 cases. The disease emerged as a localized outbreak, with most cases in various wards.*

Human contact brought the disease to the Maniktala Municipality from Calcutta; it spread via nasal, oral, and conjunctival secretions, as well as contaminated clothing. *The disease rapidly spread throughout the town, with severity lower in Anglo-Indian and affluent households. The most affected were impoverished, weakened individuals in unsanitary conditions.*

Baranagore Municipality: Calcutta area originated the May–June epidemic. *The disease outbreak from October to December was sporadic, with direct contact* *with infected individuals. The May outbreak was non-fatal, but the October outbreak resulted in fatalities due to pneumonia, especially among impoverished individuals. The spread did not directly correlate with population density, and fatalities were primarily due to neglect, exposure, and lack of medical help. The second epidemic emerged in mid-September, with infections appearing in the Rajbagan and South Mill cooly lines. New arrivals, Hindus and Muslims, were the most severely affected, followed by Bilaspuri workers.*

Someone brought the illness into Garulia Municipality from Calcutta, initially affecting the lower-class population in densely populated areas. *The town experienced severe outbreaks of a severe cholera epidemic, causing significant suffering in crowded neighbourhoods and reaching its peak severity in October.*

The disease spread from Calcutta to Barrackpur Municipality through direct contact with infected individuals. *The initial outbreak took place in June. Although the intensity of the illness diminished in August and September, it surged again in severity in October, with the most severe cases reported in the cooly lines.*

North Barrackpur Municipality: Officials recorded a few influenza cases in the second week of July, leading to its spread across several wards. *The highly contagious illness rapidly spread through air, flies, and physical contact, disproportionately affecting poorer populations. Initially mild, it became increasingly fatal in later stages.*

Tittagarh Municipality: *The disease, first introduced in July, spread rapidly throughout the municipality, affecting both affluent and impoverished residents. It intensified in July, with males being more susceptible, especially among lower socio-economic groups. The disease resurfaced in late October, with nearly all cases resulting in fatalities. The initial outbreak occurred in Khardah before spreading to Tittagarh. Workers in private bustees were more severely affected, while those in cooly lines experienced the least. Madrassis were less affected due to factors like well-ventilated homes, avoidance of physical contact, preference for fresh tap water, and daily dhotis washing. Weavers lived in densely populated bustees and dark rooms, and children of Spinning Weavers were hard hit. The disease spread quickly, affecting individuals across all demographics, regardless of gender or age. Sweepers appeared to be immune due to their work and the tendency of others to avoid contact.*

North Dum Dum Municipality: *The infection primarily spread through human interactions, with the lower socio-economic groups being the most affected.*

South Dum Dum Municipality: *The disease, first identified in Pattipukur, led to fatalities in two pneumonia-complicated cases, spreading to Nagirbazar and the municipality, affecting areas along Jessore Road.*

Naihati Municipality: During the second outbreak, only a few people reported cases, with the highest mortality occurring in November. *Gouripore Jute Mills experienced two outbreaks of a severe COVID-19 pandemic. The first outbreak was mild, causing fatigue and a severe cough, while the second was more severe, involving broncho-pneumonia. The first outbreak was traced to a woman visiting a friend in Calcutta who had contracted the virus. The second outbreak began in August, affecting those living outside the lines more than within. Middle-class* *individuals were more affected, while Europeans remained unaffected. The disease was airborne, with patient excreta, sputum, stools, and urine playing a significant role in transmission. Adult males were more affected than females, and children were more severely affected during the second epidemic.*

Halisahar Municipality: *There was no significant outbreak of influenza in this town.*

Bhatpara Municipality: The initial epidemic, occurring during June and July, was mild and uncomplicated. *A second epidemic emerged in November, more severe than the first, with the infection being transmitted from Calcutta by train commuters. The disease affected multiple members of households simultaneously and was airborne. No demographic group was immune, and sanitary conditions had minimal impact on the spread. The disease first appeared in July and persisted for two weeks, affecting a significant number of individuals but resulting in no fatalities. The second epidemic began in early November and was notably severe, often complicated by bronchitis or broncho-pneumonia. Migrant labourers from rural areas were vulnerable, and the impoverished population endured the impact. Males were more frequently affected than females, with a higher mortality rate among infected females. The second outbreak began as a mild epidemic in November, peaking in severity from the second week to the first week of December.*

Gobardanga Municipality: *Urban and rural regions experienced similar impacts, with younger people more affected. Lower socio-economic groups faced greatest hardships due to deprivation and inadequate nutrition. Baraset Municipality had a mild outbreak.*

Taki Municipality: *There were no reported cases of influenza in this municipality.*

Nadia

The first epidemic of the disease occurred in July and lasted for three weeks, primarily affecting urban areas like Krishnagar, Ranaghat, and Kushtia. The disease spread rapidly within households and was believed to originate in Calcutta. Overcrowding and inhalation of contaminated air were key factors in its transmission. The second epidemic was more aggressive and widespread, with areas that experienced the initial outbreak suffering less due to immunity gained from prior exposure. However, mortality rates were high, particularly due to complications like diarrhoea and pneumonia. The subdivisions of Sadar, Ranaghat, Hanshkhali, and Mohorpur experienced significant repercussions, while the Kushtia subdivision largely avoided the most severe effects. The reduced incidence in the Kushtia subdivision may be attributed to factors such as having already been affected during the first epidemic and being bordered by the Ganges and Gorai rivers.

Improved Gorai conditions and frequent flooding have reduced malaria cases in the area, which has previously experienced significant outbreaks. The second epidemic, which began in mid-October, was more severe due to rising costs and inadequate clothing, resulting in higher mortality rates among the impoverished. The first outbreak occurred during the peak of the rainy season, while the second outbreak began in mid-October. The first outbreak was milder, spreading through urban areas and railway stations, affecting individuals across all demographics and lasting about one month. Factors such as overcrowding, high dust levels, and contaminated air facilitated the transmission. The second outbreak was more severe, affecting the entire district, with villages experiencing greater hardship than towns. The Meherpur subdivision experienced greater hardships, while the Kusthia subdivision experienced the least impact due to its natural protection from annual floods.

Kushtia Municipality: *In July, a disease outbreak occurred in the town's commercial area, with imported cases spreading mainly. In November, the disease did not escalate to epidemic levels and there were no fatal cases. The town was free from the disease, with few cases in suburbs being imported from the heavily infected interior, exhibiting a high mortality rate.*

Kumar Khali Municipality reported no outbreaks in this town.

Krishnagar Municipality: *The disease, first originating in Calcutta, spread through human contact and was severe in its initial stages, leading to high mortality rates. The subsequent outbreaks were less severe, with the Krishnagar area experiencing greater impact due to its higher chronic malaria prevalence. Imported cases were more serious and fatal. The death toll was high in July and August.*

Ranaghat Municipality: *Influenza, characterized by intense symptoms in June and July, primarily affected poorer individuals in thatched homes and poorly ventilated spaces, while well-ventilated individuals remained unaffected.*

The disease arrived in Birnagar Municipality from Calcutta during the first week of July. *The town experienced a mild outbreak due to extensive quinine distribution and a densely populated area, with field workers and dust-exposure individuals being most affected. No fatalities occurred during the initial outbreak.*

Chakdaha Municipality: *The illness initially arrived from Calcutta and subsequently spread throughout the surrounding areas. Pneumonia cases were complicated, with some individuals avoiding it due to ventilation, while the outbreak was severe in densely populated regions and impoverished communities.*

Murshidabad: *The district experienced a similar disease outbreak, starting in July and August but not causing significant fatalities. It re-emerged in October and November, worsening in December. Hurshi thana, which avoided the outbreak, experienced a sudden double death toll.*

Berhampore Municipality: *The municipality experienced a pandemic from November 18 to December 15, affecting all parts of the town. The most severe outbreak was in Cossimbazar, with Khagra ward experiencing a milder impact. The disease was widespread across various social strata. In September, a significant epidemic in the jail affected 175 inmates, resulting in five deaths and one fatality. The disease spread rapidly in Daulatabad during October, November, and December.*

Azimganj Municipality: *Observers noted that the disease spread primarily through personal contact, with sputum and nasal secretions proving highly contagious. The outbreak, which began in August and persisted for a month in Dhulian Municipality, was primarily affecting impoverished individuals living in overcrowded, unsanitary conditions, with no fatalities reported.*

External sources introduced the illness to Kandi Municipality, initially affecting only a few families. *The disease spread throughout the town, with lower-density and isolated regions unaffected. Warmer weather significantly reduced the incidence.*

Someone brought the disease into Dinajpur town from Calcutta; the initial outbreak occurred just one week after its identification in Calcutta. *Around 25% of residences were affected by a malaria-related disease, which waned after November and December due to lack of heavy rainfall. The town is nearly free of the disease, possibly due to its isolation from the central region. Rural areas, such as Sadar subdivision, experienced the least impact, while Bechagunj, Peergunj, Razizoukoil, Raigunj, and Kusmandi were severely affected, causing significant anaemia among residents.*

Malda

A severe influenza outbreak began in Kaligram village in July, originating from a teacher from Chanchal High English School. The disease spread to over 200 villages across seven thanas, including English Bazar and Old Malda. The transmission occurred primarily through human interaction, with some less frequented areas avoiding infection. Kharba experienced the highest impact, followed by Harischandrapur and Gazal. Officials reported the disease in Manikchak, with only a few cases in English Bazar and Old Malda. In English Bazar, an influenza epidemic did not manifest, and upper classes and educated individuals remained unaffected. In Nawabganj Municipality, the illness first appeared in mid-July, with severe outbreaks in Malapara, Kasaripara, and Hukrapara. Rajarampur experienced a greater impact than other rural regions.

Darjeeling

The Indian population experienced severe cases of the epidemic, with pneumonia being the leading cause of death. Lower-income groups, particularly Nepalis and Lepchas, faced significant hardship. Poor sanitation, food insecurity, and clothing contributed to the high death toll. The disease initially affected railway staff in Kurseong, local bazaar residents, and the Indian community, with Europeans being the last to contract it. The disease spread to nearby tea gardens.

Jalpaiguri

A disease outbreak began in Jalpaiguri town in July, mainly affecting the Marwari community. It spread to impoverished and middle-class residents and trade routes across the Teesta River, affecting three major centres in August. The disease re-emerged in November, with a higher mortality rate due to colder weather. The disease did not provide immunity and meteorological factors did not influence the outbreak. The poorer segments of the population were most affected, with high mortality rates. Overcrowding in railway carriages facilitated the spread. Europeans and affluent Indians were the least affected. There was no significant epidemic within Jalpaiguri Municipality, with only a few cases reported.

Various tea estates reported the following details.

A second wave of a contagious disease outbreak occurred at Dumchipara Tea Estate, affecting a high number of individuals. The disease was highly contagious, with transmission from adjacent gardens. The severity of the illness was more pronounced among coolies from the plains, likely due to better insulation. The disease's complications significantly influenced the overall mortality rate. At Dalsinghpara Tea Estate, the disease emerged in late November and persisted until mid-December, with Nagpuris being hard hit. At Ellenbarrie Tea Estate, the disease was first identified in Bishman's lines, where Nepalis live. A second outbreak hit in November, with lower lines and coolies from the plains also affected, although the mortality rate among the latter was lower than that among the Nepali coolies.

The disease, first reported in August at Putharihora Tea Estate, spread to the Paharis or hill people, with a second outbreak in November. The disease originated in the southern region of the district and moved northward, affecting both the weak and strong, with a more severe impact in densely populated areas. The first outbreak occurred from August 7 to September 4, followed by a second outbreak from November 14 to December 18. The second outbreak began in October and affected every family in the western "dhuras". The disease spread rapidly and was severe, often complicated by pneumonia and broncho-pneumonia. Coolies in the plains experienced greater suffering than those in the hills, likely due to better clothing and smaller numbers. The New Dooars Tea Company reported that the disease initially emerged after the last Dasara holiday in lower-level tea lines, likely originating from other gardens. The lower and middle lines remained unaffected, while the upper lines, due to their higher elevation and healthier conditions, avoided infection.

The disease first appeared in August at Dailmore Tea Estate and did not escalate to epidemic levels until early October. It primarily affected the Madessias, plains' coolies, and Jainti Sankos, particularly in the western region. The Anjuman Tea Co., Ltd. reported that the disease spread from nearby areas and reached Bharatpur Tea Estate through coolies from adjacent gardens and new arrivals from Nagpur. Europeans and Babus were unaffected. The peak outbreak occurred from mid-August to the end of September, with a decline in October and December. The estate experienced a later infection due to its location on the far edges of the Western Duars.

A tea outbreak occurred in the Chalobuni Tea Estate, affecting many individuals simultaneously but causing few complications. The second outbreak had a gradual onset, affecting fewer but causing severe complications. Most affected individuals were aged 15–50. The disease began in early September and spread to Leesh River Tea Estate in early September. The most severe phase coincided with the initial outbreak in August and heavy rainfall. The illness subsided in September and October, but resurfaced in November due to excessive indulgence.

[Source: Proceedings of the Government of Bengal in the Municipal Department (Sanitation Branch) for the month of April 1919, File No. S.2D–8, Proceedings No. A. 1–20]

The epidemiological survey conducted by the British Government on the transmission of Spanish Influenza in Calcutta and nearby regions offers a detailed account of the matter. The survey outlines the onset of influenza infection in Calcutta and surrounding districts (Howrah, Hooghly, 24 Parganas, Birbhum, Bankura, Bardhaman, Murshidabad, Jalpaiguri, Darjeeling, and Malda), beginning in mid-July. Business travellers, students, and workers returning home spread the influenza virus throughout Calcutta's neighbouring districts. The districts linked by waterways saw the infection first, with elevated rates of infection. The infection initially affected only urban regions before rapidly spreading to rural areas. The impact of the infection in each municipality was severe, primarily because of close contact, sneezing, and coughing. The insufficient medical service delivery system of the British government played a significant role in facilitating the spread, with limited services available in urban or town areas and rural communities left without support (Mills, 1986, pp. 1–23). When rural residents sought treatment in Calcutta, they were unaware that they had already contracted the virus. The low death rate during the initial wave resulted in a lack of awareness regarding the illness, allowing the second wave to transform the disease from being perceived as trivial into a source of dread.

Perception of the Common Mass About the Pandemic

The Influenza Pandemic of 1918–19 in Calcutta and rural Bengal led to widespread fear, uncertainty, and susceptibility because of insufficient information regarding the virus's characteristics, spread, and seriousness. Rumours and misinformation exacerbated panic, disruption, and an overwhelmed healthcare system. In this context, the following section depicts the collective horror and superstition of the general populace during this dreadful period marked by high death rates (Times of India, October 10, 1918, p. 5).

> *The influenza pandemic that struck the city from September to December 1918 resulted in the tragic loss of nearly 5,000 lives to this previously unknown illness, causing widespread alarm throughout the community. The rapid spread of ignorance, superstition, and stigma hindered effective hygienic education. The densely populated bustee residents, living in poorly lit and ventilated conditions and in close contact with one another, became key contributors to the swift transmission of the disease. Efforts to raise awareness proved ineffective, as individuals gathered daily at the local Sitala temple, dedicated to the goddess of epidemics, seeking the charannamrito*[6] *from the priest, who assured them it would cure their ailments. The situation worsened when rural inhabitants, unknowingly infected, sought treatment, causing a severe outbreak and tragically claiming many young lives. 1919.*

Resource scarcity and isolation have influenced the influenza pandemic in rural Bengal, particularly in remote villages. Rapid spread caused distress and fear, disrupting traditional social practices and creating an atmosphere of suspicion. This shift in social dynamics added an emotional and psychological dimension to the pandemic's perception (Hardiman, 2012, pp. 644–652). The 1918–19 Influenza

Pandemic in Calcutta and rural Bengal highlighted the significance of clear communication, community support, and social resilience in managing such unprecedented crises.

Ineffective Steps of the Government and the Medical Community

This section will begin with a statistical account of the death marches that took place in various wards of Calcutta from September to December 1918, so that the reader can easily grasp the horror of death. The statistics concerning influenza-related fatalities in Calcutta from September to December 1918 present a stark illustration of the pandemic's effects. Records show 3673 deaths across various wards, hospitals, and the port area, resulting in an overall mortality rate of 4.1 per 1000 individuals. However, the severity of mortality exhibited considerable variation among different regions.

Ward XXIV emerged as the most heavily affected area, reporting an alarming 462 deaths and an extraordinarily high mortality rate of 21.4 per 1000, showing a crisis of significant magnitude. This ward experienced a far greater number of fatalities than any other locality, suggesting that factors such as overcrowding, insufficient medical resources, or substandard living conditions may have exacerbated the outbreak. Other wards with notably high mortality rates included Ward XXV, which recorded 298 deaths (6.6 per 1000), Ward XIX with 217 deaths (5.4 per 1000), Ward XXII with 286 deaths (5.2 per 1000), and Ward XXIII with 110 deaths (5.5 per 1000). We also identified these areas as critical hotspots during the pandemic. Wards XIV, X, and V showed moderate mortality rates of 3 to 5 per 1000, showing significant but less severe effects. In contrast, several wards, including Ward I, Ward II, and Ward III, reported relatively lower death rates, with figures remaining below 3 per 1000.

Hospitals also experienced considerable fatalities. Campbell Hospital recorded 128 deaths, while Mayo Native Hospital, Medical College, Sambhu Nath Pandit Hospital, and the Port Area reported fewer fatalities, suggesting either lower patient volumes or more favourable healthcare outcomes (Source: Minutes of the Meeting, Municipal Department, Calcutta Corporation, December 1918).

The significant disparities in mortality rates emphasize the unequal effects of the pandemic throughout Calcutta. The concerning statistics in Wards such as XXIV, XXV, and XIX show that vulnerable groups are probably experiencing social and environmental challenges. These trends highlight the necessity to investigate elements like population density, sanitation conditions, and access to healthcare, which may have affected the transmission and death rates during this time.

Ineffective strategies characterized the response to Spanish Influenza in Calcutta by the government and medical community from 1918 to 1919. The absence of clear protocols, insufficient healthcare facilities, absence of prophylactic medicine[7] and slow allocation of resources impeded public compliance and commitment to preventive measures, leading to widespread confusion and an increase in cases, which left many infected individuals without adequate medical support. This underscores the government's lack of readiness for the pandemic (Times of India, October 12, 1918, p. 10).

The medical community encountered difficulties in diagnosis and treatment because of limited knowledge and swift virus mutations. A lack of healthcare professionals, ineffective implementation of social measures, and an absence of a comprehensive strategy to curb virus transmission hindered the government's pandemic response. Inconsistent quarantine practices and poor enforcement of restrictions on public assemblies further obstructed their efforts (Arnold, 2019, p. 200). The Spanish Influenza outbreak in Calcutta and Bengal between 1918 and 1919 revealed flaws in governmental and medical responses, underscoring the necessity for coordinated, proactive, and informed approaches in future health emergencies. The following discussion presents an overview of the situation:

> *On July 17, 1918, at 5 p.m., a special meeting of the Health Committee convened at the Central Municipal Office, chaired by Sri Kailash Ch. Bose. Attendees included Dr. Haridhan Dutt, C L'E Colthurst, Dr. Suresh Chander Sircar, A. C. Banerjee, W.H. Phelps, J.A. Jones, and the Hon'ble Mr. W H Arden Wood. The Health Officer's report showed that the disease was spreading at an alarming rate, highlighting its highly contagious nature. They identified contact as the primary mode of transmission, noting that infected individuals could spread the illness by coughing, sneezing, or speaking, particularly in crowded, poorly ventilated areas. The risks associated with shared drinking cups, spoons, handkerchiefs, and towels were clear, and the widespread habit of spitting throughout Calcutta was likely to exacerbate the situation.*
>
> *Recommended precautions included minimizing unnecessary exposure and fatigue, avoiding travel on overcrowded trams or buses, steering clear of crowded venues, and not dismissing minor health symptoms during fever. Doctors deemed adequate bed rest essential, and advised infected individuals to isolate themselves and use boiled handkerchiefs and towels. Health Officer Dr. Crake also provided several important recommendations to prevent infection, such as using nasal douches, exercising caution with utensils and soiled linens, and discouraging spitting. He advocated for the liberal use of eucalyptus as a prophylactic and preventive measure against Spanish Flu and suggested that a saturated solution of thymol could also be beneficial.*
>
> *(Source: Minutes of the Proceedings of the Calcutta Corporation, July 1918)*

Critics targeted the government for its insufficient reaction to the second wave of the pandemic; local newspapers investigated the government's responses (Ramana, 2003, pp. 86–89). In reality, health professionals saved lives at hill stations instead of providing medical help to the general populace (Ramana, 2003, pp. 86–89). The general population was unaware of the services they may receive from the government. *The Bengalee*, on April 22, 1919, published a report titled "Influenza Epidemic: Sanitary Commissioner's Memorandum Circulated to Local Government, Shimla", where the Sanitary Commissioner strongly advised various precautions to mitigate the influenza epidemic as outlined as follows:

> *administrations transmitted a memorandum drafted by the Sanitary Commissioner addressing the management and treatment of Influenza. Considering the potential resurgence of influenza in India and responding to the urgent needs of the Government of India, we deem it essential that medical officers translate the memorandum into appropriate local languages and ensure its wide distribution.*

The initial wave of the outbreak did not acknowledge the severity of the disease. However, the second wave prompted preventive actions, since legislative measures were inadequate in most communities. The Health Department directed the Director of Public Instruction to close all governmental schools and colleges. The suggestions for educational institutions, universities, and the wider community encompassed: (i) refraining from coughing, sneezing, spitting, and hawking in public areas; (ii) upholding isolation; (iii) utilizing sprays and gargles; (xii) guaranteeing adequate disinfection; and (iv) adhering to essential quarantine protocols. The Health Department of Calcutta Corporation supplied medicines and lotions (Quinine, Sodium Benzos, Thymol, Eucalyptus oil, Cinnamon, etc.) for the prevention and treatment of influenza. Western medicine allopathic doctors prescribed various treatments for influenza, including belladonna, laudanum, camphor, creosote, and a blend of iodine and chloroform (Proceedings of the Govt. of Bengal in the Municipal Department (Sanitation) for April 1919, File No. S. 2D–80). The following prescription will detail the preventive measures recommended by Calcutta Corporation (Source: Secretary to the Govt. of Bengal, Municipal Department, January 1919, File No: S.2-D-8 (12)). The government's inability to raise public awareness about the severe influenza infection in Calcutta resulted in an increase in death severity (Source: Minutes of the Meeting, Municipal Department, Calcutta Corporation, December 1918).

Figure 1.7 will highlight the preventive measures prescribed by Dr. Crake of Calcutta Corporation.

The government's inability to raise public awareness about the severe influenza infection in Calcutta had resulted in an increase in death severity. The Sanitary Commissioner's report will highlight the immensity of the situation in a compressed manner.

The report from the Sanitary Commissioner details the number of fatalities in Calcutta because of multiple factors from September to December 1918. This time frame aligns with the severe outbreak of the Spanish Influenza pandemic, which significantly affected public health.

Overview of Mortality Trends

The statistics show a cumulative total of 13829 deaths from various causes, with the majority linked to fevers and respiratory illnesses, highlighting the substantial influence of influenza during this time.

Key Causes of Mortality and Their Trends

Cholera handled 417 fatalities, with a significant increase in cases noted towards the year's end. There were no reported cases in September; however, by December,

Medicines And Lotion Used by The Health Department, Calcutta Corporation for The Prevention and Treatment of Influenza

Tablet.

Quinine Sulph.	...	... gr. i
Ammon Carb	...	.. gr.ii
Sodi Benzoas	...	... gr.ii ½.
Ol. Thymol	...	... m. 1/8.

Mft.Tab :-

Linimant.

Liq.Ammon Fort	...	dr.	i.
Ol.Eucalyptus	...	dr.	i.
Ol Sinapis	...	Ad.oz.	i.

Ft.Lint.

Dilute Thymol solution-(1 in 1,600).

Thymol Solution(Concentrated)

Thymol-10 ozs.
KOH- 6 1/3 ozs.
Aqua-110 ozs. by volume

Dissolve caustic potash sticks in 50 ozs. of water and powder Thymol in a pestle and mortar and dissolve the same in enough alcohol. Mix the two solutions together and then make up to 110 ozs. with ordinary tap water.

Direction for use.—One tea spoonful of the Stock solution diluted with a pint of water should Be used as a nasal douche.

Mixture No.1 Sedative Expectorant.

Re.

Soda Benzoas	...	gr.	v.
Spt. Amon Arom	...	m.	xx.
Tinc. Camphor Co.	...	m.	xxx.
Vinum Ipecac	...	m.	x.
Aqua Cinnamon	...	Ad. Dr.	ii.

Adult dose--- 2 drams made up to 1 oz.

Mixture No.II---Stimulant

Re.

Spt. Amon Arom	...	m.	xx.
Spt. Aether Sulph	...	m.	xx.
Tinct. Stropenthus	...	m.	v.
Liq. Strychnine Hydrochlor	...	m.	iv.
Aqua Camphor	...	Ad. dr.	ii.

Adult does--- 2 drams made up to 1 oz.

Mixture No. III- Stimulant Expectorant

Re.

Ammon Carb	...	gr.	v.
Tinct.Scillae ...	...	m.	xv.
Tinct.Senega	...	m.	xv
Aqua Camphor	...	Ad.dr.	ii.

Adult dose----2 drams made up to 1 oz.

B.S.Prezs—1-2_1919—3800J—100---R.F.

Figure 1.7 Medicine and Lotion Used by the Health Department, Calcutta Corporation, for the Prevention and Treatment of Influenza

cholera-related deaths rose sharply to 186, suggesting a likely correlation with inadequate sanitation or contaminated water during the colder months. Smallpox resulted in 26 deaths, maintaining a relatively low yet steady presence throughout the time frame. December recorded the highest monthly toll, with 14 fatalities, showing a slight uptick in virulence. The plague, while historically important in the area, had a negligible effect during this period, with only two deaths documented, implying that control measures against the plague were successful.

Fevers and Respiratory Illnesses: The Leading Causes of Death

The category of fevers recorded 2175 deaths, closely associated with the influenza outbreak. The death toll surged dramatically in November (1017 deaths) and reached its peak in December (1112 deaths), illustrating the lethal second wave of the pandemic. Respiratory Diseases, likely encompassing pneumonia and bronchitis as complications of influenza, resulted in 1498 deaths. The notable rise in cases during November (1248 deaths) and December (1206 deaths) underscores the severe impact of respiratory complications linked to influenza.

Gastrointestinal Disorders and Other Factors

Diarrhoea and dysentery handled 1048 deaths, with a consistent increase from September to December. The peak occurred in December, with 362 deaths, showing that worsening sanitation or weakened immunity within the population may have intensified this problem. Injuries led to 183 deaths, a relatively minor figure when compared to disease-related fatalities.

Overall Mortality and Critical Periods—The monthly death toll reveals a significant spike in November (4318 deaths) and December (4119 deaths), confirming that these two months were the most lethal during the outbreak. The overall mortality rate during the four-month period reached 26.9 per 1000 individuals, a remarkably high statistic that underscores the devastating impact of the pandemic and the related health emergencies.

> *The situation reveals the seriousness of the influenza epidemic in Calcutta, especially in November and December 1918. The total number of cases from fevers and respiratory illnesses highlights the catastrophic effects of the pandemic, while simultaneous increases in cholera and diarrhoea cases show further public health issues. Contributing elements such as overcrowded housing, inadequate sanitation, and scarce medical resources probably exacerbated the situation. This data underscores the critical necessity for public health measures during outbreaks, which should include improved sanitation, enhanced healthcare infrastructure, and better preparedness for epidemics (Source: Proceedings of the Meeting, Municipal Department, Calcutta Corporation, December 1918).*

In 1919, Health Officer H. M. Crake announced a major influenza outbreak in Calcutta, reporting a fatality rate of 4.1 per thousand. The elevated death rate in Kidderpore, which was over five times the average of Calcutta, severely affected the area at 21.1 deaths per mile. Dr. Crake stated,

> *The substantial population of impoverished and uneducated coolies living in damp, dark, and filthy huts in Kidderpore seems to primarily cause the high mortality rate. This demographic presents significant challenges, as they not*

> *only hide their health issues but frequently reject any form of advice or medical treatment.*
>
> (Proceedings of the Meeting, Municipal Department, Calcutta Corporation, December 1918)

Dr. Crake also recognized that this area had many relief centres, yet they did not open promptly and were not as effective as those in other neighbourhoods. He observed that regions primarily populated by affluent Europeans had mortality rates significantly lower than the average, but he also noted,

> *Recorders measured influenza mortality rates of less than 3 per thousand individuals in Ward 2, 3, 4, 6, 8, and 11. Despite being overcrowded and exhibiting many unsanitary conditions, these wards predominantly house a significant number of middle-class residents, with the uneducated and impoverished bustee inhabitants representing a smaller segment of the population.*
>
> (Proceedings of the Meeting, Municipal Department, Calcutta Corporation, December 1918)

Crake linked high mortality rates to socio-economic status and poverty, while the government alerted the public about the virus's transmission. They advised breaking common items, such as drinking cups, tearing handkerchiefs, and avoiding spitting, as it facilitated the spread of germs. The media also endorsed these recommendations. A well-composed Bengali pamphlet titled "Epidemic Disease and their Prevention" addressed every aspect of influenza. The pamphlet informed the public in straightforward terms about how the disease affected the human body and how to fight it. Ward Health Associations distributed the pamphlets freely to every resident via door-to-door outreach (Proceedings of the Govt. of Bengal, April 1919).

The Sanitary Commissioner of Bengal regarded influenza as a minor public health issue and suggested immediate isolation, poorly ventilated residences, open-air sleeping, and clothing for disinfection. Surgeon General Lyons recommended gargling with potassium permanganate and aspirin, and hospitalizing pneumonia patients, cautioning against the use of quinine as a preventive or therapeutic drug. The authorities instructed hospitals and dispensaries to expand their capacities and use well-ventilated classroom spaces. The local press disagreed, while the government provided 66 temporary Sub-Assistant Surgeons to District Boards. Health officials sought refuge in hilly areas, but the governmental body in charge of reporting crucial incidents was ineffective. The only help from the government was the allocation of those 66 sub-assistant surgeons (Hill, 2011, p. 24). Dr. Soorya Goodeve Chuckerbutty, the District Health Officer, established relief centres in District III, staffed by volunteers. Over 100 centres managed mild cases, dispensed thymol solution, and visited local bustees for more serious cases. The 50 mobile dispensaries and over 100 centres formed an extensive network, offering guidance and treatment to various individuals. Some of the relief centres in various parts of the city included (i) Ananda Chatterjee Lane—In charge Babu C N Banerjee, (ii) 8/1 Bagbazar Street—In charge Babu B D Mullick, (iii) 23/1 Beniatola Street—In charge Dr. T K Ghosh, (iv) 83 Raja Dinendra Street—In charge Me Eleazar Ekka, and (v) 24 Girish Vidyaratna Lane—In charge Dr. S C Mitra (Proceedings of the Govt. of Bengal, Municipal Department, April 1919, File No. S. 2D-8(3)).

During the Spanish Flu epidemic, Calcutta, once the capital of British India, witnessed a significant accumulation of corpses in burning ghats and burial sites. The city confronted the grim reality of death with no one available to burn or cremate them (Minutes of the Calcutta Corporation, December 1918). The Surgeon General asserted that health officials had made efforts in Kolkata, but the local media countered this claim. The condition in neighbouring villages of Bengal was dire because of shortage of doctors, medications, and alerts. The Health Department's inadequate personnel, even with temporary Medical Inspectors, led to volunteers for lay, medical, and "open relief centres". These efforts fell short, resulting in further destruction. Despite a significant increase in staff numbers, the situation did not improve (Bankura Sanbad, October 27, 1918, p. 3). The following report will detail the treatment of influenza in rural Bengal.

Box 2.2 MR. MACPHAIL—Influenza in Rural Penge

The Influenza Epidemic in Rural Bengal—
By James M. Macphail, MB, C. MM.

People now widely recognize the influenza epidemic that swept across India in the spring of this year, but I would like to share my observations from a remote rural area, far from major population centers. Our mission station is located approximately 180 miles from Calcutta and 16 miles from the nearest railway. Initially, we learned the epidemic had reached Bombay via a mail steamer, with a few cases also reported in Calcutta. Daily newspapers chronicled its spread from province to province and city to city, and we awaited with keen interest to see if it would reach our secluded location in the jungle. Eventually, we received news that it had arrived at our closest post-town, Gobindpore, just 10 miles away, where the locals referred to it as the Belati bokhar, or "English fever." Soon after, we observed clear signs of the epidemic in our community. A native printer arrived at our station from Calcutta, exhibiting symptoms of a runny nose and cough. Although these symptoms would not typically suggest influenza, I became quite concerned, and within a few days, the epidemic had indeed reached us. I cannot definitively say whether this individual was the source of the outbreak. In our mission schools, which serve 120 students, nearly half were affected, likely reflecting the proportion of the general population that suffered. The patients consistently reported symptoms of "fever, pain in the head, and all over," with cough being the least distressing symptom for many. Prostration was notably severe. Villagers would travel from afar to the bungalow, lie down on the verandah, and remain there until their symptoms improved. Among the patients I treated, two fatalities occurred. One girl, who could walk, traveled seven miles exhibiting the usual symptoms and received standard treatment. However, two days later, I received a message showing that she had suddenly fallen gravely ill that morning with "fever and chest pain." My native assistant promptly rode to her location but arrived only to witness her passing. The other death involved a 35-year-old woman, which was evidently caused by pneumonia following influenza. Around the same time, someone reported another death in the vicinity.

In terms of treatment, for typical cases, I administered antifebrin in 5-grain doses; for severe headaches, I prescribed antipyrine in 10-grain doses. For children, I provided antipyrine in 3-grain doses because of its superior solubility. I used ipecacuanha pills and scilla to address the persistent cough often following the fever, and I gave a tonic of quinine, nitro-muriatic acid, and tincture of perchloride of iron during convalescence after severe cases. Both my native assistant and I experienced illness ourselves, and we found antifebrin to be effective. In my case, taking 5 grains three times reduced my temperature from over 102° in the morning to 99° by evening. The next day, I primarily suffered from a headache, which was eased by 10 grains of antipyrine. Some acquaintances in Calcutta reported that they found ammoniated quinine helpful in preventing impending attacks.

Recently, I worried about a resurgence of the disease when I examined four boys from the same family who suddenly developed fever, headache, backache, and cough. However, it was ultimately diagnosed as measles, which can be challenging to distinguish from influenza in patients with darker skin, as their complexion may obscure subtle symptoms.

Toonde Manbhoom
September 7, 1918

Villagers encountered a catastrophic situation with every home perishing. Medical facilities had no physicians or resources, and indigenous practitioners[8] offered help. The British government halted their actions by enacting legislation, resulting in the desperate population having difficulty adhering to regulations for their survival and income. Individuals carried the deceased to Calcutta and managed their remains without understanding the cause. The low mortality rate observed during the initial outbreak led to several fatalities in the following outbreak. The British government and health professionals remained quiet, making justifications to mask their failures and allowing the villagers to deeply feel the terror of mortality (District Statistical Handbook of Bengal, 1921).

Local Newspapers and the Voluntary Organizations

During the Spanish Influenza of 1918–19, local newspapers in Calcutta and rural Bengal helped to spread information and influence public opinion. They offered updates about the virus, prevention strategies, and advice from health officials. However, there were difficulties stemming from conflicting reports and false information, underlining the necessity for strict fact-checking. Local newspapers, even amid criticism regarding the colonial government's management of the pandemic, which resulted in legal actions aimed at curbing governmental misconduct, were vital in keeping the public updated, promoting shared responsibility, and enabling coordinated responses. Voluntary organizations in rural Bengal delivered care, established temporary medical facilities, and backed quarantine efforts. Their unwavering commitment to community health showcased the significance of grassroots actions during crises. In 1918, the Spanish Flu made its way to India, initially noted in Mumbai as "Bombay Fever", attributed to high temperatures, humidity, and a dusty environment in Bombay (Singh, 2021, pp. 35–40). This section examines how colonial authorities used weekly English reports from local newspapers between July and December 1918 to oversee and gather essential press statements regarding the government's pandemic response in rural Bengal.

War Fever: The Chaos Within Structure

1918 was a tough year for public health because of an influx of immigrants from areas affected by plague, leading to higher mortality rates, particularly from smallpox and plague. In June, an epidemic of influenza emerged, which diminished after several weeks. A severe resurgence in October persisted throughout the rest of the year and into the beginning of the next, accounting for approximately a quarter of the year's deaths. The vital statistics[9] illustrate its impact (Minutes of the Meeting of the Calcutta Corporation, July 1918). In Calcutta, on July 14, 1918, the local newspaper of Calcutta, The Bengalee on its pg. 2, released the news headline "War Fever in Calcutta–Effect on Public Health and Business", informing the residents of Calcutta that

> *all reports show that the swift spread of an epidemic of Influenza with fever in Calcutta and its surrounding districts has resulted in severe consequences not only among all segments of the public but also in public business that is facing unprecedented dislocation in the history of Calcutta.*
>
> (The Bengalee, July 1918)

In Kidderpore and Ekbalpur, the coolie and labour class lived in overcrowded, unhealthy, poorly ventilated slums, while British officials and the cosmopolitan elite lived in stylish western enclaves. *The Times of India* on October 9, 1918 stated "a fertile breeding ground" for the rapid spread of the disease, which was conveyed by insects or through human interaction.

> *On July 13th, the Amrita Bazar Patrika, an English daily based in Calcutta, reported on the swift escalation of the influenza epidemic in Calcutta and*

> *its surrounding districts. This outbreak has led to severe repercussions not only for various segments of the population but also poses an unprecedented threat to the public business sector in Calcutta. Investigations show that nearly this illness has affected every household, which, despite being perceived as short-lived, significantly undermines the overall health of those affected. The labor class, vegetable vendors, businesspeople, and students are vulnerable because of their poorly ventilated living conditions, as their coughing and sneezing contribute to the spread of the virus to those nearby.*

A comprehensive report in the Indian Medical Gazette (Bose, 1920), Epidemic Influenza in and around the City of Calcutta by Sir Koilas Chandra Bose, showed that

> *In mid-June 1918, I encountered several cases on Cross Street, which serves as both the hub of the piece-goods trade and a focal point for imported epidemic diseases. This street is typically where the germs of contagious illnesses spread throughout the city. Necessity compelled the Postal Department to reduce the frequency of letter deliveries, and in many areas, Calcutta resembled a ghost town. By early September, the death rate in Calcutta rose noticeably, and within two weeks, there was a widespread demand for medical help from all corners of the city. Medical professionals engaged in extensive discussions to determine the nature of the disease, yet no doctor or official could halt its progression.*

Infected individuals experienced fever, pain in limbs and bones, inflammation of the bronchial tubes, congestion, and pain in the eyes. *The Amrita Bazar Patrika* of June 26, 1918 stated that "Calcutta Corporation asserts the epidemic is simply an unusually widespread epidemic of influenza, which typically emerges here around August." The second wave of the influenza outbreak in British India, especially in Calcutta, led to high death rates, particularly among impoverished low-caste Hindus, as their overcrowded living situations and poverty rendered them vulnerable. The native press did not acknowledge that more women were dying than men. British India was the most severely affected region during the deadly influenza outbreak of 1918. Two consecutive waves, the first in June 1918 and the second in September, heavily concentrated migrants in Calcutta, affecting various provinces in India until April 1919.

On October 22, 1918, Dr. Turner provided conclusive proof that the disease arrived via ships in late May and spread to Delhi, Meerut, and Shimla. He observed Bombay was relatively free of infectious diseases on June 16, but by June 24, it was suffering from a devastating epidemic. Vernacular newspapers such as *Bombay Samachar* and *Jam-e-Jamshed* supported his findings, emphasizing the extensive spread of the illness in Bombay. In Calcutta, the local vernacular, *The Amrita Bazar Patrika, on July 13, reported that H. M. Crake, the Health Officer of Calcutta Corporation, addressed the contagious nature of the illness. The transmission of infectious diseases occurs primarily through contact, and traditional methods are ineffective because of various factors—(i) the challenges in making a precise diagnosis in the initial phases, (ii) the rapid and extensive spread of the infection, and (iii) the inability to manage a disease with such low mortality by itself as a dangerous infectious disease. The Board of Health advises simple avoidance measures during epidemics, which include remaining in bed until a physician permits you to rise and refraining from attempting to walk if the patient is extremely weak. The gravity of the situation causes immediate investigation.*

Inadequate Medical Relief, Civil Society, and Private Philanthropy

The local vernaculars often scrutinized the government's disproportionate actions in response to the emerging crisis, showing a lack of preparedness and obvious indifference in providing medical help because of a more severe second wave of influenza. *The Statesman*, October 18, 1918, noted that

> *We remain uncertain about the actions taken by the well-compensated government specialists to assist individuals in the districts. Even in a major city like Calcutta, it was necessary to publicize fever remedies, and Dr. Turner has had to provide medical guidance, albeit belatedly. We seek clarification on the measures the government has implemented to support the distressed population in the mofussil, which urgently requires ready-made remedies and medical advice. The public would have appreciated insights from the esteemed medical professionals employed by the government during this critical time. Currently, there is a lack of awareness regarding the services they have provided thus far. The residents of the mofussil often lack a voice in these matters. However, we hope that the government will respond more swiftly and generously to this pressing need than it has done up to this point.*

The Amrita Bazar Patrika, published on October 4, 1918, emphasizes the need for food supply and adequately ventilated housing in Calcutta amidst pestilence and famine. The article questioned whether the government had taken adequate steps to tackle food deficiencies and enhance sanitary conditions. It also proposed that the government should establish grain shops to provide grains to poorer classes at reduced prices, potentially through a loan facility, and facilitate their relocation to open spaces from their unhealthy slum areas (The Amrita Bazar Patrika, October 1918).

The 1918 Spanish Influenza pandemic notably affected Calcutta and rural Bengal, particularly in densely populated districts such as Hooghly, Howrah, and North 24 Parganas.

Local communities in India have played a significant role in delivering medical care and help during the pandemic. In Hooghly, volunteers established hospitals and quarantine facilities, while the Hooghly Relief Committee[10] managed relief activities. In Howrah, community leaders worked with district administration to create isolation wards and distribute resources. Rural districts in India, such as Murshidabad, Nadia, and South 24 Parganas, depended on grassroots movements and charitable donations. Affluent landowners and merchants contributed to support the relief initiatives, whereas awareness campaigns were essential in regions like Maldah, Birbhum, and Bardhaman. Volunteers shared pamphlets, organized public gatherings, and used traditional communication methods to disseminate information about preventive actions and early detection. Mutual aid networks in Medinipur, Jalpaiguri, and Cooch Behar delivered essential goods to at-risk groups like elderly individuals, widows, and migrant labourers during emergencies (District Statistical Handbook, 1921).

Student groups protested against school and college closures because of unemployment, emphasizing the importance of income and family help. The outbreak of the disease resulted in mental distress, prioritizing the pursuit of income over completing education. Two newspaper articles convey the public's concern and dissatisfaction regarding the Spanish Influenza outbreak in Calcutta in late 1918, with each report offering distinct viewpoints on how educational institutions are managing the situation.

> *The first letter published in the "Guardian" conveys apprehension regarding the delayed closure of City College and Ripon College in Calcutta, particularly as most other educational establishments have suspended classes because of the influenza outbreak. The writer argues that the administration of these colleges is compromising student safety and threatening public health through their noncompliance. The letter highlights the challenges faced by students, particularly those from rural areas, arising from the ambiguity surrounding the reopening timeline. The letter urges educational authorities to improve communication and act promptly, noting that students learned of the extended holiday only after returning to Calcutta. The author demands greater accountability from the administration during this public health crisis.*
>
> *The second letter, written by a student from St. Xavier's College, raises concerns about student attendance in classes amidst the ongoing influenza epidemic. The student questions the reasoning behind the continued operation of colleges, while prominent institutions and government offices have closed to control the outbreak. This correspondence emphasizes the risks associated with overcrowded classrooms, arguing that such negligence may facilitate the further spread of influenza. The student urges authorities to suspend classes for the sake of public safety and expresses dissatisfaction with the institutions for their failure to implement preventive measures promptly.*
>
> *(Source: The Bengalee, October 27, 1918)*

The two letters from Calcutta emphasize the conflict between institutional stagnation and the imperative of public safety amid the influenza outbreak. The initial report addresses administrative shortcomings that lead to student difficulties and a failure in effective communication. Conversely, the second report draws attention to the susceptibility of students and the dangers associated with overcrowded settings. Together, these letters reflect an increasing recognition of public health initiatives and a sense of frustration with institutions that prioritize standard procedures over the welfare of the community. They reveal the concerns of students, parents, and the public, pointing out deficiencies in institutional readiness and the pressing necessity for enhanced public health measures.

Reports show a hostile environment in rural Bengal, where a lack of government support led to the closure of primary schools, causing turmoil for students, parents, and the education department. This resulted in the education collapse system in rural Bengal.

> *The Spanish Influenza Ravages, the Educational Framework of Rural Bengal—Educational Institutions Close, Educators Face Challenges, and Learners Are Deprived of Educational Opportunities! The Pandemic's Hold Intensifies, Endangering the Prospects of an Entire Generation.*
>
> *(Calcutta Gazette, November 5, 1918)*

Calcutta Gazette's investigative report highlights the Spanish Influenza's role in disrupting rural Bengal's education system, resulting in school closures, teacher struggles, and students lacking essential learning opportunities. The following text aims to highlight the protest of rural Bengal teachers during the Spanish Influenza:

> *Rural Bengal Educators Protest Amidst the Turmoil of Spanish Influenza: Seeking Help as the Education System Faces Imminent Collapse.*
>
> *Following the catastrophic Spanish Influenza outbreak, the education sector in rural Bengal is experiencing unparalleled disruption, characterized by closed schools and teachers facing financial hardships. In a plea for help, educators from various parts of the region have taken to the streets, urging authorities to take immediate action. With empty classrooms and students lacking direction, these teachers are advocating for financial help, healthcare support, and a solid strategy to restore the deteriorating education system. As the pandemic continues to exert its influence, the challenges faced by rural Bengal's teachers highlight the critical necessity for prompt intervention to avert the risk of a lost generation.*
>
> (The Bengal Tribune, December 15, 1918)

The protests of teachers in rural Bengal during the Spanish Influenza outbreak generated significant concern and mobilization. The crisis underscored the difficulties confronted by educators, such as the necessity of delivering education and maintaining livelihoods. The demand for government help and a comprehensive strategy to bolster the education sector resulted in grassroots initiatives to ensure ongoing access to education (Minutes of the Meeting of the Calcutta Corporation, January 1919). Civil society organizations and community leaders in areas like Bankura, Purulia, and Dinajpur urged the colonial government to enhance their response to the 1918 Spanish Influenza pandemic. They coordinated public demonstrations, petitions, and advocacy efforts for an increase in medical help, improved sanitation facilities, and transparency in the distribution of relief funds. Despite government indifference, grassroots movements, charitable donations, awareness campaigns, and mutual aid networks took shape. The Ramakrishna Mission,[11] Red Cross Society,[12] and Hindu Satkar Samity[13] became vital sources of support, offering medical help, basic treatments, and essential supplies. The Ramakrishna Mission, a selfless organization, supplied medical aid, basic treatments, and comfort to affected communities during the turmoil, as noted in *The Bengalee* on June 27, 1918.

The Ramakrishna Mission

Famine Relief Work in Bengal During Influenza Pandemic, June 27, 1918

We are currently operating in four districts: two in Bengal and two in Bihar. Besides our existing centers at Bagda in the Manbhum district and Indpur in the Bankura district, we have recently established two new centers—Koniamara under the Gangajalghati police jurisdiction and Koalpara under the Kotalpur police jurisdiction. We have opened two additional centers at Konda and Sarwan within the Deoghar subdivision of the Santal Parganas district. By next week, we plan to inaugurate a new relief center at Bitghar in the Tippera district, which will be our fourth center opened in January. Since mid-June, we have distributed 2,000 maunds (a traditional unit of mass in British India, equivalent to approximately 37.3242 kilograms) of rice and 1,000 pieces of new clothing to around 4,000 beneficiaries across approximately 200 villages. Our weekly distribution now serves 3,765 recipients, who will require support until the end of October.

The relief efforts by the Ramakrishna Mission illustrate the monthly distribution of rice and cloth from different centres, providing an insightful overview of the humanitarian assistance efforts executed during the simultaneous crises of the 1918 influenza pandemic and the famine in colonial Bengal. The data, categorized by distribution centres—Manbhum–Bagda, Bankura–Indpur, Bankura–Koalpara, and Tippera–Koalpara—illustrates both the magnitude and focus of aid across various villages, highlighting significant differences in the extent and quantity of resources distributed. In the Manbhum–Bagda area, relief initiatives were particularly comprehensive over several months, aid reached 69 villages, benefiting 2,098 individuals through the distribution of 409 maunds of rice (MDS). The number of villages receiving clothing was lower, peaking at 32 villages with 187 garments distributed, which may indicate a prioritization of food aid over clothing or logistical challenges in textile supply. The Bankura–Indpur centre shows a consistent rise in rice distribution, reaching a significant total of 163 MDS to 640 recipients across 30 villages, while clothing distribution here varies widely, with one instance of 227 garments allocated to just 4 villages, suggesting a concentration of aid in particularly affected areas.

The Bankura–Koalpara centre provided a relatively limited amount of rice assistance, with only 7 to 18 villages receiving between 4 and 22 MDS of rice, which may indicate either a smaller number of affected individuals or constrained resources. Notably, the distribution of clothing in this region is also minimal, with no instance exceeding 5 garments, implying that the centre either had restricted access to clothing or prioritized other areas. In contrast, the Tippera–Koalpara centre distinguishes itself by serving 31 villages and 616 beneficiaries, distributing a significant 94 MDS of rice, along with clothing for 12 villages, indicating a more comprehensive approach to relief efforts. This not only shows the varying levels of famine and pandemic relief across the districts of Bengal but also emphasizes the unequal distribution of aid, influenced by factors such as logistical capacity, the severity of need, and the state of regional infrastructure. Furthermore, it draws attention to the contributions of religious and charitable organizations, such as the Ramakrishna Mission, in addressing the deficiencies of colonial administration by offering essential support during one of the most lethal global pandemics in contemporary history.

(Source: The Bengalee, June 27, 1918)

The Red Cross Society and Hindu Satkar Samity played essential roles in fighting the influenza pandemic by establishing temporary hospitals, providing urgent care, and organizing vaccination campaigns, ultimately saving lives. The Hindu Satkar Samity also took a dedicated role in cremating the deceased during the pandemic.

Many corpses overwhelm the Ganges, rendering its water nearly invisible, obscured by piles of bodies. The crematorium lacks personnel to perform the cremations, and the villagers do not have access to trains. Despite the abundance of deceased individuals, there is no one available to conduct the cremation process. Train transports the bodies to Calcutta for cremation.

(The Bengalee, October 24, 1918)

The Hindu Satkar Samity also established community kitchens and shelters to offer food and accommodation for vulnerable populations, ensuring that they could access critical resources. The information released in the local newspaper highlighted the issue more vividly—*Calcutta Herald*, November 25, 1918: "Hindu Satkar Samity Extends Lifeline Amidst Spanish Influenza Crisis",

Amidst the turmoil of the Spanish Influenza pandemic affecting Bengal, the Hindu Satkar Samity stands out as a symbol of hope and unity for those in distress. Grounded in the principles of community service and empathy, the Samity rallies its members to extend vital support to those most severely affected by the virus. Their initiatives include the distribution of medical supplies and essential goods, as well as organizing transportation for the ill to medical facilities. The relentless dedication of the Samity acts as a crucial support system for many families facing the harsh realities of the pandemic. The organization's focus on solidarity and communal harmony cultivates resilience in the face of hardship, encouraging individuals from diverse backgrounds to unite in mutual aid. As the Spanish Influenza continues to cause widespread suffering in Bengal, the Hindu Satkar Samity's steadfast dedication to humanitarian efforts exemplifies the strength of collective action during challenging times.

Another news published in the local newspaper may be recommended—

"Bengal Gazette, December 10, 1918: Death Toll Rises as Spanish Influenza Ravages Villages—Hindu Satkar Samity Extends Aid Amidst Grim Crisis",

> *As the Spanish Influenza continues to spread throughout rural Bengal, the number of fatalities rises consistently, casting a grim pall over villages and small communities. Each day brings new sorrow as families grieve for those they have lost, while entire communities confront the harsh realities brought on by the lethal virus. In this time of unprecedented hardship, the Hindu Satkar Samity stands out as a beacon of hope, reaching out to those in urgent need. Samity volunteers dedicate themselves to helping the suffering, offering solace to the grieving and support to the ill. Their efforts range from organizing respectful funerals to distributing food and medical supplies to affected families, embodying a spirit of compassion during these challenging times. The unwavering commitment of the Samity to the well-being of rural Bengal's inhabitants offers comfort and resilience to communities struggling with grief and despair. As the pandemic persists, the crucial contributions of the Hindu Satkar Samity highlight the strength and solidarity that characterize the people of rural Bengal in the face of adversity.*
>
> (Bengal Gazette, December 10, 1918)

The volunteers from the Hindu Satkar provided care, comfort, and help to the ill, grieving, and vulnerable populations, nurturing solidarity and collaboration among diverse communities during a difficult period (Annual Report of the Sanitary Commissioner, 1918–20). The Hindu Satkar Samity, being a Calcutta-based organization, supported rural communities during the pandemic, fostering community solidarity and hope. Their grassroots initiatives, which included funerals and the distribution of essential supplies, earned them trust and appreciation. Their legacy motivates future generations, exemplifying resilience and compassion in the face of extraordinary difficulties, and encouraging acts of kindness and service (Based on an analysis of Pro Quest: The Times of India Digital Database).

Conclusion

The 1918–19 influenza pandemic had a significant effect on Calcutta and the nearby districts, resulting in unmatched death rates and devastating effects. The pandemic acts as a reminder of the vulnerability of human existence during viral outbreaks and emphasizes the necessity for contemplation on lessons learned and the strength of those who survived. As we address current challenges and get ready for an unpredictable future, the reminders of the past compel us to stay alert in our endeavours to protect public health and enhance communal welfare.

Despite governmental actions, inefficiencies, bureaucratic obstacles, and lack of preparedness, the pandemic left communities in ruins and hopelessness. Grassroots movements, volunteer initiatives, community support systems, and local newspapers surfaced as crucial supports for those affected. Local newspapers and voluntary organizations were instrumental in the pandemic response, spreading information, revealing government deficiencies, and igniting discussions. An efficient pandemic response calls for a comprehensive strategy, incorporating government involvement, community participation, and media advocacy. By drawing lessons from previous errors, bolstering healthcare frameworks, nurturing grassroots resilience, and amplifying the voices of under-represented communities, we can enhance our readiness for future pandemics and ensure the welfare of all segments of society, irrespective of their social or economic status (Crosby, 2003, p. 3).

Notes

1 Rajputana—Rajputana, in western India, is renowned for its valorous Rajput rulers and vibrant cultural heritage. With majestic forts, desert landscapes, and rich history, it captivates visitors with tales of chivalry and grandeur. Renowned for its rich cultural heritage, Rajputana holds a significant place in Indian history. Today, Rajasthan, the heart of Rajputana, continues to preserve its regal legacy through its architectural marvels, colourful festivals, and enduring traditions.

2 Dengue—Dengue fever, transmitted by Aedes mosquitoes, is a viral illness prevalent in tropical and subtropical regions worldwide. Symptoms include high fever, severe joint and muscle pain, headache, and rash, sometimes leading to severe complications like hemorrhagic fever. Prevention focuses on mosquito control measures, such as eliminating breeding sites and using insect repellents. Despite efforts, dengue remains a significant public health concern, especially in densely populated urban areas.

3 Purdah System—The purdah system, prevalent in colonial India and various cultures worldwide, enforced strict segregation of genders. The purdah system secluded women from public view and often confined them to the domestic sphere. The speciality of the purdah system lies in its strict enforcement of gender segregation, particularly concerning the seclusion of women from unrelated men in public spaces. This practice aimed to preserve female honour and modesty but also limited their social and economic opportunities. Over time, the purdah system has been subject to critique and gradual reform, reflecting changing societal norms and values.

4 Bara Bazar Area—During the colonial period, Bara Bazar Area in Calcutta (now Kolkata) served as a bustling commercial hub, teeming with traders, artisans, and merchants. It was renowned for its diverse marketplaces, selling a plethora of goods ranging from textiles to spices, attracting merchants from across the world. The area reflected the vibrant cosmopolitanism of colonial Calcutta, with its narrow lanes, crowded bazaars, and dynamic interplay of cultures, making it a focal point of economic and social activity in British India.

5 Spanish Flu—The second wave of the Spanish Flu, occurring in late 1918 and early 1919, was the deadliest phase of the pandemic. It spread rapidly across the globe, overwhelming healthcare systems and causing millions of deaths worldwide. Its high mortality rate among young adults characterized this wave, unlike typical flu strains, which primarily affect older adults and young children.

6 Charanamrito—Charanamrito, also spelled as Charanamrit, is a sacred liquid in Hinduism, typically made of a mixture of water, milk, honey, yogurt, and ghee (clarified butter). Devotees receive this auspicious liquid during religious ceremonies, especially in temples. Devotees believe Charanamrito possesses purifying and sanctifying properties, and consider partaking of it a blessing and a form of divine grace. Devotees often sip a small amount of Charanamrito or use it to sprinkle on their heads or bodies as a form of spiritual cleansing and protection.

7 Prophylactic—"Prophylactic" is an adjective used to describe measures or treatments intended to prevent disease or infection. In medicine, a prophylactic approach involves taking preventative actions or administering preventive treatments to reduce the risk of illness or disease occurrence. This can include actions such as vaccinations, lifestyle changes, or the use of medications to protect against specific diseases or conditions. Prophylactic measures are crucial in public health efforts to control the spread of infectious diseases and maintain overall well-being.

8 Indigenous Practitioners—Indigenous practitioners are individuals who belong to native or traditional communities (vaidyas, hakims, etc.) and hold knowledge and expertise in traditional healing methods and practices. They often have deep cultural and spiritual connections to their healing techniques, which are passed down through generations orally or through apprenticeship. Indigenous practitioners play a vital role in providing healthcare within their communities, offering holistic approaches that integrate physical, mental, and spiritual aspects of well-being.

9 Vital Statistics—Vital statistics refer to numerical data concerning births, deaths, marriages, and other significant life events within a population. Governmental and health organizations collect and analyze these statistics to monitor population trends, assess public health outcomes, and inform policy decisions. Vital statistics provide valuable insights into demographic changes, health indicators, and social patterns within a society, aiding in the development and evaluation of public health programmes and interventions.

10 The Hooghly Relief Committee—The Hooghly Relief Committee was a notable organization established during late-19th-century colonial India to provide help during times of crisis, particularly in the Hooghly district of Bengal. Comprising local officials, philanthropists, and community leaders, its primary aim was to offer relief and support to those affected by natural disasters such as floods and famines. The committee played a crucial role in coordinating relief efforts, raising funds, and distributing aid to mitigate the impact of such calamities on the local population.

11 Ramakrishna Mission— Ramakrishna Mission is a renowned spiritual and philanthropic organization founded by Swami Vivekananda in 1897, inspired by the teachings of his guru, Sri Ramakrishna Paramahamsa. Rooted in the ideals of Vedanta philosophy, the mission aims to serve humanity by promoting spiritual growth, social welfare, and harmony among different religions. It operates through various centres worldwide, offering educational, healthcare, and humanitarian services while emphasizing the importance of selfless service (Seva) and spiritual realization.

12 Red Cross Society—The Red Cross Society, officially known as the International Red Cross and Red Crescent Movement, is a humanitarian organization founded in 1863 by Henry Dunant. It operates worldwide, helping those affected by conflict, disasters, and health emergencies. The Red Cross Society offers a range of services, including disaster relief, healthcare, blood donation, and support for refugees and migrants. Guided by principles of neutrality, impartiality, independence, and humanity, it plays a vital role in alleviating human suffering and promoting respect for human dignity across the globe.

13 Hindu Satkar Samity—Hindu Satkar Samity is a Calcutta-based Hindu charity organization responsible for the cremation of unrecognized Hindu dead bodies. Hindu Satkar Samity is the only institution that may carry the bodies of Hindus and cremate them after death. Someone founded it in 1932.

References

Books

Arnold, D. (1993). *Colonizing the body: State medicine and epidemic disease in nineteenth-century India*. University of California Press.

Crosby, A. (2003). *America's forgotten pandemic: The influenza of 1918*. Cambridge University Press.

Ramanna, M. (2003). Coping with the influenza pandemic: The Bombay experience. In H. Phillips & D. Killingray (Eds.), *The Spanish influenza pandemic of 1918–19: New perspectives* (pp. 86–98). Routledge.

Tumbe, C. (2020). *The age of pandemics 1817–1929: How they shaped India and the world*. Harper Collins.

White, N. (1919). *A preliminary report on the influenza pandemic of 1918 in India* (pp. 8–9). Government of India Press.

Articles

Arnold, D. (2019). Death and the modern empire: The 1918–19 influenza epidemic in India. *Transactions of the Royal Historical Society*, *29*, 200.

Bose, K. C. (1920). Influenza in and around the city of Calcutta. *Indian Medical Gazette*, *55*, 169.

Hardiman, D. (2012). The influenza epidemic of 1918 and the Adivasis of Western India. *Social History of Medicine*, *25*(3), 644–664.

Hill, K. (2011). Influenza in India 1918: Excess mortality reassessed. *Genus*, *67*(2), 24.

Mills, I. D. (1986). The 1918–19 influenza pandemic–The Indian experience. *Indian Economic and Social History Review*, *23*(1), 1–40.

Sen, N. D. (1920, March). Influenza as observed in The Sambhu Nath Pundit Hospital, Calcutta. *The Indian Medical Gazette*, 89–92.

Singh, M. (2021). Bombay fever/Spanish flu: Public health and native press in colonial Bombay, 1918–19. *South Asia Research*, *41*(1), 35–52.

Archival Sources

Books and Reports

Annual Report of the Health Department. (1918). *Section–I, meteorology and vital statistics.*

Annual Report of the Sanitary Commissioner with the Government of India for 1918. (1920). (pp. 5–6).

District Statistical Handbook of Bengal. (1921).

Preliminary Report on the Epidemic in India by the Sanitary Commissioner with the Government of India, File No. S.2D–8, Proceedings Nos. B27–29.

Government Documents

Minutes of the Meeting of the Calcutta Corporation. (July, 1918).

Minutes of the Meeting of the Calcutta Corporation. (December, 1918).

Minutes of the Meeting of the Calcutta Corporation. (January, 1919).

Minutes of the Meeting, Municipal Department, Calcutta Corporation. (December, 1918).

Minutes of the Meeting, Municipal Department, Calcutta Corporation. (January, 1919).

Minutes of the Proceedings of the Calcutta Corporation. (July, 1918).

Minutes of the Proceedings of the Calcutta Corporation. (September 1918).

Minutes of the Proceedings of the Calcutta Corporation. (November 1918).

Minutes of the Proceedings of the Calcutta Corporation. (December, 1918).

Minutes of the Proceedings of the Calcutta Corporation. (January, 1919).

Minutes of the Proceedings of the Calcutta Corporation. (February, 1919).

Minutes of the Proceedings of the Special Meeting of the Calcutta Corporation. (June 1918).

Minutes of the Proceedings of the Special Meeting of the Calcutta Corporation. (July 1918).

Minutes of the Proceedings of the Special Meeting of the Calcutta Corporation. (September 1918).

Minutes of the Proceedings of the Special Meeting of the Calcutta Corporation. (October 1918).

Minutes of the Proceedings of the Special Meeting of the Calcutta Corporation. (November 1918).

Minutes of the Proceedings of the Special Meeting of the Calcutta Corporation. (December 1918).

Proceedings of the Calcutta Corporation. (1919).

Proceedings of the Government of Bengal. (January 1919). Municipal Department, Sanitation Branch, File No. S. Q-5 and S. Q–2.

Proceedings of the Government of Bengal. (April 1919).

Proceedings of the Government of Bengal. (April 1919). Municipal Department, File No. S.2D-8(3).
Proceedings of the Government of Bengal in the Municipal Department (Sanitation Branch) for the month of April 1919, File No. S.2D–8, Proceedings No. A.1–20.
Proceedings of the Government of Bengal in the Municipal Department (Sanitation) for April 1919, File No. S.2D–80.
Proceedings of the Government of Bengal in the Municipal Department Sanitation, for the Month of October 1918, Prevention of the Outbreak and Spread of Influenza in Bengal, File No. S.2D-1(1).
Proceedings of the Government of Bengal in the Municipal Department, Sanitation Branch, File No. S.2D–8 (5).
Proceedings of the Meeting, Municipal Department, Calcutta Corporation. (December 1918).
Secretary to the Government of Bengal, Municipal Department. (January 1919). File No. S.2-D-8 (12).

Newspapers

Bankura Sanbad. (1918, October 27). p. 3.
Bengal Gazette. (1918, December 10). Death toll rises as Spanish influenza ravages villages—Hindu Satkar Samity extends aid amidst grim crisis (p. 4).
Calcutta Gazette. (1918, November 5).
Calcutta Herald. (1918, November 25). Hindu Satkar Samity extends lifeline amidst Spanish influenza crisis (p. 2).
The Amrita Bazar Patrika. (1918, June 26). Calcutta Corporation claims that the epidemic is merely an unusually general epidemic of influenza which he usually comes here around August (p. 5).
The Amrita Bazar Patrika. (1918, July 13). War fever in Calcutta (p. 5).
The Amrita Bazar Patrika. (1918, October 4). Necessity of adequate food supply and well-ventilated housing for people (p. 5).
The Bengal Tribune. (1918, December 15). Rural Bengal teachers rise in protest amid Spanish influenza chaos: Demanding support as education system teeters on brink of collapse.
The Bengalee. (1918, June 27). The Ramakrishna Mission famine relief work in Bengal during influenza pandemic. p. 2.
The Bengalee. (1918, July 14). War fever in Calcutta–Effect on public health and business (p. 2).
The Bengalee. (1918, October 27). Influenza epidemic: Grievance of student, guardian and postponement of university examination.
The Bengalee. (1918, October 24). Hindu Satkar Samity–Cremation of the dead bodies (p. 6).
The Bengalee. (1919, April 22). Influenza epidemic: Sanitary Commissioner's memorandum circulated to local government, Shimla.
The Hindoo Patriot. (1918, July 27). The new fever (p. 3).
The Statesman. (1918, October 18). Calcutta fever mixture (p. 3).
The Times of India. (1918, October 10). Bombay influenza (p. 5).
The Times of India. (1918, October 23). Bombay was relatively free of infectious diseases (p. 3).

2 From Calamity to Catastrophe

Spanish Influenza in Other Districts of Colonial Bengal

The Spanish Influenza pandemic of 1918–19 was a catastrophic outbreak that resulted in millions of deaths around the globe. It affected many regions in colonial Bengal, such as Khulna, Rajshahi, Rangpur, Bogra, Pabna, Dacca, Mymensingh, Faridpur, Bakarganj, Chittagong, Noakhali, and Tippera. The beginning of the pandemic in Bengal reflected its worldwide emergence, featuring sudden and extensive outbreaks. The initial cases likely emerged in early 1918, stemming from infected individuals arriving from Europe. Colonial Bengal's strategic position as a centre for trade and transport allowed for the swift spread of the virus. Ports like Chittagong acted as entry points, while Dacca and Calcutta (currently Kolkata) served as epicentres for the early transmission (Proceedings of the Government of Bengal in the Municipal Department, Sanitation Branch, for the month of June 1918, File S. 1P-3 Progs. B 151–152).

The Spanish Influenza virus rapidly spread in Bengal, leading to widespread health challenges and affecting local healthcare systems. Symptoms involved high fever, respiratory issues, and weakness. The absence of effective treatments or vaccines worsened the circumstances. The disease's progression varied across various districts, shaped by factors such as population density, socio-economic status, and healthcare access. Urban areas like Dacca and Calcutta faced elevated mortality rates because of population density and insufficient sanitation measures. The virus rapidly transmitted through rural villages and agricultural communities, such as Rangpur and Bogra, which also suffered from a lack of medical care. The Spanish Influenza propagated in colonial Bengal via established transportation routes and social networks, with travel for commerce, pilgrimage, and administrative activities aiding the spread. Mass gatherings like fairs, religious celebrations, and political demonstrations created favourable conditions for rapid transmission, particularly in densely populated regions like Khulna and Rajshahi. The Spanish Influenza significantly affected districts in colonial Bengal, worsening social and economic disparities. Disadvantaged groups, including the rural poor, labourers, and indigenous population,[1] faced inadequate healthcare and overcrowded conditions. The pandemic disturbed agricultural production, trade networks, and administrative operations (Sanitary Commissioner's Preliminary Report, 1919, pp. 6, 33, 86, 123).

DOI: 10.4324/9781003656647-3

Jurisdiction of Other Districts of Bengal

The Spanish Influenza severely affected Khulna, a significant port city, as well as Rajshahi, a region recognized for its fertile delta region[2] and markets. The district's dependence on migrant labour and the pandemic's widespread fear caused the rapid transmission of the virus. The Spanish Influenza in the rural areas of Rangpur and Bogra, predominantly agrarian districts marked by poverty and malnutrition, intensified pre-existing challenges. The absence of effective public health measures worsened the scenario, resulting in widespread agony and distress. Pabna, an essential district in colonial Bengal, encountered difficulties in dealing with the Spanish Influenza owing to its strategic position along key river routes, facilitating the movement of infected persons and complicating containment efforts, worsening the outbreak. The Spanish Influenza significantly influenced Dacca, the administrative centre of colonial Bengal, prompting widespread disease propagation due to overcrowded living conditions and inadequate sanitation. Despite the initiatives of medical staff and government representatives, the magnitude of the pandemic overwhelmed local resources, leaving many individuals to cope on their own, underscoring the necessity for improved sanitation and control practices.

The Spanish Influenza severely influenced Mymensingh, a district recognized for its agricultural yield and cultural heritage, because of its remote location, rapid transmission through trade routes, and insufficient medical facilities, leaving vulnerable groups to handle the crisis independently. Faridpur and Bakarganj in colonial Bengal encountered difficulties in combating the Spanish Influenza because of their low-lying terrain[3] and monsoon climate, which allowed for the proliferation of disease vectors. The region's dependence on river transport and agricultural labour amplified the movement of infected individuals, resulting in extensive transmission.

Chittagong, a vital port city, was susceptible to imported cases because of international travellers and cargo. Despite quarantine efforts and stringent hygiene protocols, the virus persisted in spreading unchecked, overwhelming healthcare services and generating widespread fear and uncertainty. The Spanish Influenza affected the coastal areas of Noakhali and Tippera, populated predominantly by agricultural communities. The virus proliferated swiftly through these regions, making containment attempts challenging because of the proximity of villages and limited access to healthcare services. Despite local resilience, many individuals succumbed, resulting in widespread devastation (Proceedings of the Government of Bengal, June 1918, p. 45).

The outbreak of Spanish Influenza in colonial Bengal districts of present Bangladesh serves as a powerful reminder of the severe effects of pandemics on vulnerable communities. Despite the efforts made by medical professionals, government officials, and citizens, the outbreak left enduring scars on human lives and society. Analyzing historical lessons can aid in preparing for future pandemics and in constructing a more resilient and fair society. Here, the author intends to explore the onset, progression, and dissemination pattern of the Spanish Influenza in the districts of colonial Bengal in current Bangladesh.

Onset, Course, and Spreading Pattern of the Disease in Different Districts

The remaining districts of colonial Bengal (currently in Bangladesh) witnessed unique trends in the onset, progression, and dissemination of the disease. In Khulna, Rajshahi, Rangpur, Bogra, and other northern districts, the Spanish Influenza emerged rapidly, likely because of their closeness and high population density. A quick spread characterized the disease's trajectory in these regions, resulting in notable morbidity[4] and mortality.[5]

The Spanish Influenza outbreak propagated across various districts of colonial Bengal, Bangladesh, exhibiting different onset periods, developments, and trends. Central districts such as Pabna, Dacca, Mymensingh, and Faridpur saw a later onset, attributed to superior healthcare systems and awareness initiatives. Coastal districts including Bakarganj, Chittagong, Noakhali, and Tippera experienced a gradual onset, yet a swift spread because of congested living conditions and restricted access to healthcare. It is now the present author's endeavour to outline the disease's spreading pattern in other districts of colonial Bengal succinctly.

Rajshahi Division

In Rangpur District, epidemic physicians were dispatched due to a shortage of doctors and insufficient temporary personnel. Temporary isolation hospitals were established, and public health workforces were appointed. A temporary medical team was appointed for free medicine distribution. In Pabna District, two permanent and two temporary epidemic doctors distributed essential medications, with the Sanitary Inspector, vaccination teams, and District Board staff involved.

Dacca Division

Dacca Municipality experienced a severe outbreak of a disease in July, primarily brought in by students from Calcutta. The disease spread rapidly, particularly in densely populated areas. The epidemic eventually diminished, but a second wave began in October, intensifying until peaking in November before declining again in December. The second wave was more severe but had low fatality rates. A severe outbreak in Naraingunj Municipality, primarily affecting impoverished neighbourhoods, escalated in November and receded in December, affecting educated and wealthier populations to a lesser extent. The Dacca district experienced a high-level contagion of a disease, affecting individuals from all socio-economic backgrounds, particularly young adults and middle-aged individuals. The disease affected entire households immediately, but Dacca jail and asylum were spared from the second wave. Rural areas were more affected, with mortality rates nearly tripled by November, with Narainganj and Srinagar thanas having the highest rates.

Mymensingh District

A disease was introduced from Calcutta and first appeared in Mymensingh, Tangail, and Kishoreganj in July. The disease spread to rural Muslim communities and rural residents, with dense tree cover in the suburbs being the hardest hit. The disease spread to the southeastern regions, with the northeastern, central, and riverside sections experiencing minor impacts. The poorer population was the most severely affected, with the highest mortality rates. The disease was transmitted through contact with or proximity to infected individuals. The rainy season had lower outbreak severity compared to the second wave. The town experienced less suffering than the suburbs due to better housing conditions. Occupations requiring significant exposure to cold or dusty environments were vulnerable.

Caregivers of the ill often experienced attacks, with those prone to nasal catarrh being more susceptible. The disease did not spread towards the prevailing winds, but colder weather increased the frequency and severity of attacks. Over 95% of fatalities were due to lung-related complications. The outbreak in Kishoreganj, a town and its suburbs, was identified at the Kishoreganj Fair. The disease rapidly spread to surrounding villages, causing significant hardship. Poor nutrition and inadequate clothing made individuals more vulnerable. Those living in well-ventilated homes with sufficient food and clothing were less affected. In Tangail and Bajitpur, no widespread epidemic was reported, but Chandragram village had a more virulent strain, resulting in higher mortality rates. The disease was highly contagious and severe in December, with three-quarters of fatalities among lower-class Muslims.

Faridpur District

The initial epidemic began in July with mild symptoms and low mortality rates. It was introduced into a prison on July 23 by an undertrial prisoner, resulting in 78 cases. The second outbreak began in September and was highly fatal, spreading from Calcutta and travelling along railway and steamer routes. The disease affected Khankhanapur, Rajbari, Kotwalipara thana, Shibchar, Bhedarganj, Palong, Madaripur, and Bhadraswan Char. The severity of the disease diminished around mid-December due to a sudden drop in temperature. Faridpur town was free of the disease at the time of this report, with the highest concentration of cases near the steamer station at Tepakhola. The outbreak of the disease began in July in Goalundo, affecting labourers, steamer and railway workers, and the local market population. The outbreak subsided in September, but resurgence occurred in October among emigrants heading to Assam. The disease also spread in Boalia and Pangsa, spreading along communication routes. In Madaripur Municipality, the disease first appeared in early July and remained epidemic throughout July and August. The urban population was most severely impacted, while the rural population was more significantly affected. Medical staff, including nurses, were not exempt from the outbreak. The disease affected individuals of all ages up to 50, with older adults being less susceptible.

Bakarganj District

The disease, brought to Barisal from Calcutta, began in August and severely impacted poorer classes, with no part of the town being entirely spared. The disease spread to surrounding rural areas, with Sadar subdivision and Perojpur subdivision being the most severely affected. The severity of the outbreak was closely linked to population density, with lower socio-economic classes enduring the suffering. The epidemic was not widespread in Patnakhali Municipality, lasting from November until mid-December, but mortality rates in rural areas were approximately four times higher due to poverty and lack of medical care. In Jhalakati Municipality, the disease emerged around late September and spread sporadically, with less severe effects compared to rural areas. The intensity of the outbreak increased after November and persisted until mid-December, with the southeastern part of the town remaining unaffected.

Chittagong District

The illness, brought to Chittagong Municipality from external sources, spread through direct contact with infected individuals. The initial outbreak was intense, but no additional information has been provided by the Civil Surgeon, District Magistrate, or District Board.

Noakhali District

A significant number of individuals from a district who served in the Labour Corps returned home in June, possibly contracting influenza and introducing the infection to the area. The disease first emerged in July and subsided by September, but a resurgence occurred in October and November, affecting interior regions and coastal areas. Islands like North Hatiya and Bamni thana remained unaffected, while inmates and isolated residences were spared. The most affected areas were those forced to congregate due to river erosion, leading to higher mortality rates due to poor housing and inadequate nutrition.

Tippera District

The disease began in early July, presenting in a mild form and spreading rapidly across the district. Government mail clerks and sorters contributed to the spread, with the second wave emerging in September and intensifying during October and November. This second outbreak was more severe than the first, resulting in a significant number of fatalities, with many cases progressing to pneumonia and broncho-pneumonia. No demographic, including age, sex, caste, or creed, was completely unaffected. The most vulnerable were impoverished individuals living in densely populated, poorly ventilated homes, who were also inadequately nourished and clothed. Children and young adults were hard hit.

The disease was consistently prevalent in densely populated and congested regions, while areas with lower population density remained relatively unaffected. It was believed to have been introduced to Comilla Municipality from Calcutta. The initial outbreak in August and September was mild, but the subsequent outbreak in October, particularly in November, proved to be severe, resulting in significant mortality due to complications such as pneumonia and broncho-pneumonia. Very few individuals avoided the disease, and children and adults alike, regardless of their socio-economic status, were susceptible.

In Chandpur Municipality, the initial outbreak occurred among government mail sorters who frequently travelled between Calcutta and Goalundo, and upcountry labourers working in jute offices. The disease subsequently spread throughout the town, affecting no particular area or locality, although a higher percentage of cases were reported in densely populated areas where the poorer classes live.

Chittagong Hill Tracts

A shopkeeper in Rangamati, India, reported a mild case of influenza on July 29 after returning from Chittagong. The infection spread to nearby residents and police barracks, hospitals, and boarding houses, affecting the entire town. In Ramgarh, another shopkeeper introduced the disease in August, which spread through contact and was prevalent in crowded areas. The first outbreak occurred in August, followed by a second in November, with the highest incidence in December.

[Source: Proceedings of the Government of Bengal in the Municipal Department (Sanitation Branch) for the month of April 1919, File No. S.2D—8, Proceedings No. A. 1–20].

Following the earlier account of the Spanish Influenza outbreak across the various districts of colonial Bengal, the present author has strived to present the death toll recorded in these districts from July to November 1918. An attempt has also been made to illustrate the disease and mortality rates per mile associated with various diseases in different districts of colonial Bengal during 1918–19, enabling the reader to grasp the extent of the devastation caused by Spanish Influenza in colonial Bengal.

Table 2.1 illustrates mortality statistics from the Spanish Influenza pandemic in Bengal during the period from July to November 1918, highlighting notable regional variations in death rates. The total population across the districts exceeded 45 million, with an alarming total of 734508 deaths, resulting in an average mortality rate of 16.2 per 1000 individuals. Among the divisions, Darjeeling recorded the highest mortality rate at 27.3 per 1000, followed by Jalpaiguri at 24.7, and both Bankura and Hooghly at 24.1, with Burdwan close behind at 23.8. This data indicates that certain districts within the Burdwan and Rajshahi divisions were particularly affected. Conversely, Bakargunj exhibited the lowest death rate at merely 1.09 per 1000, which may indicate potential underreporting, effective containment measures, or other local circumstances. In urban areas such as Calcutta, the overall death rate was not unimaginable (17.5), but the horror of death in certain wards was terrible. Densely populated districts like Mymensingh and Dacca reported lower rates of approximately 13 per 1000. This data emphasizes the uneven effects of the pandemic throughout Bengal, with some regions facing exceptionally high mortality rates while others encountered significantly lower figures.

Table 2.2 provides a comprehensive overview of significant disease outbreaks and mortality rates in the districts of colonial Bengal during the years 1918 and 1919, with a particular emphasis on cholera, smallpox, plague, and fever. A comparative

Table 2.1 Total Mortality Caused by Spanish Influenza for the Period From July to November 1918

Districts	*Population*	*Total Deaths From July to November 1918*	*Ratio of Deaths per 1000 Population*
Burdwan Division			
Burdwan	1538371	36685	23.8
Birbhum	935473	19447	20.8
Bankura	1138670	27393	24.1
Midnapore	2821201	49937	17.7
Hooghly	1090097	26316	24.1
Howrah	943502	13047	13.8
Presidency Division			
24 Parganas	2434104	31521	12.9
Calcutta	896067	14693	17.5
Nadia	1617846	37217	23.0
Murshidabad	1372274	31799	23.2
Jessore	1758264	19534	11.1
Khulna	1366766	20979	15.3
Rajshahi Division			
Rajshahi	1480587	24525	16.5
Dinajpur	1687863	28569	16.9
Jalpaiguri	902660	22310	24.7
Darjeeling	265550	7246	27.3
Rangpur	2385330	39207	16.4
Bogra	983567	16136	16.4
Pabna	1428586	17200	12.0
Malda	1004159	17419	17.3
Dacca Division			
Dacca	2960402	39356	13.3
Mymensingh	4526422	58172	12.8
Faridpur	2121914	23827	11.2
Bakargunj	2428911	26617	1.09
Chittagong Division			
Chittagong	1508433	32876	21.8
Noakhali	1302090	22951	17.6
Tippera	2430138	29499	12.1
Total for Bengal	**45329247**	**734508**	**16.2**

Source: Proceedings of the Govt. of Bengal, Municipal Department (Sanitation), April 1919

analysis of the two years indicates a general rise in both disease prevalence and death rates in 1919, which may be attributed to vulnerabilities following the influenza pandemic, as well as disruptions in environmental conditions or public health systems.

Cholera exhibited a significant increase in most districts in 1919, with notable rises in Birbhum (from 1.89 to 6.79), Darjeeling (from 0.16 to 4.7), and 24 Parganas (from 2.28 to 5.9). This trend may imply a deterioration in water sanitation or heightened population mobility in the aftermath of the pandemic. Similarly, cases

Table 2.2 Disease and Death Rate per Mile From the Major Diseases Occurred in Different Districts of Colonial Bengal During 1918–19

District	*Year*	*Cholera*		*Smallpox*		*Plague*		*Fever*	
		Disease	*Death Rate*	*Disease*	*Death Rate*	*Disease*	*Death Rate*	*Disease*	*Death Rate*
24 Parganas	1918	5565	2.28	523	.21	35	.01	46342	20.5
	1919	14360	5.9	1143	.5	80	.03	49949	23.0
Calcutta	1918	1526	1.70	545	.60	210	.23	5997	6.69
	1919	3688	4.1	1870	2.1	334	.4	6324	7.1
Nadia	1918	2192	1.35	123	.07	1	.0006	75028	46.37
	1919	5071	3.1	803	.5	2	.001	56576	35.0
Murshidabad	1918	3659	2.66	16	.01	1	.0007	67093	48.99
	1919	5983	4.4	205	.1	–	–	57092	37.0
Jessore	1918	2572	1.46	108	.06	–	–	43933	24.98
	1919	3215	1.8	158	.1	–	–	44944	25.6
Khulna	1918	2530	1.85	26	.01	–	–	30658	22.43
	1919	4950	3.6	87	.1	–	–	38980	28.5
Burdwan	1918	3241	3.3	417	.3	–	–	64985	42.24
	1919	5040	.7	819	.5	–	–	63114	41.0
Birbhum	1918	1769	1.89	5	.005	1	.001	40567	43.36
	1919	6352	6.79	269	.28	–	–	48247	51.57
Bankura	1918	456	.40	58	.05	–	–	47154	41.41
	1919	1300	1.1	209	.2	–	–	33361	29.3
Midnapore	1918	5127	1.81	209	.07	–	–	84506	29.35
	1919	7947	2.8	932	3	–	–	87805	31.1
Hooghly	1918	1059	.97	48	.04	3	.002	29215	26.8
	1919	1477	1.4	675	.6	1	.001	27248	25.0
Howrah	1918	2362	2.50	146	.15	2	.002	14505	15.37
	1919	3067	3.3	1483	1.6	5	.01	14261	15.1
Rajshahi	1918	1018	.68	86	.05	–	–	52575	35.50
	1919	3107	2.1	525	.4	–	–	52382	35.4
Dinajpur	1918	992	.58	1033	.61	–	–	65203	38.63
	1919	2042	1.2	7511	4.5	–	–	61712	36.6
Jalpaiguri	1918	1975	2.18	190	.21	–	–	39125	43.34
	1919	3793	4.2	538	.6	–	–	29357	32.5
Darjeeling	1918	44	.16	92	.34	–	–	11047	41.60
	1919	1252	4.7	222	.8	–	–	8288	31.2
Rangpur	1918	3044	1.27	1616	.67	–	–	81140	34.01
	1919	3754	1.6	6250	2.6	–	–	68136	28.6
Bogra	1918	1116	1.13	264	.26	1	.001	26587	27.03
	1919	1338	1.4	1910	1.9	–	–	21372	21.7
Pabna	1918	2066	1.44	2260	1.58	–	–	46471	32.52
	1919	4370	3.1	26.2	1.8	–	–	42196	29.5
Malda	1918	1429	1.42	161	.16	–	–	37468	37.31
	1919	1948	1.9	760	.8	–	–	32815	32.7
Dacca	1918	3774	1.28	92	.03	–	–	73117	24.69
	1919	5538	1.87	1867	.63	–	–	56377	19.04
Mymensingh	1918	11435	2.52	225	.04	5	.001	107057	23.65
	1919	9942	2.2	2856	.6	–	–	95183	21.0
Faridpur	1918	4585	2.16	62	.02	10	.004	51634	24.33
	1919	3282	1.5	646	.3	–	–	46018	21.7

(Continued)

Table 2.2 (Continued)

District	*Year*	*Cholera*		*Smallpox*		*Plague*		*Fever*	
		Disease	*Death Rate*	*Disease*	*Death Rate*	*Disease*	*Death Rate*	*Disease*	*Death Rate*
Bakargunj	1918	2410	.99	43	.01	22	.009	55022	22.65
	1919	5431	2.2	208	.1	–	–	57231	23.6
Chittagong	1918	5540	3.67	6	.003	–	–	57764	38.29
	1919	6675	4.4	125	.1	–	–	52790	35.0
Noakhali	1918	6474	4.97	81	.06	–	–	39534	30.36
	1919	4032	3.1	463	.4	–	–	31905	24.5
Tippera	1918	4419	1.81	252	.10	–	–	52619	21.65
	1919	5995	2.5	2276	.9	–	–	49927	20.5

Source: Proceedings of the Govt. of Bengal, Municipal Department (Sanitation), April 1919

and fatalities from smallpox also escalated, particularly in Dinajpur, where the death rate surged from 0.61 to 4.5, and in Tippera (from 0.10 to 0.9), indicating potential shortcomings in vaccination programmes or issues related to overcrowding.

While plague remained relatively uncommon, its presence in urban centres such as Calcutta (increasing from 0.23 in 1918 to 0.4 in 1919) and a slight rise in 24 Parganas are significant, suggesting ongoing urban sanitation challenges. The most prevalent disease regarding both incidence and mortality was fever, likely including malaria and other febrile conditions. Districts such as Murshidabad, Birbhum, Rajshahi, and Jalpaiguri experienced alarmingly high fever death rates, often exceeding 40 per mile in 1918, although some areas saw a slight reduction in 1919. For example, Murshidabad's rate decreased from 48.99 to 37.0, while Birbhum experienced a notable rise from 43.36 to 51.57, indicating ongoing environmental or health infrastructure challenges. Urban areas like Calcutta reported comparatively lower influenza fever death rates (6.69 in 1918 and 7.1 in 1919), likely due to improved access to medical care. In contrast, rural districts such as Nadia, Burdwan, Dinajpur, and Midnapore faced significantly higher influenza fever-related death rates, with Nadia reaching a peak of 46.37 in 1918. This trend highlights the disparity in healthcare access and public health measures between rural and urban regions.

In summary, the data illustrates a complex interaction of endemic diseases exacerbated by vulnerabilities following the pandemic, revealing distinct regional differences. Districts in western and northern Bengal appeared to suffer the most from influenza fever-related fatalities, while cholera and smallpox spread more extensively and severely in 1919, reflecting a deteriorating public health situation in the wake of the Spanish Flu.

Utilizing the two comprehensive statistical tables presented—Table 2.1, which details total mortality attributed to the Spanish Influenza from July to November 1918, and Table 2.2, which outlines disease and death rates from significant illnesses during 1918–19—we can construct a clear and thorough understanding of the demographic effects, extent of destruction, and the human toll experienced by colonial Bengal during the influenza pandemic.

Demographic Impact and Nature of Devastation

The mortality statistics presented in Table 2.1 reveal an alarming death toll of 734508 individuals in Bengal over a mere five-month period, resulting in an average death rate of 16.2 per 1000 inhabitants. This figure is notably high, particularly as it reflects only the officially documented fatalities. Specific districts such as Darjeeling (27.3), Jalpaiguri (24.7), Murshidabad (23.2), Nadia (23.0), and Burdwan (23.8) exhibit especially severe effects, suggesting that certain areas experienced mortality rates nearly double the provincial average. The disparities in mortality rates further indicate localized susceptibility, potentially attributable to factors such as population density, famine-like conditions, inadequate health infrastructure, and restricted access to medical care.

The demographic crisis becomes increasingly evident when we examine Table 2.2, which sheds light on other simultaneous diseases such as cholera, smallpox, plague, and fever, under which influenza-like illnesses were frequently classified. Significantly, deaths attributed to fever surged in almost all districts during 1918 and 1919, with certain regions like Nadia (46.37), Murshidabad (48.99), Birbhum (43.36), Jalpaiguri (43.34), and Darjeeling (41.6) experiencing alarmingly high fever-related mortality rates in 1918. Given that Spanish Influenza was often categorized as "fever", these statistics bolster the hypothesis that the true number of influenza-related fatalities was considerably greater than what was officially documented in Table 2.1. The most notable observation is the significant increase in disease incidence and mortality rates from 1918 to 1919 across various districts. For instance, the smallpox death rate in Calcutta rose from 0.60 in 1918 to 2.1 in 1919, with comparable patterns evident for cholera and other illnesses. This situation illustrates the compounded health challenges and diminished immunity following the influenza outbreak, potentially resulting in an uptick in secondary infections and comorbidities. Furthermore, the public health systems' failure to respond effectively contributed to extended suffering and recurring episodes of illness.

Human Cost and Broader Implications

The human toll extended beyond mere statistics of fatalities, manifesting in a profound societal disintegration. The pandemic had a disproportionate impact on working-class individuals, women, and children, who frequently faced barriers to healthcare and were more vulnerable to malnutrition and secondary infections. The economic repercussions, characterized by labour shortages, an increase in orphaned minors, and overwhelmed cremation and burial facilities, culminated in a humanitarian crisis. Socially, reports indicated that entire communities were abandoned, with unburied bodies left for days and mass graves becoming a frequent occurrence. Furthermore, the sociocultural ramifications were severe, marked by widespread grief, disruption of familial structures, and pervasive psychological distress. The absence of colonial medical support highlighted the weaknesses in British public health policy, which predominantly focused on urban areas while neglecting the suffering in rural regions.

In a nutshell, the demographic statistics from the districts of colonial Bengal illustrate the devastating effects of the influenza pandemic of 1918–19. The scale of mortality, along with subsequent disease outbreaks, indicates a health crisis of extraordinary severity. These figures signify not merely a biological occurrence but also a significant humanitarian and systemic breakdown, where governmental neglect, insufficient infrastructure, and socio-economic weaknesses converged to produce one of the most lethal periods in Bengal's colonial past.

Perception of the Common Mass About the Pandemic

Local context, socio-economic conditions, and the outbreak's severity shaped perceptions of the Spanish Influenza pandemic across Khulna, Rajshahi, Rangpur Bogra, Pabna, Dacca, Mymensingh, Faridpur, Bakarganj, Chittagong, Noakhali, and Tippera. Rapid onset districts, like Khulna, Rajshahi, and Rangpur, experienced fear, panic, and heightened urgency because of the sudden surge in cases and high mortality rates. People witnessed the disease's rapid spread first-hand, leading to deep-seated apprehension about the severity and unpredictability of the situation. Conversely, in districts like Dacca, Mymensingh, and Faridpur, where the pandemic spread gradually, initially, people may have exhibited scepticism or complacency. However, as cases increased and the pandemic's impact became more apparent, attitudes shifted towards a more serious understanding of the virus's danger. These communities were likely adapted by adopting preventive measures like mask-wearing, good hygiene, and avoiding large gatherings, as the virus's impact became more apparent.

Geographical location and socio-economic conditions have influenced the Spanish Influenza pandemic's spread in coastal districts like Bakarganj, Chittagong, and Noakhali. Some individuals may have underestimated the severity of the situation, especially in remote communities with limited access to information or healthcare services. People who had done this before may have been more careful to protect themselves and their families. This mixed perception of the pandemic's severity may have influenced responses (Proceedings of the Government of Bengal, January 1919, p. 23).

During the Spanish Influenza pandemic in Bangladesh, blindly respecting religious and cultural traditions[6] and superstition led to widespread religious dependence and unscientific practices among the common masses. These beliefs deeply influenced people's perceptions of illness and responses to the pandemic. Some individuals turned to religious leaders or clerics for guidance and protection, believing prayers and rituals could ward off the disease or mitigate its effects. This reliance on religious figures often caused gatherings or events where people did not observe social distancing measures, thus inadvertently spreading the virus. Various unscientific practices based on religious superstition emerged during this time. For example, some people resorted to using amulets, charms, or talismans believed to possess protective powers against the influenza virus. Others adhered to traditional healing methods or folk remedies[6] promoted by religious healers, despite the lack of scientific evidence supporting their efficacy. Religious practices, by diverting attention and resources from public health, fueled misinformation and superstition. In spite of the dangers associated with viral transmission, religious gatherings and festivals persisted, as religious duties frequently outweighed public health considerations (Nicholas, 1981, pp. 35–44). Religious traditions in districts led to gatherings becoming hotspots for the spread of the Spanish Influenza, worsening the already dire situation. The following news published in the local newspaper of Rajshahi may be a point of apprehension:

Local Gazette: The Rajshahi Chronicle, Date: March 15, pg. 2., 1918
Title: Religious Dependence Amidst Spanish Influenza Outbreak

> *The outbreak of Spanish Influenza in Rajshahi has resulted in an increased reliance on religious beliefs among the local population, raising alarms regarding its implications for public health. Despite initiatives aimed at promoting awareness of preventive strategies and scientific guidance, a significant number of residents have resorted to religious rituals and superstitions to safeguard themselves and their families. Attendance at local mosques and temples has surged, with congregants seeking divine help. However, these gatherings frequently overlook the social distancing protocols advised by health officials, which may contribute to the virus's transmission. According to Biswas et al. (2021, pp. 3, 7, 9), there are unscientific practices based on religious superstition, including the use of amulets, charms, and talismans. Despite the absence of empirical support for these practices, some members of the community persist in their adherence, complicating efforts to mitigate the disease's spread. In navigating these difficult circumstances, it is essential to balance faith and rationality, integrating religious convictions with informed choices, and comply with evidence-based public health recommendations. Collaborative efforts and vigilance are vital in overcoming the pandemic and fortifying the community.*

We can also mention another news—

The Bogra Herald, September 28, pg. 3., 1918
Title: Amidst Pandemic, Religious Devotion Prevails

> *The Spanish Influenza pandemic has prompted a notable increase in religious fervor in Bogra, as residents turn to faith for comfort and safety. Devotees, adorned in traditional clothing, gather outside the historic Shah Sultan Mosque,[7] praying for divine help in the face of the challenges posed by the virus.*

Religious reliance and unscientific methods intensified the Spanish Influenza outbreak in various regions of colonial Bengal (currently in Bangladesh). Belief can offer solace during emergencies, yet its indiscriminate use without scientific backing can lead to harmful effects. Tackling these challenges causes a comprehensive strategy that incorporates community involvement, education, and cooperation with spiritual leaders. The understanding of the pandemic in these regions evolved, shaped by elements such as the intensity, rapidity, availability of information, socio-economic conditions, and cultural values. Anxiety, ambiguity, and shared responsibility significantly influenced community perceptions and reactions to one of the most catastrophic pandemics in history.

Funeral Practices, Religious Interventions, and Civil Society Responses During the Spanish Influenza

During the devastating outbreak of the Spanish Influenza pandemic from 1918 to 1919 in colonial Bengal, the practices of burial and cremation were significantly challenged, especially in the districts of Rajshahi, Rangpur, Bogra, Pabna, Dacca, Mymensingh, Faridpur, Bakarganj, Chittagong, Noakhali, and Tippera. These regions witnessed an extraordinary number of deaths, with thousands perishing within weeks. Government mortality reports and colonial medical bulletins documented a rapid increase in death tolls, leading to frequent disruptions or complete abandonment of traditional religious and social funeral protocols.

In the regions of Rajshahi, Rangpur, and Bogra, rural Hindu families traditionally conducted open-air cremations along riverbanks. However, the overwhelming number of deaths resulted in overloaded pyres, leading to many bodies being cremated in mass without the customary rituals such as mantra chanting or sacred bathing. In certain cases, corpses were quickly incinerated in group pyres to mitigate the risk of disease transmission. Conversely, for Muslims residing in Pabna, Dacca, and Faridpur, where burial is the established religious practice, graveyards became inundated. Reports from these areas indicate the presence of shallow and overcrowded graves, with multiple bodies interred in a single trench, frequently without the Janazah (funeral prayer) due to the unavailability of religious leaders or the apprehension of contagion (Arnold, 2019, p. 210). In coastal districts such as Bakarganj, Chittagong, Noakhali, and Tippera, the heavy monsoon rains exacerbated the situation. The waterlogged conditions not only postponed burials and cremations but also resulted in distressing scenes of partially submerged or decomposing bodies. Colonial accounts characterized these as "unsanitary and demoralizing" sights, while local newspapers condemned the inhumane treatment of the deceased (Klein, 2020, p. 56).

In rural Bengal, despite the colonial government's insufficient and largely apathetic response, religious organizations and private individuals took the initiative to provide assistance. Local Hindu temples and Muslim madrassas endeavoured to offer support by repurposing school buildings and dharmashalas into temporary shelters. In Dacca and Mymensingh, Muslim charitable trusts (waqf) and Hindu social reform organizations reportedly coordinated funeral services and distributed essential medicines such as quinine and herbal treatments. Missionary-operated clinics, particularly in Chittagong and Faridpur, provided limited medical aid, although they were ill-equipped to manage the extensive needs (Chakrabarti, 2012, pp. 176–179). Furthermore, local NGOs played a significant role; in Rajshahi and Pabna, certain landowning families facilitated mass cremations and financed relief kitchens (Arnold, 2020, pp. 289–291). Female volunteers, often from reformist Brahmo or Christian backgrounds, extended support to widows and orphans. Nevertheless, these efforts, while commendable, were inconsistent and grossly insufficient given the magnitude of the epidemic. Overall, the response to the widespread fatalities during the influenza pandemic in these Bengal districts was marked by urgency, makeshift solutions, and profound religious compromise. The disintegration of traditional funeral customs and the dependence on private and religious assistance underscored not only the humanitarian crisis but also the shortcomings and failures of the colonial public health system.

Indigenous Practitioners and the Colonial Government

The Spanish Influenza pandemic of 1918–19 represented a catastrophic worldwide health emergency, resulting in millions of fatalities and significant social repercussions. In colonial Bengal, under British governance, the pandemic unfolded against a backdrop of tense relations between local populations and colonial authorities. Exploitation by colonizers, cultural oppression, and economic subjugation intensified the pandemic's effects on local communities. The treatment of local medical practitioners during the pandemic highlights the harshness of colonial brutality and the cruel actions taken against their traditional knowledge and healing methods (Chandavarkar, 1998, p. 234).

Indigenous medical practitioners[8] in colonial Bengal were essential in delivering healthcare and healing to their communities well before colonial powers (Hochmuth, 2006, pp. 40, 43, 49, 53, 70–72). These healers, commonly known as vaidyas, hakims, ojhas, or kabirajas, were recognized for their extensive understanding of traditional remedies, herbal medicines, and holistic therapies (Christian, 2006, pp. 45–50). They were respected in their communities, and people frequently sought their health counsel. However, with the onset of British colonial rule in Bengal, the prominence of indigenous medical practitioners diminished as the colonial government introduced and favoured western practices (Anshu & Supe, 2016, pp. 256–259). The colonial encounter reshaped indigenous knowledge systems, including traditional medicine, as western powers regarded these practices as primitive and superstitious compared to the scientific supremacy of western medicine (Kumar, 1998, pp. 78–79). Colonial authorities systematically marginalized indigenous medical practitioners, branding them as unscientific and attempting to supplant them with western medical techniques and pharmaceuticals, driven by a negative viewpoint (Sharma, 2012, pp. 16–41). There were several reasons contributing to this colonial mindset towards indigenous practitioners.

A Eurocentric[9] perspective, favouring western knowledge and practices, frequently led colonial rulers in Bengal to be wary of indigenous methods. The colonial notion of superiority and a civilizing mission legitimized the enforcement of western systems and standards, solidifying this belief. Colonial administrators commonly regarded indigenous practices with suspicion and bias, viewing them as primitive or superstitious. This mindset was further amplified by a lack of understanding and appreciation of the cultural and social contexts within which indigenous healing traditions function (Arnold, 1996, p. 1076). Colonial authorities prioritized western scientific approaches and medical practices, perceiving them as rational and progressive. Economic motivations fueled the colonial agenda, and western medicine suited commercial and industrial goals. Western medical professionals advanced their practices at the expense of indigenous healers, pushing them into the margins (Kanagarathinam, 2018, pp. 182, 190–195, 201–204). The colonial administration in Bengal aimed to consolidate power over the indigenous population by dismantling local institutions and authorities, including indigenous healers and practitioners. This resulted in the discrediting of indigenous knowledge systems, allowing colonial rulers to impose western governance and control. The lack of trust in indigenous practices stemmed from colonial attitudes of superiority, economic interests, and the desire for control over the colonized populace (Kumar & Basu, 2013, pp. 1–22).

During the Spanish Influenza pandemic, tensions between indigenous medical practitioners and the colonial administration escalated. Indigenous healers, using centuries-old knowledge, provided care and support to those affected by the disease, using herbal remedies, dietary advice, and spiritual practices (Hardiman, 2009, pp. 265–275). However, colonial authorities viewed indigenous medicine as a barrier to western medical practices. In response, the colonial administration implemented measures to control the spread of the disease and manage healthcare resources, often marginalizing and harassing indigenous medical practitioners. Colonial officials, influenced by racist and paternalistic attitudes, targeted indigenous healers as scapegoats for the failure of their public health initiatives, blaming them for the pandemic's persistence and presenting them as obstacles to progress and modernization (Report on the Administration of the Bombay, 1920, p. 11).

During the Spanish Influenza pandemic, colonial officials eliminated civic benefits, harassed indigenous healers, and suppressed their practices. These healers, already pushed to the margins, experienced heightened scrutiny and surveillance. Bias, rather than facts, often propelled allegations of disseminating misinformation, fraud, or witchcraft against them. Colonial authorities, attempting to reinforce their control over healthcare, arrested, detained, and occasionally physically assaulted and tortured them. The impact of the Spanish Influenza pandemic on colonial Bengal involved the persecution of indigenous medical practitioners, endangering the health of the general populace. The effects of the pandemic pushed traditional healers into the shadows or made them operate underground, isolating them from essential healthcare resources. The colonial administration's emphasis on western medical practices undermined trust between colonial authorities and the indigenous community, worsening tensions and fueling resentment and opposition. Local newspapers have already covered this matter.

> *The Bengal Gazette*, September 15, 1918, pg. 4, published the news, *Colonial Authorities Clamp Down on Indigenous Healers Amidst Influenza Outbreak—In a recent development that underscores the colonial administration's perspective on indigenous medical practitioners, authorities in colonial Bengal have taken steps to diminish the influence of traditional*

healers during the ongoing Spanish influenza outbreak. The friction between the colonial government and indigenous healers is clear, with traditional medicine practitioners facing accusations of quackery and superstition. Colonial officials have expressed doubts regarding the efficacy of indigenous healing methods, labeling them as outdated and inferior to modern medical practices. A senior colonial administrator has stressed the importance of Western medical techniques and pharmaceuticals in addressing the influenza virus, asserting that dependence on traditional healers obstructs containment efforts. This crackdown has sparked protests among local communities that rely on traditional medicine, leading to the marginalization and persecution of indigenous practitioners, as evidenced by reports of arrests and harassment. As the pandemic continues, the colonial administration's stance highlights persistent colonial attitudes towards traditional knowledge and cultural practices, raising concerns about finding a balance between western medicine and indigenous healing in the face of the ongoing crisis.

Another news published in the local newspaper of Mymensingh is notable—

The Mymensingh Chronicle, December 7, 1918, pg. 3, reported a news titled, "Colonial Authorities Target Indigenous Healers in Spanish Influenza Response"—

In a contentious decision that has ignited significant debate within the local community, colonial officials in Mymensingh have escalated their efforts to curtail indigenous healing practices in response to the Spanish influenza outbreak. The intensified actions against traditional healers have provoked a strong backlash from residents, many of whom depend on these time-honored medical practices for their health care. Indigenous healers, who are integral to the cultural landscape of Mymensingh and possess an extensive knowledge of herbal treatments and holistic approaches, are increasingly facing marginalization and condemnation from colonial authorities. Recent reports of arrests and intimidation directed at these practitioners have heightened tensions between the indigenous community and the colonial government.

The Khulna Tribune, October 25, 1918, pg. 6, reported a news, "Colonial Authorities Crack Down on Indigenous Healers Amid Influenza Crisis"—

Recent reports highlight an escalating divide between colonial authorities and traditional healers, who are increasingly subjected to hostility and persecution. The colonial administration, reflecting sentiments prevalent in other parts of Bengal, has raised questions about the effectiveness of indigenous medical practices in addressing the influenza outbreak. Earlier this week, a colonial official remarked, "It is essential that we focus on implementing modern medical methods to tackle the current public health crisis." The recent arrests and harassment of indigenous healers have intensified the friction between the local population and the colonial government. In a striking incident, a well-regarded healer from a rural community was apprehended

> *on allegations of witchcraft and disseminating false information regarding the influenza virus. Such measures have only intensified the mistrust and animosity towards colonial governance among the local community.*

Another local newspaper of Dacca, *The Dacca Daily News*, August 12, 1919, pg. 5, reported the news, "Colonial Authorities Accuse Indigenous Healers of Spreading Influenza Misinformation"—*In a contentious decision that mirrors colonial perspectives on indigenous healing methods, colonial authorities in Dacca have charged indigenous healers with disseminating false information about the Spanish influenza pandemic. Recent remarks from colonial officials show an increasing skepticism towards traditional healers and their contributions to managing the outbreak. Colonial administrators have expressed worries about the proliferation of what they term "misleading information" concerning the influenza virus, partially blaming indigenous healers for this issue. A representative of the colonial government remarked, "There is a troubling pattern of misinformation being spread by certain individuals within indigenous communities. We cannot allow superstition and rumors to jeopardize our efforts to control the pandemic." This accusation has incited anger among local populations, many of whom regard traditional healers as reliable sources of wisdom and support.*

Apart from the news of these local newspapers of colonial Bengal, the most important news will remain unknown if we do not mention it here. This news from the *Amrita Bazar Patrika* is, without a doubt, a clear sign of the brutal atrocities committed by the colonial government against the indigenous practitioners.

The Amrita Bazar Patrika, August 20, 1918, pg. 4, "Indigenous System of Medicine and Government"

> *We have previously addressed the Government's responsibilities concerning indigenous medical practices in these columns. To date, there has been no sign of any actions the Government intends to undertake regarding this issue. However, a recent discussion in the Madras Legislative Council has raised significant concerns about the official stance on the matter. Sir Alexander Cardew and Surgeon General Col. Gifford, representing the Government of Madras, not only displayed a lack of support for indigenous medical systems but also made dismissive remarks. Sir Alexander claimed that "indigenous systems were extinct," while Col. Gifford, exhibiting a blend of ignorance and arrogance, expressed pity for those who adhere to these traditional practices. Reports suggest that the non-official members of the Madras Council were shocked by this display of official insensitivity. One of the most detrimental aspects of a bureaucratic government is the arrogance and sense of superiority it fosters. It is widely recognized among our populace that many cases deemed incurable by practitioners of mainstream medicine are effectively treated by our kavirajas and hakims. Public knowledge is often unknown to those in official positions.*
>
> *We do not wish to assume that the Government of Bengal harbors the same biases as that of the Madras province. It would be beneficial for some*

non-official members of the Bengal Council to bring this issue to the forefront in a Council meeting, in order to determine the Government's stance on the matter and the actions it intends to pursue, considering the country's pressing need for more qualified medical professionals.

The Amrita Bazar Patrika, September 20, 1918, pg. 5, Ayurveda in Madras Council–Kaviraj Jogindra Nath Sen's Letter

Box 2.1 *In response to the recent criticism of Ayurveda by Sir Alexander Cardew and Surgeon General Gifford during the Madras Legislative Council, Vaidyaratna Kaviraj Jogindra Nath Sen has addressed a letter to Vaidyaratena Pandit D Gopalacharlu, the Principal of Madras Ayurvedic College, dated September 15, 1918.*

My Dear Brother,

I have received your letter and find it perplexing that you place such significant weight on the unfounded criticisms of Sir Alexander Cardew and Surgeon General Gifford, both of whom lack expertise in Ayurveda. They possess little understanding of this system, yet you feel compelled to seek evidence supporting the notion of 'Ayurveda as a Science' in response to their denunciations. Such disparagement from individuals outside the field should be dismissed with the disdain it warrants. The status of Ayurveda as a science remains intact, regardless of the vehement opposition from many laypersons. Have these two individuals presented any substantial arguments to back their claims, apart from outright condemnation? I question how they could make such defamatory statements about a system that is highly respected by esteemed figures within their own circles, such as Sir Pardey Lukis.

Regardless of its classification as a science, the truth remains constant. The foundational principles of Ayurveda are intricate and enduring, proving effective in the diagnosis and treatment of ailments. In contrast, the theories of Western medicine are still in an experimental phase, lacking finality and undergoing constant revision. Notably, after years of misguided efforts, Allopathic medicine has reached similar conclusions regarding certain conditions—such as the goal-oriented treatment of tuberculosis and the recommendation to avoid salt and water in cases of ascites—without acknowledging their origins in Ayurvedic practices. Should we pursue the truth or chase after ephemeral theories that may be discredited tomorrow? Why, then, attempt to align the profound and nuanced principles of Ayurveda with the ever-evolving theories of Western medicine? The principles of Anatomy, Physiology, Midwifery, Surgery, and other aspects of Ayurveda surpass those of contemporary medical practices. This is clear in their lack of awareness regarding the seven layers of skin, the 'Sukrasmari,' and the 'Marmas.' Even today, Ayurvedic surgeons find it easier to treat surgical cases and perform operations within the Ayurvedic framework. These factors serve as compelling evidence of our advanced surgical techniques.

For these reasons, I cannot support the current notion of enhancing the Ayurvedic system based on modern scientific standards. If the essence of science is defined by adherence to empirical evidence and a lack of fixed principles, while neglecting the fundamental issues of accurate diagnosis and improved treatment of diseases, then I must reject such a definition of science. I am pleased to note that the Madras Government has provided no subsidies to promote Ayurveda, as I believe that such financial support could have potentially compromised the standing of Ayurvedic practitioners. I have no objections if you send this letter to press.

Yours Affectionately

Kaviraj Sudhindra Nath Sen, Joint General Secretary Sd. Jogindra Nath Sen, Ayurveda Sabha, Calcutta has also endorsed the above opinion.

Local newspapers in colonial Bengal expressed their discontent regarding the harsh treatment of Ayurvedic practitioners by the British authorities. The colonial administration not only disseminated negative news about indigenous practitioners but also enacted legal measures to prohibit their practice. During the period of colonial governance in India, the Registration of Medical Practitioners Act[10] (RMPA) served as a crucial tool used by the British rulers to undermine indigenous medical practices. The 1916 RMPA sought to solidify British dominance over Indian society, encompassing healthcare, by positioning western medicine as the primary system and diminishing the status of indigenous healing traditions (Kalpagam, 2002, pp. 35–40, 49–52). The stringent registration and licensing stipulations of the RMPA for medical practitioners, which typically benefited those educated in western medical institutions, created obstacles for indigenous healers lacking formal western medical credentials. This marginalization resulted in many traditional healers being excluded from the official medical profession, despite their vast expertise and knowledge in indigenous healing practices (Sriram et al., 2021, pp. 3, 5, 9).

Colonial authorities used the RMPA to create regulatory institutions in India, supervising medical practices. These institutions frequently functioned with biases favouring western medicine, sidelining indigenous healers. Indigenous practitioners attempting to maintain their traditional practices encountered harassment, persecution, and legal repercussions. The RMPA also aimed to regulate medical education in India, requiring western curricula and standards, further sidelining indigenous knowledge systems (Ramanna, 2006, pp. 3321–3323). The British colonial authorities in India controlled medical education to cultivate medical professionals indoctrinated in western medical ideologies, sustaining British colonialism in India. Despite opposition from indigenous communities and nationalist movements, the RMPA remained an influential instrument in asserting control over healthcare, undermining indigenous healing traditions and reinforcing colonial supremacy. The impact of the RMPA continues to influence present-day India, as the nation contends with the persistent effects of colonialism within its healthcare system (Scott, 1995, pp. 191, 211–215, 219).

This severe incident eliminated and classified the practices of Ayurvedic physicians, kavirajas, and hakims as "irrelevant". The Bombay government closed Pune Ayurvedic Dispensaries in 1915 because of the Registration of Medical Practitioners Act (RMPA), claiming that the medical officers were under-qualified. However, Ayurvedic physicians in Calcutta made significant contributions to the preservation and practice of Ayurveda despite colonial rule and the RMPA. They advocated for the recognition and legitimacy of Ayurveda as a distinct medical tradition, documenting and affirming traditional knowledge, conducting studies to enhance its scientific credibility, and founding educational institutions for future practitioners (Rai, 2020, pp. 4–6). Ayurvedic physicians in Calcutta, dedicated to maintaining Ayurveda's legacy and community healthcare, played an essential role in ensuring the continuity and resilience of India's traditional healing system. This resulted in countrywide demonstrations organized by Ayurvedic groups, accompanied by extensive media coverage and public gatherings, including a petition in Pune that involved Bal Gangadhar Tilak[11] (Ramanna, 2006, pp. 3324–3326). Clearly, the urgent battle to prevent mass casualties from influenza outbreaks interrupted these conflicts. The suppression of indigenous medicine during the influenza pandemic intensified colonial dependence on institutions and pharmaceutical companies, reinforcing colonial dominance over healthcare in colonial Bengal. This undermined indigenous healing practices and advanced western medical authority, fostering colonial exploitation and marginalization in the area (Verma, 1995, pp. 130, 133–137).

The Spanish Influenza pandemic in colonial Bengal revealed the cruelty and savagery of colonial governance. Colonial authorities subjected indigenous healers with their traditional knowledge to harassment, detention, and oppression. This suppression not only robbed communities of essential healthcare resources but also heightened tensions between the indigenous population and the colonial authorities. The legacy of colonial cruelty towards indigenous medical practitioners underscores the lasting effects of colonialism on the health, well-being, and autonomy of marginalized communities globally.

> *It is important to highlight the accessibility of indigenous practitioners to the villagers, even in the face of the British brutality. To exemplify this, I will refer to a particular incident involving the renowned poet Rabindranath Tagore and his efforts to protect his students at Santiniketan from a severe infection through indigenous remedies.*
>
> *"During this crisis, the fever spread to the guru kula school established by Tagore in Santiniketan, Bolpur, West Bengal, where medical resources were severely limited. In a letter, Tagore noted, 'This place [Santiniketan]*

has only Kshitimohan Babu [the grandfather of Nobel Laureate Amartya Sen, who possessed an extensive knowledge of Ayurveda] and I for doctor.' With a lifelong interest in medicine, the poet felt it was his duty to apply his knowledge to the well-being of the students. He visited check on the health and hygiene of those affected. Tagore prepared an Ayurvedic remedy known as 'Panchatikta Panchan,' which comprised teuri (banana roots), neem leaves, gulancha, nishinda (Nirgundi or Vitex negundo), and thankuni (Centella asiatica or Indian pennywort), and he ensured all students received this treatment."

(Sri Ramakrishna Math, 2020)

Ineffective Steps of the Government and the Medical Community

Bengal's districts of Khulna, Rajshahi, Rangpur, Bogra, Pabna, Dacca, Mymensingh, Faridpur, Bakarganj, Chittagong, Noakhali, and Tippera encountered a significant crisis during the 1918–19 Spanish Influenza pandemic because of insufficient responses from government authorities and the medical community. Insufficient healthcare infrastructure, a lack of preparedness, and shortages in medical supplies aggravated the crisis. The government's response was characterized by indecisive actions towards public health measures, resource mismanagement, corruption, and inefficiency, resulting in the neglect of vulnerable populations and an unfair distribution of aid (Barry, 2005, p. 297). History shows the necessity of taking prompt and collective action to manage public health emergencies. It is crucial for everyone to be treated equitably and included. Indian and British doctors carry the significant burden of combatting the flu, yet their approaches contradict contemporary scientific understanding. They depend on nursing care for survival; however, India does not have sufficient doctors to coordinate extensive relief efforts.

Medical personnel possess no special immunity to the disease and the fact that their calling brought them into closer contact with infection than any other, resulted in a large percentage of them becoming incapacitated, when their services were most in demand.

(Sanitary Commissioner's Preliminary Report, 1918, p. 6)

Doctors recommend a range of treatments such as oral antibiotic gargling, but these remedies prove to be ineffective. Dr. Crake proposes the use of topical ointments, inhalations of oils like eucalyptus, and small amounts of alcohol as nourishment, yet these techniques do not work effectively during critical situations. This section seeks to show these initiatives.

(Source: Minutes of the Meeting of the Calcutta Corporation, January 22, 1919, H M Crake)

I. The circulatory type is uncommon and generally starts with a high fever, chills, and shivering, along with a quick and erratic pulse, and a propensity to faint from the beginning, frequently resulting in a lethal outcome in a brief timeframe.

II. (a) The onset is like the Febrile type of nasal and throat catarrh, along with limb pain, but besides these symptoms, nausea, diarrhoea, and abdominal pain arise. The diarrhoea is of the septic variety, with stools occasionally resembling those seen in enteric cases. The disease follows a viral progression. In this type, bronchopneumonia complications are rather frequent.
(b) Begins with diarrhoea and general symptoms characteristic of the Febrile type, but by the third or fourth day, dysentery emerges accompanied by cramps and frequent stools containing blood and mucus. The duration is extended; occasionally, hiccups may also be present.

III. The onset is akin to the Febrile type but occurs much more abruptly. The fever escalates significantly with delirium from the outset; the patient becomes agitated and maniacal, and the coma arrives, leading to death within two to three days.

Complications—The subsequent complications have been noted:

(a) (i) Otitis—in two instances; (ii) Parotitis—in two instances; (iii) Hematuria—in one instance; (iv) Dysentery and Diarrhoea—in several instances; (v) Keratitis—in one instance; (vi) Epistaxis—in two instances; (vii) bleeding from the throat and gums.
(b) The fever begins with cough and bronchial catarrh and occasionally with a sore throat and hoarseness. The duration is typically around a week, featuring daily temperature fluctuations between 99°F and 102°F. No specific lesion is identified in any system.

IV. The onset is as mentioned earlier, but subsequently, the catarrh extends downwards and progresses into bronchitis, which can last from a few days to two weeks along with fever. Afterwards, loose expectoration begins, the lungs become clear, and fever along with other symptoms diminish.

This hospital's patients predominantly belong to this category, and the hospital admitted many patients with advanced disease. The illness begins as the Febrile type, but later Broncho-pneumonia emerges, with patch after patch of dullness developing along with heightened symptoms as another new patch is involved. In nearly all cases, they show pleurisy. This type has a prolonged course with a high mortality rate because of extreme exhaustion, which shows minimal response to any stimulating treatment.

Line of Treatment Suggested

The text presents a thorough description of Dr. Crake's actions during the Spanish Influenza in various regions of colonial Bengal, now known as Bangladesh.

Khulna District

The most significant impact was felt by the impoverished population. In the Khulna Municipality, the prevalence of the disease was highest among the lower-income groups, likely because of inadequate clothing and negligence in care.

Rajshahi District

According to the Civil Surgeon, the disease predominantly affected the under-privileged community, whose health had deteriorated because of a lack of food, clothing, and other essential resources, exacerbated by rising prices. The onset of the cold season contributed to many cases of lung-related issues, particularly among the poor. The Chairman of the District Board noted that rural impoverished individuals were the hardest hit, while urban areas and railway hubs experienced comparatively fewer cases, as the diseases afflicted those who were malnourished, poorly dressed, and inadequately housed more than those in better circumstances.

Rangpur District

In Rangpur Municipality, the lower-income groups faced significant hardships because of poverty and lack of adequate clothing.

Bogra District

The Civil Surgeon reported that in certain areas, younger individuals were more affected than older adults and frail. The highest mortality rates were observed among the poorer classes and women who were exposed to cold and damp conditions. He noted, "The disease has a severe impact on the heart, which is why the poorer classes and women are vulnerable." Creosote in various forms was beneficial.

Pabna District

The Civil Surgeon reports that the disease predominantly impacted individuals from lower socio-economic backgrounds, although a notable number of cases were also found among wealthier individuals. Key factors contributing to the vulnerability of the poorer population included insufficient nutrition, unsanitary living conditions—especially inadequate ventilation and overcrowding—and a lack of proper warm clothing. In contrast, the police force and inmates experienced a relatively lower risk, as they were provided with adequate warm clothing and superior nutrition compared to the public. Dr. Crake's tablets, which contain Quinine, Sodium Benzoin, Ammonium Carbonate, and Thymol, proved to be effective during the early stages of the illness.

Dacca District

Civil Surgeon—It is recommended to administer general diffusible expectorant stimulants, particularly Tincture Strephantiu, starting with full doses every hour or every two hours if the pulse is rapid and soft. Essence of cinnamon is also beneficial. Quinine is effective only when there is a concurrent malarial infection. Subsequently, Tincture Ferri Perchlor and Liquid Strychnine are the most effective in alleviating depression.

Dacca Municipality—The incidence and mortality rates are notably higher among the lower socio-economic classes, as they neglect fundamental hygiene principles and preventive measures. They often live in small, unsanitary huts, and face significant poverty.

Mymensingh District

Tangail Municipality—Implementation of stimulants systematically.

Bajitpur Municipality—The use of Anarash or Kamranga has proven effective in 75% of cases.

The Civil Surgeon—Reports show that lower-income groups are disproportionately affected, exhibiting higher mortality rates, likely because of a lack of understanding regarding the illness.

Tangail Municipality—Individuals such as farmers, artisans, labourers, and women, particularly those who are excessively exposed to cold or who gather in large numbers in enclosed spaces at night, have been the most severely impacted.

Mymensingh Municipality—The lower socio-economic groups living in rural areas and their adjacent regions have been the most affected. The impoverished population has suffered because of inadequate clothing and lack of proper care.

Kishoreganj Municipality—Individuals who are poorly dressed and inadequately nourished, particularly those impacted by the devastating consequences of the recent flood, have experienced the greatest suffering.

Faridpur District

Faridpur Jail Hospital—All patients received treatment with Quinine, which proved to be highly effective. The Assistant Surgeon at Rajbari Hospital reports that farmers and labourers were the most affected. The primary factors contributing to the decline in health include exposure to cold, overcrowding, unsanitary conditions, and lack of adequate rest, which explain the higher prevalence of the disease in these groups.

Bakargunj District

Assistant Surgeon, Barishal Hospital—The use of calcium salts is particularly recommended in cases of pneumonia.

Jhalakati Municipality—The thymol nasal douche has not gained popularity. However, a stimulant expectorant with some antiseptic properties has proven beneficial. In severe cases, inhaling steam with Tincture Benzoin Co. has shown significant effectiveness.

Barishal Municipality—Farmers, labourers, and individuals from lower socio-economic backgrounds have experienced considerable hardship because of poverty and inadequate clothing.

Jhalakati Municipality—Those who were poorly nourished, lived in adverse conditions, and maintained unsanitary habits have suffered the most.

Chittagong District

In Chittagong Municipality, the underprivileged labouring population experienced the most severe hardships because of inadequate rest and unsanitary living conditions. Attempts to ease their suffering with influenza medication were unsuccessful.

Noakhali District

In Noakhali, older adults, children, and impoverished individuals, who had diminished resistance, were particularly affected by severe complications, resulting in higher mortality rates among these groups. Areas with high population density and overcrowded housing faced significant challenges.

Tippera District

According to the Civil Surgeon, the disadvantaged communities living in densely populated, poorly ventilated, and unsanitary homes, along with inadequate nutrition and clothing, were the most adversely affected.

Brahmanbaria Municipality

In Brahmanbaria Municipality, the less fortunate segments of the population endured considerable suffering, exacerbated by overcrowding, which increased their vulnerability to illness.

Comilla Municipality

In Comilla Municipality, the impoverished population faced severe difficulties because of a lack of adequate food, care, and clothing. Pregnant women who contracted influenza experienced miscarriages.

[Source: Proceedings of the Government of Bengal in the Municipal Department (Sanitation Branch) for the month of April 1919, File No. S.2D—8 (13)]

The outbreak has impacted families, particularly elderly individuals, who are vulnerable because of the widespread influenza. Limited availability of quality care, such as food and nursing services, has complicated the help for caretakers. This situation has led to the rapid spread of the infection, making it challenging for people to grasp the situation. The opacity of the disease also hindered medical experts. F. Norman White[12] expressed uncertainty about whether the influenza bacillus they discovered was the actual cause of the illness and documented:

> *It is unequivocal that the influenza virus is a living organism that can be directly transmitted between individuals. The influenza bacillus was consistently found in the cases examined during the second severe wave of the epidemic in India; however, it does not seem to have been as frequently identified during the initial mild phases of the outbreak.*
>
> (Preliminary Report, 1918, p. 24)

Norman White gives a detailed summary of the influenza's spread and the difficulties in clarifying its transmission. He shows certain bacilli that were typically present during the second wave, while noting a correlation between the first and second waves and the absence of bacilli in the first wave. Dr. Crake's microbiological findings are significant, as they identified influenza via nasal swabs and sputum tests. His discoveries include the following details—*Dr. Crake's bacteriological report offers comprehensive insights into the microbiological investigation of the 1918 influenza outbreak. It outlines the processes of specimen collection, examination, and analysis from infected patients, emphasizing the scientific methods employed to identify the pathogen responsible for the outbreak. The study used swabs and sputum samples from the West, along with blood smears and bronchial secretions, which were examined using Gram staining techniques. The findings revealed Gram-positive streptococci, some arranged in long chains and others as diplococci. A Gram-negative diplococcus similar to Moraxella catarrhal was identified in one sample, suggesting the potential for secondary bacterial infections. Small Gram-negative bacilli were detected in all specimens.*

A research investigation involving samples from influenza patients revealed the bacteria belonged to a category of hemophilic bacteria linked to B. influenzae, now known as Haemophilus influenzae. The observed colonies varied in size and appearance, from small, transparent bluish forms to larger, white, and opaque ones, suggesting the existence of several bacterial strains. The smaller colonies, akin to those seen in the initial smears, failed to grow when transferred to fresh agar, showing either their non-viability or dependence on specific growth conditions. Dr. Crake's report initially attributed the primary cause of influenza to Haemophilus influenzae before the viral nature of the illness was confirmed. His findings were consistent with a report from the Health Officer of Bombay dated July 15, 1918, which associated the influenza-like organism found in nasal secretions with pneumococci and a notable rise in respiratory-related fatalities. This situation illustrates the uncertainty among medical professionals regarding the true cause of the Spanish Influenza, which was ultimately identified as viral. The identification of bacterial agents such as B. influenzae and Streptococcus pneumoniae highlights the significant role of secondary bacterial infections in increasing mortality rates during the pandemic. Data from the Bengal Presidency shows a marked increase in mortality rates from July to November 1918, underscoring the severe impact of the influenza outbreak.

This report provides an in-depth examination of the extensive bacteriological studies performed during the 1918 influenza pandemic. While the identification of Haemophilus influenzae as the primary cause was later discredited, the emphasis on bacterial complications presents valuable insights into the complex relationships between viral and bacterial pathogens during major respiratory outbreaks. Dr. Crake's findings illuminate the scientific uncertainties of that time and emphasize the prompt measures implemented by health authorities to observe and document the pandemic's impact in colonial India (Source: Minutes of the Proceedings, held at central Municipal Office, Wednesday, July 17, 1918).

In the fall of 1918, India encountered a significant healthcare crisis caused by a deficiency of medical personnel, a scarcity of specialists, and the lack of clinics in rural regions. Accounts of the flu pandemic underscored the endeavours of medical authorities to tackle these challenges, reflecting grievances about understaffed facilities without directly addressing the matter (Arnold, 2000, pp. 19–56).

Lt-Col C. MacTaggart[13] reported that in areas lacking public health officers,[14] influenza death rates varied from 30.4 per thousand to 114.21 per thousand. Regions with health officers, despite serving a much smaller population, reported death rates of 8.17–115.39 per thousand (Taubenberger, 2006, pp. 86, 97–100, 109–112). The overall average mortality rate for both groups was 68 per thousand, with a median of 60 per thousand in areas with health officers and 75 per thousand in places without health officers. Surviving the epidemic called for more than mere access to health officers, along with transportation and connectivity to other regions (United Provinces Report on Influenza Pandemic, 1918, p. 23).

Mac Taggart was against nasal sprays and masks for infection control, referencing their efficacy in plague and smallpox vaccinations. IMS devoted considerable resources and time to influenza vaccine development, notwithstanding doubts, leading to unsuccessful attempts to create effective vaccines (Kent, 2013, p. 26). Norman White's feedback on vaccine research condemned the public's misunderstanding regarding vaccine production. He reiterated Mac Taggart's scepticism, emphasizing the reservation of 300000 doses for the flu vaccine that was sanctioned in December 1918. The protection was only effective for a limited segment of the population, leaving the majority at the mercy of the outbreak. This illustrates the difficulties encountered by British doctors in India during and in preventing prospective epidemics. Mac Taggart's troubled past showcased the necessity of treatment access to reduce fatalities. Despite doubts regarding the flu vaccine's efficacy, the government persists in manufacturing and controlling its distribution. The vaccine is obtainable for public surgeons and healthcare providers, yet its effectiveness in prevention or treatment remains ambiguous. Despite scepticism, the government continues to produce vaccines. There are deliberately ineffective antibiotics (Brimnes, 2004, pp. 199, 213–219).

In this situation, as a precaution, Dr. Crake arranged influenza vaccinations, yet the public had little trust in this vaccination. The subsequent details outline the vaccination dosage.

Box 2.2 *Dr. Crake suggested the dosage for the influenza vaccine as recommended by the Central Research Institute in Kasauli. The Institute recommends two doses of the influenza vaccine for optimal effectiveness, with a gap of seven to ten days between them. If a single dose is not workable, the larger second dose is recommended as the only vaccination to enhance protection, as per the table's guidelines.*

This table classifies the recommended vaccine dosages into six specific age categories: 4–6 years, 6–8 years, 8–10 years, 10–12 years, 12–14 years, and 14 years and older. The dosage increases progressively with age to correspond with the individual's immune system development and size.

For 4–6 years, the recommended dosage is 0.15 CC for the first dose and 0.3 CC for the second dose.

For 6–8 years, the dosage rises to 0.2 CC in the first dose and 0.4 CC in the second dose.

For 8–10 years, the suggested dose increases to 0.25 CC and 0.5 CC, respectively.

For 10–12 years, the dose is 0.3 CC for the first shot and 0.6 CC for the second.

For 12–14 years, the recommended doses are 0.4 CC and 0.8 CC.

For individuals aged 14 years and upwards, the maximum dosage is 0.5 CC in the first dose and 1 CC in the second dose.

This incremental strategy reflects a carefully crafted plan that administers lower doses to younger children while offering higher doses to older adults to optimize their immune response. The differences in dosage highlight the consideration given to age-related immunity and body weight.

The note at the bottom specifies that these dosage recommendations pertain only to vaccines developed by the Central Research Institute in Kasauli, underlining the distinct nature of vaccine formulations and their effectiveness. This disclaimer serves to inform healthcare professionals that vaccines from other manufacturers may have different formulations, which may require adjustments in dosage. Overall, it can be said that this structured dosage chart illustrates the scientific diligence involved in tailoring vaccination protocols during the influenza pandemic. It showcases a commitment to achieving a balance between efficacy and safety by proposing appropriate dosing strategies for different age groups (Source: Proceedings of the Government of Bengal in the Municipal Department (Sanitation) for the Month of January 1919, File No. S.2D–1 (3) Proceedings No. A.18–19).

In this context, another letter published in the Indian Medical Gazette is worth mentioning.

> *A correspondence addressed to the editor of the Indian Medical Gazette by Debendranath Sen, a pathologist at Sambhu Nath Pandit Hospital in Calcutta, provided insights on isolating Pfeiffer's Bacillus. He observed that, similar to many of his contemporaries, he could not detect the bacterium in internal organs. He shifted his focus to "the various recesses communicating with the nasal cavity," where he identified a "mucoid substance containing yellowish lumps." These lumps were found to harbor bacteria "identical to Pfeiffer's bacillus," presenting a new research direction for his colleagues as they sought to combat the disease (Sen, 1919, p. 241)*
>
> *In another letter, Cecil Webb Johnson from the Royal Army Medical Corps (R.A.M.C) at the British Station Hospital in Calcutta wrote to the editor of the Indian Medical Gazette, emphasizing that the foremost requirement in cases of influenza is complete rest from the onset of the illness. He advised against any food intake until the fever subsides, dismissing the outdated notion that increasing nourishment would bolster strength. Given the high incidence and risks of heart failure associated with influenza, he urged medical professionals to determine whether it is more prudent to preemptively address this complication or to await mitral incompetence to manifest. He recommended that the chest be rubbed twice daily with a rubefacient to enhance peripheral circulation. Should pneumonia develop despite all precautions, the patient should be seated in an armchair for four hours each day (Johnson, 1919, p. 3)*
>
> (Source: Minutes of the Meeting of the Calcutta Corporation, January 22, 1919, H M Crake)

The medical community in India struggled with influenza treatment because of limited knowledge and effectiveness. Preventive plans were only effective for a small percentage of the population, leaving the rest vulnerable to the pandemic (Misra, 2021, pp. 467–469). Most people in colonial Bengal and India did not trust or depend on the vaccine's efficacy. Despite this, the government manufactured and created rules for its distribution, making the vaccine available to Civil Surgeons, health officers, and private practitioners upon request. The government continued manufacturing the vaccine despite fewer people's acceptance (Watts, 1999, pp. 174–186).

> *The Spanish influenza outbreak in Bangladesh during 1918–1919 revealed critical deficiencies in the responses of both government and medical authorities across multiple districts. There was a failure to establish unified public health strategies, including quarantine measures and the effective communication of information, which resulted in unpreparedness and worsened the transmission of the virus. The healthcare system faced challenges because of insufficient infrastructure and resources, leading to an overwhelming number*

of patients. This historical event underscores the necessity for prompt and coordinated efforts from both governmental bodies and healthcare providers in times of public health emergencies.

During the 1918–19 Spanish Flu epidemic, areas in present-day Bangladesh, such as Khulna, Rajshahi, Rangpur, Bogra, Pabna, Dhaka, Mymensingh, Faridpur, Barkarganj, Chittagong, Noakhali, and Tippera, showed little response to the worldwide pandemic. As communities struggle with the pandemic, public demonstrations have arisen in reaction to governmental actions. Local newspapers have been essential in advocating for action. Growing public discontent over insufficient medical care, lack of supplies, and government actions remains a concern (Dicke, 2015, pp. 195, 200, 211–217).

Local newspapers serve a critical role in spreading information, backing public sentiment, and inspiring the populace. They offer updates on the epidemic, guidance for prevention, and accounts of those affected and their families. Journalists delve into reports, reveal governmental shortcomings, and hold officials accountable. They amplify the voices of under-represented communities, drawing attention to socio-economic disparities. Local newspapers foster communication among communities, exchanging resources, information, and support systems. They encourage solidarity and combat depression, promoting social cooperation and togetherness. In summary, local newspapers help to advance public opinion and address the crisis. Many local newspapers denounced the government's neglect and inability to prevent horrific fatalities. Following are some news headlines that underscore the significance of the situation:

Public Discontent Regarding the British Government's Ineffectiveness in Addressing the Spanish Influenza, The Bengal Chronicle, November 15, 1918, p. 3 . . . in a passionate expression of dissatisfaction, residents throughout Khulna and Rajshahi.

Rangpur and several other districts have mobilized to express their discontent with the British government's insufficient response to the Spanish influenza pandemic. Thousands of demonstrators gathered to articulate their anger over the delayed actions taken to mitigate the spread of this lethal virus, which has resulted in many fatalities within our communities. During the protests, speakers emphasized the authorities' shortcomings in delivering adequate medical support, establishing quarantine centers, and supplying essential resources to the impacted regions. The lack of organized initiatives to inform the public and implement preventive strategies has intensified the crisis, rendering communities exposed and defenseless.

Anger Grows in Districts as British Officials Struggle to Address Influenza Crisis, The Rajshahi Times, December 3, 1918, p. 5. Reports from various regions, including Bogra, Pabna, and Dacca, show a rising tide of frustration among residents as the Spanish influenza continues its lethal advance without restraint. Faced with insufficient government action, communities are compelled to confront the relentless spread of the virus on their own.

Daily protests are emerging in towns and villages, with citizens expressing their outrage over the ineffectiveness and indifference of colonial officials in managing this public health crisis. Demands for prompt action echo through the streets, as families grieve for those lost and worry for their own safety amid growing uncertainty. In conversations with The Rajshahi Times, local leaders criticize the lack of preparedness and resources dedicated to tackling the pandemic, highlighting the necessity for a comprehensive and coordinated response to halt its progression. With hospitals overwhelmed and medical supplies running low, the situation is becoming increasingly critical, emphasizing the pressing need for intervention from British authorities.

Public Outrage Intensifies as Spanish Influenza Devastates Communities, Government Criticism Grows, The Chittagong Gazette, January 12, 1919, p.2 Amidst the relentless spread of the Spanish influenza, frustration among the residents of Chittagong, Noakhali, and Tippera reaches a critical point as the British government's failure to manage the crisis faces severe criticism. With each day, the number of fatalities continues to rise, exacerbating the suffering of the affected populations. In various villages and towns throughout the region, protests are mounting as citizens call for immediate action from colonial officials to tackle the severe lack of medical resources, insufficient healthcare infrastructure, and the ineffective implementation of containment strategies. Anger is palpable in the streets, driven by a sense of neglect and apathy from those in authority. In conversations with The Chittagong Gazette, local activists express their dismay over the lack of preparedness and foresight shown by British officials, accentuating the urgent need for intervention to avert further casualties. As makeshift hospitals become overwhelmed with patients and burial sites struggle to accommodate the deceased, the magnitude of the tragedy becomes increasingly clear, highlighting the critical nature of the situation.

Communities Affected by Spanish Influenza: British Authorities Confront a Crisis, The Bogra Chronicle, February 27, 1919, p. 3. In the aftermath of the Spanish influenza pandemic, Bogra, and its neighboring areas are experiencing an unprecedented health emergency, as the British government struggles to manage the outbreak. With hospitals inundated and medical resources severely depleted, residents are left to navigate this crisis on their own amid growing despair. Public discontent has escalated into protests, with citizens demanding accountability from colonial officials for their insufficient response to the pandemic. Alarming reports of widespread infections and increasing death tolls highlight the urgent need for effective measures to address the devastation caused by the virus. In an interview with The Bogra Chronicle, community leaders voiced their anger over the government's neglect of citizen welfare, urging immediate action to remedy the critical lack of medical supplies and healthcare workers. As families mourn their losses and confront the fear of illness, the pandemic's impact on the community becomes increasingly clear. As the situation worsens, residents remain determined to hold authorities responsible for their inaction and insist on prompt measures to ease the suffering of those impacted. The time for excuses and hollow assurances has ended; only through unified efforts and strong leadership can we hope to navigate this challenging period in our history.

Dacca and Mymensingh Face Ongoing Battle Against Influenza, Residents Call for Government Action, The Dacca Dispatch, March 15, 1919, p. 3.

In Dacca and Mymensingh, the fight against the Spanish influenza continues relentlessly, as communities contend with the severe consequences of the pandemic. Despite the dedicated efforts of healthcare professionals and volunteers, hospitals are inundated, and critical medical supplies are scarce, leaving residents at risk from the virus's effects. Public frustration is growing, with citizens demanding immediate intervention from colonial authorities to tackle the worsening situation. Protest marches and demonstrations fill the streets as families grieve for lost loved ones and worry for their own safety amid an increasingly precarious future. In an interview with The Dacca Dispatch, local leaders criticize the government's slow response to the crisis, emphasizing the urgent requirement for more resources and support to enhance healthcare systems and curb the virus's spread. Each day reveals the pandemic's escalating impact on our communities, highlighting the pressing need for decisive measures to address this extraordinary public health crisis. As residents come together in solidarity against the shared threat of the influenza pandemic, they remain resolute in their calls for accountability and transparency from colonial officials. The period of complacency and inaction has long since ended; only through unified efforts and effective leadership can we hope to navigate the challenges that lie ahead.

The articles from local newspapers in different districts during the Spanish Influenza pandemic of 1918–19 illustrate the extensive devastation and public reaction to the emergency. They accentuate the gravity of the situation and the inadequate response from British colonial authorities. The articles showcase the collective struggle and resilience of the people facing hardship, highlighting the pressing need for decisive action, accountability, and transparency from those in power. They also function as historical records, illuminating a critical moment in the region's history and stressing the necessity of effective public health measures and responsive governance in crises. During the Spanish Influenza pandemic across various districts, local newspapers were vital in social mobilization and reporting. They served as the sole media outlet to present public protests to the government and broadcast information to the public, empowering communities and spurring action to address the challenges posed by the disease.

Conclusion

This chapter examined the crippling famine and despair that impacted the various communities in colonial Bengal. The story emphasizes the sharp contrast between the fertile land of Khulna and the vibrant urban areas of Rajshahi and Dacca, where commerce once flourished. In regions like Rangpur, Bogra, and Pabna, where rural life previously resonated with harvest and festivity, famine altered the scenery into a barren tableau. The fear of starvation compelled families to make dire choices between hunger and survival.

The urban areas of Mymensingh, Faridpur, and Chittagong are experiencing a catastrophic famine, with hunger and disease taking lives with brutal efficiency. Even with the attempts of local relief committees and charitable organizations, the extent of the crisis exceeds their ability to provide aid. The "mountain of corpses" rises in areas such as Bakarganj, Noakhali, and Tippera, serving as a stark reminder of the human cost of colonial exploitation and administrative neglect. Despite the hopelessness, instances of resilience and solidarity emerge from the darkness, as communities unite to assist each other via mutual aid and collective action. These instances of shared humanity provide a flicker of hope amidst overwhelming despair. The chapter acts as a poignant reminder of the human cost of colonialism and the lasting resilience of the common mass in the face of unspeakable suffering. The chapter urges us to witness the horrors our ancestors faced and to ensure their stories remain alive. By honouring their legacy and striving for a more just and fairer world, we pay homage to the many lives lost and reaffirm our determination to create a future where such atrocities may never transgress again.

Colonial Bengal faced extensive destruction and despair because of the Spanish Influenza, as highlighted in the chapter. Fear and panic spread in districts like Rangpur, Bogra, and Pabna because of the outbreak, which strained healthcare systems and intensified famine and poverty. The ill and dying filled the streets of Dacca and Mymensingh, as makeshift hospitals struggled to manage the surge of patients and a lack of medical supplies. The pandemic revealed the resilience of the Bengali people through acts of solidarity and compassion, as shown in communities in Faridpur, Bakarganj, and Chittagong. These communities showcased the strength of the human spirit during hardship. However, the narratives also reveal the inadequacy of colonial governance in safeguarding the welfare of its subjects, particularly in districts such as Noakhali and Tippera. The legacy of the Spanish Influenza pandemic in colonial Bengal acts as a reminder of the interconnectedness of human suffering and the lasting resilience of the human spirit. We must remember the lives lost and learn from past errors, working towards a future where all have fair access to healthcare and social justice.

Notes

1 Indigenous Population—The term "indigenous population" refers to the original inhabitants of a particular region, often characterized by a deep connection to the land, distinct cultural practices, and historical continuity within that territory. Diverse indigenous populations inhabit the globe.

2 Fertile Delta Region—A fertile delta region is a geographical area formed at the mouth of a river where it deposits sediment, creating a triangular or fan-shaped land mass. Rich soil and high agricultural productivity characterize these regions because of the deposition of nutrient-rich sediments carried by the river.

3 Low-lying terrain—Low-lying terrain refers to areas of land that are at relatively low elevations compared to surrounding regions, often close to sea level or in basins prone

to flooding. These areas have flat or mildly inclined terrain and are along coastlines, river deltas, or in zones with high water tables.

4 Morbidity—Morbidity refers to the state of being diseased or unhealthy within a population. We often use it to measure the prevalence and impact of illnesses, injuries, and other health conditions within a specific group or community. We usually present morbidity rates as the number of cases of a particular disease or condition per unit of population over a specified period, such as per 1,000 individuals per year.

5 Mortality—Mortality refers to the occurrence of death within a population. It is a fundamental measure of the health status and well-being of a community, providing insights into the frequency and causes of death within a population over a specified period. We usually express mortality rates as the number of deaths per population unit over a specified period, often standardized to a specific time frame, such as per 1,000 individuals per year.

6 Cultural traditions and beliefs strongly root folk remedies, and these remedies often reflect historical experiences, knowledge, and values of a particular community. This knowledge has been transmitted across generations within a particular community or culture. These remedies often involve the use of natural ingredients, such as herbs, plants, roots, and other substances found in the local environment, to address various health conditions and ailments.

7 Shah Sultan Mosque—The Shah Sultan Mosque, also known as the Sultan Masjid or Shah Sultan Masjid, is one of the most iconic and important mosques in Bangladesh. They named Sultan's Mosque after the first Sultan of Singapore, Sultan Hussein Shah. Sultan Hussein Shah himself, with a grant from the East India Company built around 1824 the Mosque. Denis Santry of Swan & Maclaren designed it in Saracenic style and incorporated domes, minarets, and balustrades. A special feature of the Mosque is the base of its dome which is formed out of many glass bottles.

8 Indigenous Medical Practitioners—Indigenous medical practitioners are individuals within a community or culture who possess traditional knowledge and skills in diagnosing, treating, and preventing illnesses and injuries using methods passed down through generations. The practices of indigenous medical practitioners are often deeply rooted in cultural beliefs, spirituality, and holistic views of health and well-being.

9 Eurocentric World View—The Eurocentric World View refers to a perspective that places Europe and European culture at the centre of historical, cultural, political, and economic narratives, often to the exclusion or marginalization of other regions and cultures. This worldview emerged during the period of European colonial expansion and dominance, which began in the 15th century and impacted global history and geopolitics considerably.

10 Registration of Medical Practitioners Act—During colonial rule in India, the British administration implemented various regulations to govern the practice of medicine and ensure standards of medical care. One significant piece of legislation related to the registration of medical practitioners was the Medical Act of 1858, also known as the Indian Medical Act of 1858. The Indian Medical Act of 1858 established the framework for the registration and regulation of medical practitioners in British India. The Act established a system of licensing for medical practitioners, requiring individuals to receive a license from a specified medical authority for the practice of medicine.

11 Tilak—Bal Gangadhar Tilak, often referred to as Lokmanya Tilak, was a prominent Indian nationalist, freedom fighter, and social reformer who played a crucial role in India's struggle for independence from British colonial rule. Born on July 23, 1856, in Ratnagiri, Maharashtra, Tilak emerged as one of the leading figures of the Indian nationalist movement in the late 19th and early 20th centuries.

12 Frederick Norman White—Frederick Norman White served as the Sanitary Commissioner in British India during the colonial period. As Sanitary Commissioner, White played a crucial role in implementing public health measures aimed at improving sanitation and preventing the spread of diseases in various regions of British India.

13 Lt. Col.C Mac Taggart—Lieutenant Colonel C. Mac Taggart was a significant figure in British India during the colonial era. Taggart served in various capacities within the British military administration, contributing to the maintenance of colonial rule and the management of British interests on the Indian subcontinent. Colonel Hon. C. Mactaggart, C.S.I., C.I.E., served as the Inspector-General of Prisons and Civil Hospitals in the United Provinces, India, and was awarded the British War Medal for his service during the period 1914–20.

14 Public Health Officials—Public health officials isolate and restrict individuals exposed to contagious diseases but not yet showing symptoms to prevent the spread of those diseases. One of the earliest documented instances of quarantine dates back to the 14th century in the Republic of Ragusa (present-day Dubrovnik, Croatia). Ragusa established a quarantine system in 1377 to prevent the spread of the plague.

References

BookArnold, D. (2019). *Colonizing the body: State medicine and epidemic disease in nineteenth-century India*. University of California Press.

Arnold, D. (2000). *Science, technology, and medicine in colonial India*. Cambridge University Press.

Barry, J. M. (2005). *The great influenza: The story of the deadliest pandemic in history*. Penguin Books.

Chakrabarti, P. (2012). *Medicine and empire: 1600–1960*. Palgrave Macmillan.

Chandavarkar, R. (1998). *Imperial power and popular politics: Class, resistance, and the state in India, c. 1850–1950*. Cambridge University Press.

Kent, S. K. (2013). *The influenza pandemic of 1918–1919: A brief history with documents*. Bedford/St. Martin's.

Klein, I. (2020). *Forgotten pandemic: The influenza in colonial India*. In H. Bashford & R. W. Sullivan (Eds.), *Health and empire* (pp. 50–60). Cambridge University Press.

Kumar, A. (1998). *Medicine and the raj: British medical policy in India*. Sage Publications.

Kumar, D., & Basu, R. (2013). *Medical encounters in British India*. Oxford University Press.

Rai, S. K. (2020). *In search of indigenous medicine: Medical pluralism and the ayurvedic movement in colonial India* (pp. 1–22). Occasional Paper History and Society, New Series 104. Nehru Memorial Museum and Library.

Sanitary Commissioner's Preliminary Report. (1918). *United provinces report on Spanish influenza 1918*. Government Monotype Press.

Sanitary Commissioner's Preliminary Report. (1919). *The influenza pandemic of 1918 in India*–The Sanitary Commissioners with The Government of India. Government Monotype Press.

Sharma, M. (2012). *Indigenous and western medicine in Colonial India*. Cambridge University Press.

Watts, S. J. (1999). *Epidemics and history: Disease, power and imperialism*. Yale University Press.

White, F. N. (1919). *A preliminary report on the influenza pandemic of 1918 in India*. Government Monotype Press.

Articles

Anshu, & Supe, A. (2016). Evolution of medical education in India: The impact of colonialism. *Journal of Postgraduate Medicine*, *62*(4), 255–259.

Arnold, D. (1996). The rise of Western medicine in India. *Department of Medical History*, *348*(9034), 1075–1078.

Arnold, D. (2020). Pandemic India: Disease, death and political crisis during the 1918 influenza. *Past & Present*, *249*(1), 271–300. https://doi.org/10.1093/pastj/gtaa023

Biswas, D., Chatterjee, S., & Sultana, P. (2021). Stigma and fear during COVID-19: Essentializing religion in an Indian context. *Humanities and Social Sciences Communications*, *8*(130), 1–10.
Brimnes, N. (2004). Variolation, vaccination and popular resistance in early colonial South India. *Journal of Medical History*, *48*(2), 199–228.
Christian, H. (2006). Patterns of medical culture in colonial Bengal, 1835–1880. *Bulletin of the History of Medicine*, *80*(1), 39–72.
Dicke, T. (2015). Waiting for the flu: Cognitive inertia and the Spanish influenza pandemic of 1918–19. *Journal of the History of Medicine and Allied Sciences*, *70*(2), 195–217.
Hardiman, D. (2009). Indian medical indigeneity: From nationalist assertion to the global market. *Social History*, *34*(3), 263–283.
Hochmuth, C. (2006). Patterns of medical culture in Colonial Bengal, 1835–1880. *Bulletin of the History of Medicine*, *80*(1), 39–72.
Johnson, C. W. (1919). Treatment of influenza. *The Indian Medical Gazette*, *54*(1), 3–4.
Kalpagam, U. (2002). Colonial governmentality and the public sphere in India. *Journal of Historical Sociology*, *15*(1), 35–58.
Kanagarathinam, D. V. (2018). Indigenous and western medicines in colonial South India: Nature of discourses and impact. *Indian Journal of History of Science*, *53*(2), 182–204.
Misra, S. (2021). A quick overview of medical services and disease prevention in colonial India: Public health in British India. *International Journal of Applied Research*, *7*(1), 467–469.
Nicholas, R. W. (1981). The Goddess Śītalā and epidemic smallpox in Bengal. *The Journal of Asian Studies*, *41*(1), 21−44.
Ramanna, M. (2006). Systems of medicine: Issues and responses in Bombay presidency. *Economic & Political Weekly*, *41*(29), 3321–3326.
Scott, D. (1995). Colonial governmentality. *Social Text*, *43*, 191–220.
Sen, D. (1919). A note on the influenza bacillus. *The Indian Medical Gazette*, *54*(6), 241–242.
Sriram, V., Keshri, V. R., & Kumbhar, K. (2021). The impact of colonial-era policies on health workforce regulation in India: Lessons for contemporary reform. *Human Resource Health*, *19*(100), 1–10.
Sri Ramakrishna Math. (2020, May). Rabindranath Tagore and the 1918 influenza pandemic. *The Vedanta Kesari*, *107*(5), 162–167.
Taubenberger, J. K. (2006). The origin and virulence of the 1918 'Spanish' influenza virus. *Proceedings of the American Philosophical Society*, *150*(1), 86–112.
Verma, R. (1995). Western medicine, indigenous doctors, and colonial medical education: A case of desire for 'hegemony' in conflict with demands of 'colonial partiality'. *Itinerario*, *19*(3), 130–141.

Archival Sources

Books and Reports

Minutes of the Proceedings, held at Central Municipal Office, Wednesday, 17th July , 1918.

Government Documents

Proceedings of the Government of Bengal in the Finance Department (Medical), File 2A -2, Proceedings B 110–111, January 1919.
Proceedings of the Government of Bengal in the Municipal Department (Sanitation Branch) for the month of June 1918, File. No. S–2. D–8 (3).
Proceedings of the Government of Bengal in the Municipal Department (Sanitation Branch) for the month of June 1918, File S.1P-3 Progs. B 151–152.

Proceedings of the Government of Bengal in the Municipal Department (Sanitation Branch) for the month of April 1919, File No. S.2D–8, Proceedings No. A. 1–20.
Proceedings of the Government of Bengal in the Municipal Department (Sanitation Branch) for the month of April 1919, File No. S.2D–8 (13).
Proceedings of the Government of Bengal in the Municipal Department (Sanitation) for the Month of January 1919, File No. S.2D–1 (3) Proceedings No. A.18–19.
Report on the Administration of the Bombay Presidency, 1918–1919. (1920). Government Central Press (p. xi).

Newspapers

Chittagong Chronicle. (1918, October 12). Sounds alarm as Spanish influenza grips the city. Panic ensues as the deadly virus spreads like wildfire (p. 5).
The Amrita Bazar Patrika. (1918, August 20). Indigenous system of medicine and government. (p. 4).
The Amrita Bazar Patrika. (1918, September 20). Ayurveda in Madras Council–Kaviraj Jogindra Nath Sen's letter (p. 5).
The Bengal Chronicle. (1918, November 15). Public outcry against British government's inefficiency in Spanish influenza response (p. 3).
The Bengal Gazette. (1918, September 15). Colonial authorities clamp down on indigenous healers amidst influenza outbreak. p. 4.
The Bogra Chronicle. (1919, February 27). Communities besieged by Spanish influenza from British authorities grapple with crisis (p. 2).
The Bogra Herald. (1918, September 28). Amidst pandemic, religious devotion prevails (p. 3).
The Chittagong Gazette. (1919, January 12). Public outcry escalates as Spanish influenza ravages communities, government response criticized (p. 5).
The Dacca Daily News. (1919, August 12). Colonial authorities accuse indigenous healers of spreading influenza misinformation (p. 5).
The Dacca Dispatch. (1919, March 15). Dacca and Mymensingh struggle against influenza onslaught, residents demand government intervention (p. 5).
The Hindu. (1918, September 19). The famine and the flu (p. 5).
The Hindu. (2018, June 26). From the archives June 26, 1918. Curious fever epidemic in Bombay.
The Khulna Tribune. (1918, October 25). Colonial authorities crack down on indigenous healers amid the influenza crisis (p. 6).
The Mymensingh Chronicle. (1918, December 7). Colonial authorities target indigenous healers in Spanish influenza response (p. 3).
The Rajshahi Chronicle. (1918, March 15). Religious dependence amidst Spanish influenza outbreak (p. 2).
The Rajshahi Times. (1918, December 3). Anger mounts across districts as British authorities fail to quell influenza crisis (p. 6).
Times of India. (1918, September 28). Influenza pandemic: Health officer's appeal.

Other Documents

Cardew, Note. (1918, September 15). T.N.A., G.O. 593, Rev. (Spl.) (Conf.), 13 October 1918.
Lokopakari. (1918, September 23). In Native Newspaper Reports; *Indian Patriot,* 10 September 1918, cutting in T.N.A., G.O. 922, Public (Conf.), 8 October 1918.
Wood, R. B. (1918, September 15). Director of Civil Supplies to Secretary, Rev. (Special). T.N.A., G.O. 841, Rev. (Spl.), 5 December 1918.

3 When Famine Met the Spanish Influenza

This chapter delves into the devastating convergence of the 1918 influenza pandemic and a concurrent famine[1] in colonial Bengal, illuminating a twin catastrophe that, though scarcely explored in scholarship, left profound and lasting repercussions. It traces the development of famine policies, notably the Bengal Famine Code of 1913, and analyzes the evolving responses of the colonial government in the early 20th century. The study reveals how systemic neglect, socio-economic disparities, and ecological vulnerabilities converged during a period of severe hardship. The chapter examines the underlying factors contributing to food shortages, labour displacement, and crop failures during the pandemic, demonstrating how the influenza outbreak exacerbated existing challenges (McAlpin, 1983, pp. 161–190). It critically assesses the effectiveness of the colonial state's interventions and their ripple effects on agrarian communities and marginalized populations. Through this analysis, the chapter provides a historical perspective on the intricate relationships between public health, governance, and humanitarian efforts in colonial India. The final section emphasizes the lasting impact of these crises, advocating for the establishment of equitable and resilient systems to address interconnected disasters.

In the records of history, the year 1918 acts as a grim reminder of the convergence of several crises that swept across the planet, leaving destruction in their aftermath. During World War I, the world encountered armed conflict, flu pandemic, and famine, notably in colonial India, where famine's ominous presence trailed behind the virus's unrelenting spread (Ghosh, 1944, pp. 3–14). F Norman White, the Sanitary Commissioner of Bengal, aware of the ongoing tragedy, drew a direct link that highlighted the significant obstacles presented by the simultaneous crises. He emphasized the interaction between the famine and the flu pandemic, observing that the failure of the monsoon[2] exacerbated food scarcity, resulting in malnutrition and increased vulnerability to diseases like influenza (Sanitary Commissioner Report, 1919, p. 68). The failure of monsoons triggered a disastrous event in India, creating a series of consequences. By early autumn, prices surged because of a reduced harvest, increasing susceptibility to the influenza virus. The pandemic swept through communities already weakened by hunger and deprivation, leading to a higher death toll, especially among those on the verge of starvation (Mishra et al., 2019, pp. 2075, 2081–2083). Local newspapers depicted the

DOI: 10.4324/9781003656647-4

British as ruthless oppressors, uncaring of the Indian people's suffering. Here, it is crucial to emphasize the report published in the *Dainik Basumati. The Dainik Basumati* (Calcutta) of August 30, 1918, p. 5 published the following report:

Box 3.1 *Bengal is currently in such a dire situation that it raises whether discussing politics or social issues is even relevant anymore. What significance do these matters hold for those who are facing death? The daily reports we receive from the rural areas make it increasingly difficult for us to maintain our composure. Some time ago, the government imported standard cloth to ease the suffering of the populace. However, for reasons that remain unclear, the actions to deliver these supplies to Bengal have not been executed. The price of rice has now exceeded Rs. 10 per maund, and it continues to escalate. Dealers are raising prices both in the morning and evening, yet no solutions are being offered. We are receiving alarming reports of starvation-related deaths from rural regions. There are accounts of individuals weakened by three days of hunger, collapsing in the fields; others have reportedly gone insane from lack of food, and some have fallen ill after consuming wild plants and leaves. This situation is reminiscent of the catastrophic famine of 1176. There is a real risk of looting and civil unrest. What desperation might starve individuals resort to? What words can soothe those tormented by hunger? If the Bengal Government had forgone its retreat to the hills during this challenging year and instead focused on Eastern Bengal, the funds saved could have been used to assist the public. Further delays are unacceptable. The government must prioritize the urgent task of saving its people.*

British authorities in India, comprising the Indian Medical Service (IMS) and the Government, faced a considerable dual crisis in dealing with famine and disease. They emphasized famine as a key element in the propagation of the influenza pandemic (Davis, 2001, pp. 23, 117, 311). The British administration deemed the 1918 famine in India a success, while the Indian population associated it with failures of British imperialism. The Legislative Council[3] demanded greater intervention than what the British will offer, revealing the deep-rooted tensions and disparities that characterized colonial governance in India. The relationship between the pandemic and famine complicated the official response, resulting in confusion and conflicting viewpoints (Chhun, 2020, pp. 96–130).

Amartya Sen's notion of "entitlement", as explained in *Poverty and Famine* (1981), provides critical perspectives on the fundamental mechanisms of famines. Sen contends famines arise not from a lack of food but from insufficient access, as illustrated by the 1943 Bengal famine, accentuating the necessity for government involvement (Sen, 1981, pp. 39–44). The 1918 pandemic, a consequence of World War I, severely impacted India's resources and personnel, undermined

British morale, and strained the resources of the Indian Medical Service[4] and army. Despite some experience with influenza, the pandemic's magnitude and mortality rate left the medical service with little time for preparation. The short-lived nature of the pandemic, which vanished in less than three months, complicated efforts to effectively manage its aftermath (Arnold, 2019, pp. 181, 191–200).

In contrast, the British colonial government possessed substantial experience in famine preparation, evidenced by the well-established Famine Codes,[5] a system of provincial protocols for officials to adhere to (Brennan, 2012, pp. 95–100). The British, notwithstanding the strains of war, considered themselves well-prepared to manage a minor famine in 1918. However, the flu and famine presented new challenges, leading them to prioritize famine relief efforts despite the complexities of the pandemic (Arnold, 1993b, pp. 385, 399, 403). The centralized bureaucracy of the Indian government and its dependence on local administrations for immediate relief intensified the pressure on response efforts. Institutional oversights resulted in an uneven emphasis on famine relief, as the flu represented a new challenge, with the death toll enabling wealthy British officials to disregard its effects (Brennan, 1984, pp. 34–69).

The incidents of 1918 in colonial India serve as a glaring reminder of the interconnectedness of famine and disease, along with the significant ramifications of colonial governance in the lives of millions. The twin disasters of the flu pandemic and famine exposed the inequalities and injustices ingrained in colonial rule, revealing the callous disregard of British officials for the suffering of the Indian populace. As we contemplate this dark chapter in history, it is crucial that we address the legacies of empire and strive for a fairer and more just world for everyone.

History of Famine in Colonial Bengal

Famine has long been a spectre haunting the historical narrative of India, especially during the time of British colonial domination. During British colonial domination, India went through many famines, resulting in widespread hardship, loss of life, and economic turmoil. British policies intensified these crises, although the fundamental reasons often extended beyond their influence. British actions frequently aggravated the situation, prioritizing imperial interests over the welfare of Indian populations (Taylor, 1873, pp. 143–145, 165–167, 180–182). The chronicles of famine in colonial Bengal represent a brief but significant history that the British government concealed to avert the risk of their empire's collapse. Economic tactics, environmental influences, and administrative shortcomings shaped the history of famines in colonial Bengal, marked by many disasters from the late 18th century to 1947 (Brennan et al., 1984, p. 18). The Great Bengal Famine, a disastrous famine in 1770, impacted the Bengal Presidency, which included Bangladesh, West Bengal, Bihar, and parts of Odisha. Historian Mike Davis links the calamity to colonial economic strategies enforced by the British East India Company. Heightened land taxes and cash tax obligations compelled small farmers to deplete their grain reserves; concurrently, traders stockpiled supplies to manipulate prices.

This resulted in a marketplace devoid of food and a weakened populace. Bengal endured several significant famines after the 1770 disaster, including those in 1783, 1866, 1873, and 1897, primarily because of inadequate agricultural methods, poor irrigation, and British economic measures.

Introducing a railway system by the British eased the flow of goods and relief efforts, yet it also led to the relocation of food supplies abroad, frequently leaving the local populace in hunger. The famine of 1918, influenced by the Spanish Influenza epidemic, is often neglected because of the British government's refusal to classify it as a famine. The most catastrophic famine in Bengal's history occurred during World War II. The Bengal Famine of 1943 was a catastrophic natural disaster in Bengal's past, worsened by British strategies and wartime circumstances (Greenough, 1980, p. 223). The British government rerouted resources to fuel the war effort, causing a severe food shortage. The Japanese invasion of neighbouring Burma severed essential food supplies, resulting in approximately 3 million fatalities because of starvation and malnutrition. The famines disrupted societal structures, led to mass migrations, and critically weakened Bengal's agricultural economy, hindering recovery from repeated famines. British colonial policies, economic exploitation, and administrative failures were primarily responsible for the Bengal famines (Padel, 2012, pp. 26–28). The British government placed more importance on financial profit than on the well-being of local populations, which resulted in poor management of resources and increased vulnerability (Stahl, 2016, pp. 169–184). This underscores the need to comprehend the causes of food shortages and emphasizes the significance of fair and environmentally sustainable development to avert future disasters (Famine Commissions Reports, 1770–1943, pp. 4–144).

Examining the origins of these famines shows that British colonial authority in India significantly transformed land ownership, agriculture, and commerce, thus impacting food security. Imposing exploitative land revenue systems, such as the Permanent Settlement in Bengal[6] and the Ryotwari system in certain areas of South India, disrupted traditional farming and introduced indigo[7] cultivation which left farmers susceptible to economic exploitation (Kumar, 2018, p. 518). The British approach prioritized revenue generation over sustainable agricultural practices, which led to land degradation and diminished capacity for food production. The encouragement of cash crops for export further compromised food self-sufficiency (Kumar, 2016, p. 56). The British established market-driven policies that disrupted conventional food exchange systems and imposed colonial monopolies, leading to disparities in food availability across regions. British trade regulations also favoured the exportation of food grains from India, further diminishing domestic food resources and driving up local market prices (Tiwari & Sharma, 2023, pp. 25, 27).

British strategies in India resulted in famines during the 19th century, which marginalized and deprived vulnerable populations of access to vital food supplies (Blair, 2006, pp. 67–90). The Great Bengal Famine of 1770,[8] which occurred during British governance, led to approximately 10 million deaths, making it one of the most devastating famines in documented history. The British colonial administration instituted measures to ease the consequences of recurring famines, such as the Orissa Famine of 1866 and the Great Famine of 1876–78, affecting Indian communities (Bhatia, 2006, pp. 238–270).

One such measure was the establishment of the Famine Codes in the 1880s, which aimed to create a systematic governmental approach to famine management in India (Report of the Indian Famine Commission, 1880, p. 86). As highlighted by Amartya Sen in *Poverty and Famines*, the mere existence of these codes did not ensure their effective execution. Sen asserts the frameworks established by imperial authorities for managing food distribution could frequently worsen famine conditions by either facilitating or restricting access to essential resources (Sen, 1983, p. 21). The Famine Codes should prevent famines in India, but faced obstacles such as bureaucratic inefficiencies, corruption, and political unwillingness. The latter part of the 19th century witnessed a notable rise in famines, especially following British colonial dominance. Factors such as land tenure systems, agricultural policies, and trade practices contributed to widespread food shortages, exacerbating the problem (Bhatia, 1963a, p. 58).

Mike Davis, in "Late Victorian Holocausts",[9] explores the horrific human cost of famines in India during the late 1800s, estimating that from 1876 to 1902, between 12.2 and 29.3 million individuals lost their lives. Davis contends that British policies that favoured imperial gains over the well-being of Indians resulted in an immense death toll. He underscores the connection between famine and illness, as malnutrition undermines immune systems and exposes people to outbreaks. British famine camps, which traded food for labour, fostered the spread of infectious pathogens,[10] resulting in additional fatalities. Widespread malnutrition and compromised immune systems rendered even those not in the camps vulnerable to contagious pathogens. The 1918 flu epidemic in India, aggravated by a terrible famine, intensified the already dire plight of at-risk populations. The virus took advantage of the weakened condition of malnourished individuals, illuminating the relationship between famine and illness, serving as a tragic reminder of the failures of colonial governance and imperial neglect (Roy, 2002, pp. 109, 113, 121; Chhun, 2015, p. 100).

The record of famine in British India illustrates the severe effects of colonialism on food security and human well-being. British policies intensified food scarcities, resulting in widespread anguish and deaths. The recurring famines of the 19th century, associated with sickness, underscore the wrongs of colonial administration and the pressing need for a fairer system of global food governance.

The Bengal Famine Code of 1913 and the Development of Famine Policy From 1900 to 1918

The Famine Codes in British India were a crucial response to food scarcity, providing a systematic framework for addressing the issue (Report of the Indian Famine Commission, 1898, p. 113). The Famine Codes provided both indirect and direct relief measures to stricken populations during the pandemic. Indirect relief included suspending revenue demands and providing loans to ease financial strain. Direct relief focused on immediate needs, such as establishing poor houses, community kitchens, and employment opportunities. These measures aimed to prevent widespread destitution and impoverishment. The codes also detailed procedures for different stages of famine, from early warning signs to full-blown crises (Wood, 1918, p. 45). For instance, the revised edition of the Bengal Famine Code of 1913 stands as a testament to the British colonial administration's efforts to address the recurring threat of famine in the region. This colonial document outlined procedures for managing food scarcity and coordinating relief efforts, providing a road map for officials in crisis management.

Here, an attempt has been made to highlight the major concern of the Bengal Famine Code of 1913 in a compressed manner—

> *The first chapter outlines the necessary preparatory and precautionary measures that must be consistently upheld during normal conditions. The second and third chapters focus on the actions to be taken when information suggests an impending scarcity or famine. The subsequent fifteen chapters of the Code address the responsibilities of various officials and the different relief strategies to be implemented when scarcity or famine is occurring. Following these chapters are six appendices that provide additional rules and instructions that complement those established in the main body of the Code. The final section of the Code includes the forms required for managing relief efforts, with each type of form assigned a letter of the alphabet to show its specific purpose.*

The Bengal Famine Code emphasized early warning systems and data gathering, which allowed officials to pinpoint regions vulnerable to famine and enact proactive measures. This allowed authorities to expect food shortages and to allocate resources accordingly. The code also included provisions for relief measures, which were categorized into public works and village works overseen by civil officers and private individuals. By February 15, the District Engineer, District Officers, and Executive Engineer must prepare and present a public works programme to the Superintending Engineer. Village works comprise enhancements to tanks, wells, drainage systems, irrigation, channels, roads, and sanitary facilities. Authorities may also enforce special regulations during famine to ensure the safety of the community. The code included provisions for relief works. Special rules can also be enacted during famine (railway project in the relief works programme, district liabilities where the railway traverses, permanent protection of the district via railway, the number of individuals for whom relief works may be necessary for severe famine, the number of individuals for whom suitable work can be provided by the railway, etc.).

Relief works executed strategies such as halting revenue demands, offering loans, and establishing relief initiatives like poorhouses and community kitchens to ease economic burdens and offer immediate help. The Bengal Famine Code outlined the initiation of detailed relief work measures during famine, which is as follows—Whenever a severe famine occurs, authorities will implement comprehensive relief measures. The local government will typically appoint a Famine

Commissioner. When the Local Government confines famine conditions to a division, it may appoint an Additional Commissioner.

Once the Local Government announces famine conditions, it will enhance the system of village inspections.

- The Circle Officer, along with his superiors, shall meticulously review the preliminary gratuitous relief lists. This initial selection must be executed strictly by the Circle Officer and his superiors.
- Should any district experience unusual strain because of a supply of food grains or fodder that may be imposed on any railway administration, the District Officer will inform the Commissioner of the Division on the matter. The Commissioner will convene a meeting to determine the best approach to meet the demands and assist the railway.
- In urgent situations, the District Officer shall have the authority to open relief works ahead of receiving official sanction, notifying his actions via telegram to the Commissioner and the Local Government.
- Immigrants from native states should not interfere except—(a) if they lack the strength to complete the journey, (b) if the destination cannot sustain them, and (c) when they would roam aimlessly.

When migration numbers are significant, a regular network of relief depots should be established. Those who can afford it will buy and sell crops only. Immigrants should not be pressured to return home. Political agents should facilitate their return to their homeland.

- Local authorities shall not import any grain into any relief work without prior authorization.

We will facilitate all necessary measures for the unobstructed operation of private trade during famine. The Indian government will lower railway fees for the transportation of grains.

- If there is a shortage of supplies in any relief work or area, the District Officer may support private trade by providing recoverable loans to grain merchants, with or without interest, and must report his actions to inform the Local Government.

The Bengal Famine Code highlighted the necessity of proactive planning and readiness. The Bengal Famine Code required ongoing preparations and annually updated assessments of relief needs, ensuring officials were equipped to address famine emergencies. Officials classified relief efforts into allowed and urgent projects, giving priority to the former for execution. The colonial administration implemented measures to address famines and support at-risk populations.

The code also tackled issues related to maintaining social stability during periods of scarcity. It specified methods for monitoring any rise in criminal activity linked to inflation or food shortages, underscoring the government's commitment to averting social turmoil. By observing and managing potential sources of disorder, the authorities have aimed to ensure stability and safety in regions affected by famine. The 1913 Bengal Famine Code represented a comprehensive framework for handling famines in British India. By instituting logical procedures and guidelines, the code empowered officials to expect, react to, and lessen the effects of food insecurity on vulnerable communities. Although there were some shortcomings, the code showed the colonial government's dedication to addressing the challenges posed by famine and safeguarding the welfare of the populace under its jurisdiction (The Bengal Famine Code, 1913, pp. 13–53).

However, as scholars such as James C. Scott have observed, bureaucratic frameworks might overly simplify intricate societal dynamics, resulting in gaps in comprehension and action (Haggis et al., 1986, pp. 1435–1445). The Famine Codes hassled that contingency planning and preparedness were vital elements of famine management. Regions susceptible to famine faced increased oversight, with ongoing preparations and annually updated estimates to expect relief needs. Officials distinguished relief efforts into approved and emergency projects, giving priority to the former for execution. Colonial leaders actively strategized to manage famines and safeguard at-risk individuals. Interestingly, the Famine Codes also highlighted the significance of sustaining the morale of impacted populations. Acknowledging the psychological impact of food scarcity, the codes emphasized the necessity for proactive preparations to build confidence and avert moral decline among the public. This dimension of the codes emphasizes the colonial authorities' appreciation of the significance of psychological health during crises (Famine Inquiry Commission Report, 1918, p. 43). The Famine Codes dealt with worries surrounding social stability during periods of scarcity. The government promptly monitored rises in crime linked to escalating prices or food deficiencies, concentrating on averting social disorder. The thorough documentation and reporting protocols established in the codes showed a deliberate effort to observe and manage potential instability sources (Felix, 2012, p. 123).

Besides relief initiatives, the Famine Codes delineated long-term approaches for famine prevention and alleviation. These approaches encompassed programmes to enhance agricultural productivity, encourage crop diversity, and improve infrastructure for water management and irrigation. By investing in strategies to bolster agricultural resilience and lessen reliance on single crops, the British administration sought to diminish the likelihood of future famines (Simonow, 2023, p. 78). The Famine Codes represented a comprehensive and visionary strategy for combating food shortages in British India. Despite their shortcomings and occasional setbacks, these codes illustrated the colonial authorities' dedication to handling famine emergencies and easing their social and economic impacts. The careful planning, data gathering, and contingency strategies outlined in the codes emphasized the British administration's attempts to exert control over famine scenarios and shield vulnerable populations from the ravages of starvation and deprivation.

Between 1900 and 1918, the famine policy in India largely followed the guidelines displayed in the Famine Codes and the recommendations of the 1901 Famine

Commission, which were incorporated into the Provincial Famine Codes (Report of Famine Programmes, 1906–18, pp. 16, 33, 79). While officials removed the idea of a "minimum" wage, compliance with the Commission's requirements—such as a personalized help for the vulnerable and job assignments based on workers' abilities—was still compulsory. We closed the gender wage gap, but the gap for dependents persisted. The Provincial Famine Codes permitted a 25% deviation from the regular famine wage, contingent on specific criteria. Local governments employed convenient strategies for choosing candidates for relief work. Despite the concerns raised by the 1901 Famine Commission regarding the effectiveness of free kitchens, the Government of India allowed for their implementation in relief programmes under certain precautions. It supported the Commission's proposal to appoint a Famine Commissioner during imminent famine situations or large-scale relief operations, as well as shifting to single officer supervision for each relief initiative, as suggested by the Commission (Report of Famine Programmes, 1902–03, pp. 11, 17–29).

In response to the Commission's recommendations concerning fodder supply during famines, the Government enforced certain regulations in September 1903. These regulations opened grazing lands that were typically restricted for cattle and vice versa, prioritizing the export of grass while ensuring local cattle were adequately fed. They instituted strict rules for grazing in forested areas and regions designated for plantations or regeneration. Acknowledging the effect of inadequate railway infrastructure on food grain costs and losing agricultural cattle, the government directed local administrations to maintain prompt communication with railway officials when famine threats were detected. The government mandated collaborative meetings among civil, railway, and commercial leaders to tackle supply demands. The government supported the Famine Commission's recommendation to provide generous revenue suspensions and remissions during widespread disasters. These allowances were to be determined based on communal village losses rather than individual taxpayers' situations, with provisions established for reducing interest in advances in particular cases (Miller, 1902–03, p. 147).

The 1918 Famine and the Spanish Flu: Connectivity, Causes, and Consequences

The pathological interconnectivity between the 1918 famine and the Spanish Flu in colonial Bengal shows how malnutrition, immune system vulnerabilities, and environmental factors collectively exacerbated the pandemic's effects (Greenough, 1980, pp. 266–271). The famine, marked by extreme food shortages and declining living conditions, severely weakened the population's immunity. Arnold (1993a) shows that individuals having malnutrition often faced deficits in crucial nutrients like vitamin A, zinc, and protein, all of which are vital for maintaining immune function. These nutritional deficiencies impaired the mucosal defenses in the respiratory tract, making individuals more prone to influenza infections and their complications. The famine resulted in the overcrowding of relief camps, where poor sanitation conditions facilitated the rapid spread of the influenza virus

(Chakrabarti, 2012, pp. 1–18). The Spanish Flu, well-known for its severe impact on the respiratory system, particularly targeted those with compromised immune systems, often resulting in secondary bacterial infections such as pneumonia. Harrison (1994, pp. 202–220) highlights that the interplay of malnutrition, insufficient hygiene, and limited medical resources in famine-impacted Bengal raised mortality rates during the pandemic. Colonial relief measures were frequently slow and insufficient, failing to address the nutritional deficiencies that put the population at risk. This convergence of biological and social elements emphasizes that the virulence of the virus alone did not lead to the devastating consequences of the Spanish Flu in Bengal; the vulnerabilities created by famine played a significant role in shaping them. Understanding this relationship provides valuable insights into how social determinants of health can amplify the effects of pandemics, a lesson that remains relevant in contemporary global health discussions.

In 1918, India faced the ongoing consequences of the First World War alongside the challenges posed by a deficient South-West Monsoon.[11] The monsoon was notably weak in both northern and southern regions, falling short of average levels by 19%. Crops experienced widespread failure in various areas, including Gujarat, Bombay, the Deccan, Berar,[12] Rajputana, the southern portions of the Central Provinces, Orissa, and the United Provinces. Despite these difficulties, the official declaration of famine and the commencement of relief efforts occurred only in the Central Provinces and the United Provinces, while other impacted regions remained under observation and preliminary assessment (Williams, 1985, p. 92).

Box 3.2 *Colonial Bengal in 1918 faced famine alongside the Spanish Flu because of the combination of various factors (Arnold, 1979, pp. 111, 127, 133, 139, 144). Initially, the lack of monsoon rains in various regions of Bengal and nearby areas resulted in severe crop failures, particularly harming rice, the region's main food source. This decline in agricultural output led to severe food shortages and heightened the population's susceptibility to famine situations (Turner, 1918, p. 56). Colonial strategies and economic frameworks worsened the effects of crop failures. The British colonial approach, which included land tenure systems, taxes, and trade laws, prioritized the needs of colonial powers and landlords over the local population's welfare, resulting in uneven resource distribution and increased food insecurity (Fagan, 1999, p. 112). The Spanish Flu pandemic in 1918 aggravated the global crisis, leading to widespread hunger, malnutrition, and outbreaks of diseases. The interrelation of colonial governance, environmental factors, and public health consequences highlights the necessity for comprehensive solutions (Lokopakari, September 23, 1918, p. 10). Here, I feel compelled to reference the news published in the Dainik Basumati on September 3, 1918, which will aid in understanding the gravity of this famine—*"Hungry I am"–Famine in Bengal: ***The Dainik Basumati*** (Calcutta) of September 3 writes—*The specter of famine looms over Bengal, with the populace welcoming death as a release from their suffering. The people of Bengal find themselves with no option but to succumb to starvation. Our fears are materializing, as widespread looting and pillaging are occurring. In various areas of East Bengal, groups of beggars are visiting homes, demanding, "You must provide us with something before taking anything." There is a growing concern about potential looting in the markets. Have we assessed the total rice reserves at Hatkhola and Chetla? Are the current fluctuations in prices during the morning and evening driven by a shortage of rice or by merchant activities? Is it possible that the mahajans, who are selling rice at the market rate of Rs.10 per maund, are profiting by purchasing it at Rs.4 per maund from their own stock? An investigation into this situation has fallen under the influence of a few affluent merchants who are manipulating the circumstances to their advantage. The government must understand that without importing rice from Burma, the rice shortage in Bengal cannot be eased, even for the month of September. Why were proactive measures not taken to address this crisis in advance? The government states, "We hope to arrange for the import of rice." A definitive commitment from them regarding the importation of rice, along with confirmed arrangements, would likely have pressured the mahajans to lower their prices.*

The Collector of Chittagong addressed the Chairman of the local Municipality, complaining about the prolonged suffering of the starving population in Bengal. He questioned how much longer these individuals could depend on mere hope, emphasizing that even a single day's delay could lead to dire consequences, including death. He warned that the seeds of Bolshevism, which modern civilization fears, could take root in Bengal. It is only natural for those who suffer from hunger to break societal bonds and resort to theft from the affluent in order to satisfy their needs. He urged our leaders to take immediate action to address the food scarcity currently affecting Bengal. A warning was issued to the Government, the wealthy, and our leaders to act swiftly to avert a significant disaster that could affect everyone.

Households cannot spare even a handful of rice for beggars at their doorsteps. The struggling middle-class individuals in the province will not benefit from introducing Burmese rice, as they are reluctant to consume it because of health concerns. Therefore, it is essential for the authorities to ensure that local rice is available at more affordable prices. Reports have been concealed regarding the starvation and famine affecting impoverished villagers, which have severely disrupted their livelihoods. If this situation persists, it will become increasingly difficult for the law-abiding citizens to safeguard their dignity and property. The Government must take prompt action to rectify this crisis.

Source: Dainik Basumati, September 3, 1918, p. 6

Specifically, in 1918, the monsoon failures in multiple areas, especially in the north and the west, motivated the British government to take swift action to prepare for the impending threat of famine or, at the very least, scarcity. Yet, this concentrated focus on famine management resulted in a blind spot regarding the response to the influenza pandemic (The Hindu, September 19, 1918, p. 5). Despite the obvious link between the famine and the flu's death rate, as repeatedly showed by sanitary commissioners throughout the subcontinent, archival documentation regarding the impact of the 1918 famine remains somewhat limited. This shortage of records was likely influenced by the overlapping flu pandemic and ongoing wartime conditions. The relatively minor severity of the 1918 famine compared to earlier crises may have also contributed to the limited documentation (Cardew, 1918, p. 35). The Bombay Famine Report from that period even remarked, "The most notable feature of the latter year was that it never produced in any district visible signs of emaciation or aimless wandering. There was no famine in the sense of starvation among the people." Despite its comparatively mild effects, the famine held a considerable place in the British officials' concerns, often overshadowing the far more lethal flu pandemic (Maharatna, 1992, p. 78).

The United Provinces Famine Report of 1918–19 documented relief projects that provided work and improved areas, emphasizing the "of permanent utility" principle to ensure lasting community benefits (Famine Relief Report, 1918, pp. 23–33). The British government prioritized infrastructure development and community development, selecting relief works to provide employment and address long-standing infrastructure needs, reflecting their belief in the value of productive labour (Famine Proceedings, 1874–1919, pp. 11, 21–67).

Prior to 1918, famines in late 19th-century India were catastrophic, even with the belief that railways would ease food shortages. Historian Mike Davis contends railways were used to move grain and enable price manipulation, worsening the effects of famines due to improved communication networks (Davis, 2001, p. 111). The 1896 grain riots in India revealed the government's failure to manage escalating food prices and execute effective relief strategies, intensifying the famine's effects (Sahu, 1978, pp. 808, 810). In 1918, India faced a famine because of failed monsoons, akin to the crisis in the United Provinces in 1907, leading to widespread hardship and distress (Tabor, 1910, pp. 295, 299). The 1907 famine prompted a change in government management approaches, emphasizing decentralized relief activities and infrastructure enhancements, resulting in reduced mortality rates when compared to earlier crises (Matthews, 2008, pp. 1189, 1201–1203).

The 1907 Indian famine represented a crucial transformation in the nation's history, shifting attention from drought to food pricing. The government prioritized tackling soaring food costs and guaranteeing access to affordable food, concentrating on transport for supplies rather than on employment for those affected by famine. This showed a dedication to addressing the root causes of food scarcity (Passmore, 1951, p. 303).

The 1918 famine in India, worsened by the influenza pandemic, underscored the intricacies of managing famine and relief initiatives under British colonial authority. Despite failed monsoons and food shortages, the British government enacted relief measures. Insufficient documentation shows the necessity for further investigation (Famine Inquiry Commission Report on Bengal, 1945, p. 73).

Colonial Government's Response

In 1918, India encountered a combination of crises that deeply impacted its citizens and exposed the shortcomings of colonial rule. The collapse of monsoons in various areas, along with the emergence of the Spanish Flu pandemic, resulted in a severe scenario that tested the British colonial administration's competency in responding effectively (Tirmizey, 2020, pp. 59, 77). Amid the backdrop of World War I and its economic consequences, India struggled with challenges related to famine, public health, and economic turmoil. This section will examine the interlinked nature of these crises, the actions taken by the British colonial government, and the broader effects on India's social, economic, and political landscape (Kaur, 2022, pp. 24, 31, 41).

The failure of the monsoons in 1918 was a crucial precursor to the famine and deprivation that followed in various regions of India, especially in the northern and western parts. The monsoon season is vital to India's agricultural cycle,[13] and its failure often results in crop failures, food shortages, and economic hardship (Chhun, 2019–2020, pp. 1–11). In 1918, the monsoon failure worsened pre-existing vulnerabilities in India's agrarian economy, where most of the population depended on agriculture for their livelihoods. The lack of rainfall led to reduced crop outputs, causing skyrocketing food prices and widespread scarcity.

As the British government acknowledged the failure of the monsoons, fears about impending famine or deprivation intensified. Initiatives to mobilize relief efforts and reduce the impact on vulnerable groups characterized the response to these crises. However, the emphasis on famine relief created a gap where the response to the Spanish Flu pandemic should have been. Despite the correlation between the famine and the flu pandemic, the British colonial administration inadequately addressed the public health crisis (Srivastava, 1968, pp. 285–324).

The Spanish Flu pandemic, which spread globally in 1918, resulted in millions of deaths worldwide, including a substantial number in India. The swift transmission of the virus, exacerbated by crowded living conditions and insufficient healthcare facilities, caused an overwhelming mortality rate. The flu pandemic had a significant impact on rural populations, restricting access to medical care and worsening existing health inequalities. The British colonial government's reaction to the flu pandemic was insufficient and overshadowed by its emphasis on famine relief initiatives. Even with the devastating effects of the virus on India's populace, the government did not allocate adequate resources to curb the disease's spread. The negligence in investing in public health systems, combined with restrictive policies concerning health crises, highlighted the colonial administration's indifference towards the welfare of India's people. The context of World War I further complicated India's difficulties. The war resulted in a notable rise in defense spending, funded through war loans and a reconfiguration of India's financial infrastructure.

Increasing taxes and stagnant export prices for Indian agricultural goods further burdened the economy. The looming scarcity because of failed monsoons exacerbated these financial pressures as prices climbed throughout the nation.

The economic effects of World War I, coupled with the failure of monsoons and a flu pandemic, created significant difficulties in India. The nation's agricultural economy, which was already susceptible because of colonial policies and structural inequalities, was poorly prepared to handle the repercussions of these crises. The response of the British colonial administration to these issues showed its limited perspective, focusing on sustaining control and safeguarding colonial interests instead of prioritizing the welfare of India's populace (Arnold, 2022, pp. 129–157). Faced with these interrelated crises, members of the Legislative Council expressed worries about the government's spending priorities and its inability to tackle the fundamental causes of famine and public health emergencies (Proceedings of the Govt. of Bengal, December 1918). Appeals for the redirection of funds from large-scale projects to ease the widespread suffering caused by rising prices emphasized the necessity for a more thorough and fair approach to governance. Mr. Kamini Kumar Chanda's[14] critical comments highlighted the imbalance in government focus, recognizing provisions for famine relief while accentuating the extensive suffering brought about by inflated prices (Proceedings Govt. of India, 1919, p. 33). His critique of the government's neglect of prioritizing health initiatives and offering sufficient relief measures emphasized the pressing need for reform. Chanda's reproach of the government's misguided spending priorities and restrictive policies regarding public health emergencies mirrored the wider sentiment of disillusionment with colonial administration. Addressing India's complex challenges would demand a united effort to prioritize public health, invest in infrastructure, and implement fair relief strategies (Arnold, 2021, p. 187). This would require a departure from the limited focus on famine relief towards a more comprehensive approach that tackles the root causes of vulnerability and fosters resilience within communities. Encouraging stronger collaboration among government agencies, private entities, and local communities would be vital in efficiently responding to future emergencies (Woodhead Committee Report, 1918, pp. 11, 26).

The colonial government's reaction to the 1918 Bengal famine in British India included relief initiatives, administrative actions, and economic strategies. These actions encompassed food distribution, relief camps, and public works projects. Detractors criticized these actions for their insufficiency and failure to confront the crisis's fundamental causes, leading to widespread agony and death (Foodstuffs and Transport Board, August 2, 1918, p. 17). The British government implemented the Famine Codes to direct famine relief efforts, but bureaucratic inefficiencies and logistical hurdles hindered effective aid distribution. Economic strategies, including elevated taxes and trade limitations, worsened the famine's effects, resulting in escalating food prices and scarcity. The government's focus on revenue generation over famine relief further exacerbated the predicament (Bagchi, 2014, pp. 5–13). The Spanish Flu pandemic prompted public health initiatives like quarantine and vaccination campaigns, but limited resources and insufficient infrastructure impeded effective management. This resulted in high mortality rates and widespread public protests, highlighting deep-rooted grievances and dissatisfaction with colonial governance (Tambolkar et al., 2022, pp. 642–643).

In summary, the crises of 1918 revealed the interconnected nature of India's socio-economic and public health issues and underscored the shortcomings of colonial governance. India faced a succession of crises: failed monsoon seasons, the Spanish Flu, and the economic impacts of World War I. The British colonial administration's response to these challenges showed its narrow focus on maintaining control and safeguarding colonial interests, rather than prioritizing the welfare of India's populace. Addressing India's vulnerabilities would cause a holistic and fair approach to governance, one that prioritizes public health, allocates resources towards infrastructure development, and enacts measures to ensure inclusive growth (Ojo, 2020, p. 1023).

Reaction of the Local Press and Public Discourse

Local newspapers in colonial Bengal probably expressed outrage and disapproval towards the injustices of the colonial government during the Spanish Influenza and famine episodes in 1918–19. They helped to share information and articulate public sentiment, bringing attention to the distress of the people, and criticizing the government for its negligence, incompetence, or manipulation of events. There may have been calls for accountability. Local newspapers amid the 1918–19 Spanish Influenza and famine crises denounced the government's sluggish reaction, deficient public health system, and misallocation of resources. They urged for swifter actions, effective distribution, and prompt communication. Their articles revealed the colonial government's misdeeds, swaying public opinion against the British government and stressing the importance of transparency and wise resource management. Various writings regarding these significant impacts published in different newspapers were gathered from the Report on Native Papers–State Archives—Education Records Department, 1918, Part–2, which are:

August 31, 1918, p. 850

Prospects of the Crops and Condition of the People

98. The Jasohar (Jessore) dated August 3rd draws the government's attention to the pressing issue that the nation is on the brink of a serious crisis because of the unprecedented increase in the cost of essential goods, coupled with a significant decline in the prices of jute and minor commodities.

99. The Jamhur (Calcutta) on August 22, in discussing the conference chaired by Sir Claude Hill in Nagpur, states that the assembly ought to have featured individuals such as Mr. Gandhi, the Raja Sahib of Mahmudabad, Mr. Jinnah, and Mr. Tilak, rather than being only made up of Europeans. In regions experiencing significant scarcity, the following measures should be implemented—

1. Revenue should not be collected from the zamindars.

2. Sufficient taccavi loans must be provided to the farmers.

3. The current practice of collecting subscriptions for the war loan alongside revenue in certain districts should be discontinued immediately.
4. Measures should be implemented to ensure the availability of railway wagons, and freight charges should be promptly lowered to ease the transportation of food items.
5. The export of wheat, rice, and barley must be immediately banned.
6. The government should establish price controls for all food items and caution grain merchants against hoarding grain supplies.

September 7, 1918, pg. 873–874

Prospects of the Crops and Condition of the People

85. The Moslem Hitashi (Calcutta) published on August 30th highlights the dire situation faced by the peasantry in Bengal, attributing it primarily to the excessive greed of moneylenders and zamindars. The cultivators' own wastefulness and the declining fertility of the land further exacerbate their plight. Therefore, we propose each zamindar establish an agricultural bank to provide loans to their tenants at a low interest rate. They should educate their tenants on frugality and assist them in implementing modern agricultural techniques. The government must also extend support to the cultivators, as their downfall would inevitably lead to the country's decline.

87. The Jagram (Bagerhat) dated August 25, and the Sanjay (Faridpur) from August 23 express concern that the recent surge in rice prices has significantly worsened the hardships faced by the populace, urging the government to address this issue promptly.

90. *The Bengali (Calcutta) edition dated September 1st discusses the devastating floods that have inundated sections of Bogra town and nearby rural areas. The local population is experiencing significant hardship, and Rai A C Sen Bahadur is actively involved in providing help. The entire region along the railway line between Santahar and Kahanu stations is submerged. Currently, rice is being sold at a rate of 10 or 11 seers per rupee. There is an urgent need to organize public relief efforts. The same publication reports on the flooding affecting parts of Faridpur town and its surrounding villages, with water levels continuing to rise.*

November 9, 1918, pg. 1060

Prospects of the Crops and Condition of the People

44. The Calcutta Samachar, in its edition dated October 30, reports a severe famine affecting the nation, causing significant distress among the populace because of rising food prices. The government must act swiftly to address this issue by appointing competent officials to oversee relief efforts. Despite the government's regulation of kerosene and salt prices, the impoverished are not reaping the benefits, as vendors cannot sell these essential items at the established rates. Therefore, it is crucial to assign officers to ensure compliance with government directives.

45. A correspondent for the Bangali, writing on November 3rd, highlights the dire famine conditions in Manbhum and certain areas of Bankura. Many individuals from respectable backgrounds are facing starvation, and laborers are departing in search of work elsewhere. The situation has led to an increase in criminal activity, and it is imperative that relief initiatives, particularly the excavation of tanks, be started without delay.

December 14, 1918, pg. 1148

Prospects of the Crops and Condition of the People

67. The Viswamitra (Dacca) on December 2 appeals to the Government to promptly import rice from Rangoon to avert a potential increase in prices locally.

68. The Hitavadi (Calcutta) of the December 6 invites attention to the severe distress now prevailing in the mufassil owing to the inordinate rise in prices and asks Government to take prompt steps in the matter.

December 21, 1918, pg. 1166

Prospects of the Crops and Condition of the People

The Bengali (Calcutta) edition from December 11th states that the three calamities—pestilence, famine, and war—that can devastate a nation are currently prevalent in both Europe and Asia. Only God knows the extent of the devastation these conditions will bring. In our modest province of Bengal, while there is no active conflict, the effects of famine and disease are wreaking havoc that is far more severe than war.

Box 3.3 In 1919, the Spanish Influenza and famine persisted in inflicting considerable pain and deaths in Bengal. The famine was caused by colonial economic strategies, agricultural failures, and disruptions of war. The Spanish Flu pandemic devastated the at-risk population, leading to higher death rates because of heightened vulnerability to the virus. The workforce was impacted, and agricultural output remained stagnant. These calamities caused significant harm to Bengal's social structure, populace, and economy, highlighting the deficiencies of colonial rule and inadequate governance. Local newspapers were equally outspoken in their reporting against the British government. The brutality of the British Government to whatever extent it reached can be understood from the news published in the following daily newspapers. Some of the news are mentioned as follows as examples:

The Bengalee (January 23, 1919)

The report critiques the Bengal Government for its lack of action regarding cloth prices, contrasting this with the proactive stance taken by Bihar and Orissa. It shows that forthcoming decisions on standardized cloth sales in Bengal will be shaped by market fluctuations, perpetuating economic distress. The report expresses dissatisfaction with the government's sluggish response and urges for decisive measures to regulate prices and mitigate economic hardship, in stark contrast to the commendable initiatives of neighboring states.

The Mussalman (January 24, 1919)

This report sheds light on the challenges faced by the impoverished due to escalating cloth prices. To tackle this issue, the government established a Cloth Control Committee and set fixed prices for specific types of dhotis and saris. However, this led cloth dealers to lower their prices to evade the consequences of the standardization, resulting in a temporary price drop that ultimately dissuaded the government from further intervention. Prices surged back to levels that are unaffordable for middle and lower-income families. The report stresses the urgent need for government action to ensure that essential goods, such as rice and cloth, remain accessible, particularly in rural areas where rice prices are high. It highlights the severe economic challenges confronting rural communities.

The Tippera Guide (Comilla, May 13, 1919)

This report emphasizes the efforts of the Burma Government to stabilize rice prices through price controls, raising concerns about the Bengal Government's delayed response. It posits that timely intervention could ease economic burdens in Bengal. The report suggests that public discontent regarding the government's inaction on food price inflation is prompting Bengal to consider adopting Burma's strategies.

The Dainik Basumati (Calcutta, May 14, 1919)

This article addresses the economic crisis in Bengal, which is associated with widespread poverty and increasing prices of textiles, while also condemning the government's inadequate measures. It shows that labor shortages in England and disruptions in supply chains have prevented the expected drop in cloth prices. The report emphasizes the necessity of importing rice from Burma to Bengal, cautioning that a lack of adequate supplies could lead to famine. It urges for prompt interventions, such as reducing freight charges and controlling rice exports, to stabilize local food prices.

(Source: Report on Native Papers–State Archives: Education Records Department, 1918–19)

These reports collectively underscore the significant economic turmoil experienced in Bengal in 1919, marked by soaring prices for food and textiles. Each document calls for government action to ease the worsening situation. While *The Tippera Guide* suggests adopting the proactive strategies implemented in Burma, The *Dainik Basumati* consistently highlights the critical necessity for adjustments in freight rates, regulation of food prices, and comprehensive economic stabilization. The recurring theme of public dissatisfaction and the threat of social unrest emphasize the serious repercussions of continued governmental inaction during this time. All the reports reflect the growing public frustration with government inefficiency and highlight the urgent need for proactive measures to ensure economic stability.

Examining the core of the news released in all the aforementioned local newspapers, the Spanish Flu, and famine in colonial Bengal and India were not caused by natural events but because of the colonial government's disregard and absence of initiatives. The absence of effective famine relief and rising prices of goods resulted in individuals succumbing to their inability to afford essentials. The British Government's severe negligence and poor administration were the primary contributors to the crisis.

Entangled Catastrophes: Dual Attack of Famine and Influenza

The simultaneous occurrence of famine and the 1918 influenza pandemic in colonial Bengal can be described as an entangled catastrophe, where two separate yet interconnected disasters exacerbated each other's impact. This entanglement was not merely a matter of timing but also structural, highlighting the profound interconnection between biological susceptibility and sociopolitical neglect during colonial rule. Using Michel Foucault's notion of bio-politics (Foucault, 2008, p. 75), which illustrates how modern states exert control over life by regulating populations through health, sanitation, food supply, and mortality management, this dual crisis reveals the shortcomings and failures of colonial governance. The British administration in Bengal practiced selective bio-political governance, prioritizing economic extraction and civil order over the safeguarding of indigenous lives. Relief efforts for the famine were minimal and contingent, while public health responses to the pandemic were sporadic and inadequate. The famine weakened individuals through extended malnutrition and chronic undernourishment, creating conditions that allowed the influenza virus to thrive with increased lethality (Arnold, 2019, pp. 181–195).

The pandemic severely weakened the economic and logistical capabilities of rural Bengal. Agricultural work was disrupted, transportation routes were hindered, and networks for distributing relief collapsed. The colonial government's pre-existing famine regulations, such as the Bengal Famine Code of 1913, were inadequately implemented, highlighting a bureaucratic reluctance to protect local lives during concurrent crises. Viewed from a Foucauldian perspective, the situation exemplifies how colonial bio-politics functioned through a strategy of "letting die"—a passive exercise of power that left vast segments of the population vulnerable to disease and starvation. The intersection of famine and influenza was not merely a natural occurrence but was politically influenced, shaped by the imperial governance framework that regarded the native populace as expendable (Tirmizey, 2020, pp. 1–2). Therefore, this dual catastrophe should be recognized as more than a mere coincidence; it was a historically interconnected event that revealed the structural violence inherent in colonial policies. The intertwining of hunger and disease, along with physical deterioration and governmental neglect, created a devastating scenario where the lines between death from starvation and death from infection became tragically indistinct.

In 1918, colonial Bengal confronted a significant famine and a crisis because of the Spanish Flu pandemic, resulting in great pain and evaluating the endurance of both the people and the colonial government (Srivastava, 1985, pp. 285–324). The collapse of the monsoon triggered food scarcity and famine, while the influenza virus ravaged communities, leading to a significant humanitarian catastrophe and placing colonial Bengal in a dire fight for existence (Sen, 1977, pp. 33, 49, 53). In 1918, colonial Bengal endured a simultaneous disaster: famine and the Spanish Flu pandemic. This merging of emergencies caused widespread distress and assessed the durability of both the populace and the colonial authority. The breakdown of the monsoon resulted in severe food shortages, with basic food grains reaching famine-level prices and a decline in fodder availability lowering milk supply. Escalating costs for items such as blankets and warm clothing worsened the predicament significantly. The influenza virus, a lethal illness, inflicted extensive damage and intensified the humanitarian disaster in colonial Bengal, presenting unprecedented difficulties and intricacies. The lingering question is: this catastrophic virus resulted in the death of how many individuals?

According to various historical sources, such as government reports and contemporary accounts, the famine of 1918 in Bengal was severe and led to considerable human suffering (Bengal Famine Report, 1918, p. 23). Although sources differ, estimates suggest that the famine's death toll reached the tens, if not hundreds, of thousands. One major difficulty in accurately assessing famine deaths arises from the very nature of the crisis itself. Mortality associated with famine often goes beyond direct starvation, encompassing issues like malnutrition, disease outbreaks, and social disruption, complicating efforts to attribute deaths solely to food shortages. The historical record-keeping during colonial Bengal was not as thorough or systematic as modern data collection techniques, further complicating the determination of accurate figures (Bengal Secretariat Report, 1918, p. 61). The 1918 famine in Bengal was a catastrophic event, resulting in extensive suffering and elevated mortality rates. The crisis particularly impacted vulnerable groups, such as the impoverished, elderly, and children, which led to destitution, starvation, and mass displacement. The historical evidence highlights the significance of effective governance, disaster preparedness, and humanitarian help in alleviating future catastrophes, reinforcing the necessity for disaster preparedness and humanitarian actions (Bhatia, 1963b, p. 33).

The article in *The Hindu* (2018, p. 3) shows a connection between the pandemic and famine, illustrating a population at risk of disease outbreaks because of food scarcity and elevated prices. The interplay between socio-economic factors and public health crises is intricate, with economic difficulties heightening vulnerability to infectious diseases. Malnutrition, worsened by famine, raises susceptibility to influenza, affecting at-risk groups such as the malnourished poor and young adults. This dual vulnerability intensified the crisis's severity and contributed to the tragic death toll in Bengal (Brainerd & Siegler, 2003, pp. 3, 5, 23, 33). The flu and famine in Bengal stemmed from systemic issues, including colonial policies and socio-economic factors. The combined impacts of war, monsoon failure, and economic strain created famine-like circumstances and heightened susceptibility to disease outbreaks. Food shortages and increasing prices worsened the condition, resulting in widespread malnutrition and fatalities (Mills, 1989, p. 222). The Bombay Famine Report of 1918–19 emphasized Bengal's resilience compared to earlier famines, credited to the adaptive abilities and coping mechanisms of its agricultural population. The crisis was significant, with Bengal enduring a disproportionate share of misery. Elements like malnutrition resistance and scarcity of food grains contributed to the staggering death toll in India, illustrating the complex dynamics and multifaceted character of the crisis (Bhatia, 1963a, p. 47).

Ultimately, the 1918 famine and Spanish Flu in colonial Bengal serve as a case study of how socio-economic vulnerabilities and public health emergencies intensify human suffering. It underscores the necessity for comprehensive crisis responses, resilience building, community support, and adaptive approaches for recovery following disasters.

Critical Appraisal of the Government Response About Famine

The colonial government's response to the famine of 1918 in colonial Bengal, occurring concurrently with the Spanish Flu pandemic, warrants critical appraisal from various perspectives, including effectiveness, equity, and responsiveness (Arnold, 1988, pp. 73–91).

Effectiveness

Critics criticized the colonial administration's inadequate reaction to the famine. Help efforts, such as relief camps[15] and food aid, were inadequate, resulting in overcrowding and insufficient resource allocation. Bureaucratic inefficiencies and logistical issues obstructed the distribution of aid to impacted regions, further emphasizing the difficulties encountered by the government (Simonow, 2015, p. 21).

Equity

Critics condemned the colonial government's inequitable crisis response, citing reports of favouritism and corruption in relief distribution.

Responsiveness

Critics criticized the colonial government's slow and inadequate reaction to famine and the Spanish Flu pandemic, despite prior warnings. The government failed to plan effectively, secure adequate resources, or possess sufficient medical expertise, resulting in many deaths and widespread hardship. The deficiency in medical knowledge and infrastructure further intensified the crisis (Fagan, 1999, p. 41).

To be more explicit, 1918 represented a crucial turning point in the history of colonial Bengal, as the area encountered the catastrophic impacts of famine and the

Spanish Flu pandemic (Dyson, 1989, pp. 222–260). The dual crises of 1918 and the Permanent Settlement of 1793 revealed weaknesses in colonial governance frameworks and socio-economic disparities within the Indian subcontinent. Colonial policies, such as land revenue systems, concentrated land ownership among affluent landlords and exploited tenant farmers, resulting in poverty and restricted access to resources and economic development for rural Bengalis (Blyn, 1966, pp. 3–13).

In 1918, the failure of monsoon rains aggravated the agricultural crisis, leading to crop failures and food scarcity. The shortage of food grains drove up prices, rendering essentials unaffordable for many. Starvation spread, forcing millions to confront hunger and destitution, particularly in rural regions. The colonial government started relief efforts, such as establishing relief camps in Bengal to provide food help and employment opportunities. However, these initiatives were often inadequate, and many individuals continued to suffer from hunger and malnutrition (Report of the Indian Famine Commission, 1901, pp. 51–71). Meanwhile, the Spanish Flu pandemic, which began in America, then in Europe, swiftly spread to colonial Bengal in 1918, leading to a breakdown of the healthcare system and many deaths because of inadequate sanitation and malnutrition (Mills, 1986, pp. 1–20). A deficiency in resources, medical knowledge, and infrastructure obstructed the colonial government's response to the crisis. Illiteracy and misinformation resulted in hospitals being overwhelmed and public health initiatives failing. As the crises of famine and flu unfolded, public discourse in colonial Bengal increased, with dissenting individuals blaming colonial officials for negligence, incompetence, and indifference towards the suffering of the Indian population, especially the rural poor (Kalpagam, 2002, pp. 39–43).

One of the primary issues was the unequal allocation of relief resources; corruption and favouritism led to allegations of profiteering and exploitation by local officials and merchants. There are demands for enhanced representation and structural reforms to tackle poverty and vulnerability. Despite these obstacles, resilience, solidarity, and grassroots mobilization have emerged in response to the famine and flu pandemic, with local communities, charitable organizations, and religious institutions playing vital roles in providing relief and help (Report of the Indian Famine Commission, 1918, p. 73). Critics criticized the colonial government's reaction to the 1918 famine and Spanish Flu pandemic in colonial Bengal for its lack of effectiveness, fairness, and responsiveness. Relief efforts were frequently inadequate, unjust, and poorly organized, underscoring the systemic shortcomings of British colonial governance in dealing with humanitarian emergencies. These occurrences also underscored the strength and unity of the Indian people, as communities united to help one another amid challenges. The responses to these crises emphasized the pressing necessity for reforms to tackle socio-economic disparities and vulnerabilities (Chhun, 2020, pp. 115–128).

Conclusion

This chapter examines the tragic events of 1918 that devastated colonial Bengal with both famine and the Spanish Flu pandemic. The chapter offers an extensive overview of the famine and influenza pandemic in Bengal, emphasizing their significant effects on the local population. Poor rainfall, elevated food prices, and widespread malnutrition resulted in a severe famine, putting millions in jeopardy of starvation and illness. Despite initial warnings, the colonial administration's response was marked by inefficiency, inequality, and a lack of responsiveness. Bureaucratic obstacles, corruption, and delays frequently tainted relief efforts to provide aid, worsening the plight of those in distress. The government's failure to effectively tackle the Spanish Flu pandemic because of insufficient medical knowledge and infrastructure further intensified the humanitarian crisis and resulted in an overwhelming death toll. The chapter underscores the systemic shortcomings of colonial governance in responding to humanitarian crises and advocates for reforms to tackle socio-economic disparities. It draws attention to the human costs of inaction and urges policymakers to focus on the welfare of all individuals, especially in times of emergencies.

The "March of Death" in colonial Bengal stands as a testament to perseverance. The Indian government prioritized dealing with the Spanish Flu pandemic over the famine because of its perceived manageability, despite the flu's rapid transmission. This viewpoint influenced the shift in focus, where famine was a controllable matter, while the flu represented a more uncontrollable challenge. The government's dependence on local governments and private charities for relief was practical, but the widespread effects of the flu overwhelmed local relief capacities. The flu presented an immediate danger to everyone, resulting in a shift of priorities towards the more controllable issue of famine, even with the flu's extensive impact. This emphasizes the vital priorities and decision-making dynamics of the Indian government during that era. The British authorities' view of their effectiveness in controlling the famine was not entirely accurate. Many news outlets reproached the Government for overlooking the people's suffering, although there was some variation in assigning culpability. Some attributed responsibility to Indian representatives for not adequately conveying the struggles of their populace to the Government, while others criticized the Government itself. The swift emergence of the flu in India caused British officials to redirect their attention to the famine, which resulted in an obsession with death figures instead of focusing on ways to avert future outbreaks. As news circulated, mentions of influenza diminished, and it became just a minor detail in historical narratives. This underscores the difficulties in deciding during crises and the biases that affect how resources are allocated and relief is delivered. The transition from flu to famine illustrates the inclination to give precedence to issues deemed more controllable, frequently neglecting more urgent problems.

Notes

1 Famine—Many factors combine to cause famines. Geographically, they are brought on by natural calamities such as floods and droughts that impair agricultural output and cause food shortages. Socio-economic factors such as poverty, income inequality, political unrest, and economic crises make food inaccessible and expensive for vulnerable

groups, which contributes to famine. A vicious cycle of food insecurity, malnutrition, and humanitarian crises is produced by the interaction of these variables.

2 Monsoon—The monsoon is a seasonal weather pattern that brings heavy rainfall to certain areas for a predetermined amount of time because of a change in wind direction. In many parts of the world, particularly in South and Southeast Asia, it is an important phenomenon. The difference in temperature between the sea and the land causes low-pressure zones to form over land masses, which attracts humid air from the oceans and causes the monsoon. This humid air rises and cools, releasing copious amounts of precipitation that are vital to agriculture, water resources, and the general health of the ecosystem.

3 Legislative Councils—An essential part of the legislative process is the Legislative Council, sometimes referred to as the upper house or second chamber of a bicameral legislature. The Legislative Council's members are frequently chosen or appointed according to a variety of standards, guaranteeing representation from a range of social groups. Legislative review and amendment, acting as a check on government actions, and minority or regional interest representation are among the Council's primary responsibilities.

4 Indian Medical Service (IMS)—In India's medical history, the Indian Medical Service (IMS) has played a pivotal role. One of the nation's first organized medical services, it was founded in 1772 by the British East India Company. Throughout the colonial era, the IMS was essential in providing medical care to the Indian populace. The service comprised doctors, surgeons, and pharmacists who worked in different parts of India. They were to establish hospitals, offer medical support to the British military, perform medical research, and provide the local populace with healthcare services.

5 Famine Code—One important piece of legislation passed in India during the colonial era was the Famine Code. The British government instituted it in 1883 as a solution to the nation's ongoing famine problems. A framework for famine relief and prevention was established by the Famine Code. During times of famine, it included provisions for the creation of relief camps, the distribution of food and supplies, and the execution of public works initiatives. To effectively respond to food shortages and lessen the effects of famine, the code also stressed the significance of early warning systems, effective administration, and coordination between various government departments.

6 Permanent Settlement in Bengal—The second Governor-General of Bengal, Lord Cornwallis, established the Permanent Settlement, also referred to as the Permanent Settlement of Bengal, in 1793. It was a substantial land revenue system. Under this system, land revenue was fixed for a set amount of time, usually in perpetuity, and usually at a high rate. The Permanent Settlement promoted agricultural productivity, offered stability, and brought in money for the Company. But the effects were far-reaching. It was harmful to the peasants even though it benefitted the zamindars (landlords), who acquired hereditary rights over land and served as middlemen between the peasants and the British government.

7 Indigo—Indigo has a noteworthy role in colonial India's history. The plant, known as indigo, or Indigofera tinctoria, was used to make a vivid blue dye. Bengal and other regions of India saw the rise of indigo cultivation as a significant cash crop during the British colonial era. The indigo cultivation system was imposed by the British planters, who made the Indian farmers cultivate indigo on a portion of their land. The 1859–1860 Indigo Revolt was a notable rebellion against these repressive customs.

8 The Great Bengal Famine 1770—During the British East India Company's rule, one of the worst famines in Indian history occurred during the Great Bengal Famine of 1770. This devastating event, which occurred between 1769 and 1773, claimed the lives of about 10 million people, or almost one-third of the region's total population. A combination of human and natural factors contributed to the famine; in Bengal, a severe drought caused crop failures, but British economic policies made matters worse.

9 Late Victorian Holocausts—The term "Late Victorian Holocausts" describes a string of catastrophic famines that struck late-19th-century European colonies, mainly Brazil, China, and India. Millions of people died because of these tragedies, which had severe long-term socio-economic effects and were aggravated by colonial powers' exploitative economic policies and El Niño weather patterns. The phrase emphasizes the scope and human cost of these catastrophes, comparing them to a holocaust because of their immense destruction and the political choices made by humans that contributed to their severity.

10 Infectious Pathogens—Infectious pathogens are organisms that cause diseases in their hosts, including viruses, bacteria, fungi, and parasites. These pathogens can enter, survive, and multiply within the host body, leading to infections that can range from mild to life-threatening. Viruses, such as the influenza virus and SARS-CoV-2, are tiny, simple organisms that require living cells to replicate. Bacteria, like Streptococcus and Escherichia coli, can often survive independently and may benefit or harm their hosts depending on the species.

11 South-West Monsoon—A major meteorological phenomenon, the South-West Monsoon, brings vital rainfall to the Indian subcontinent from June to September, sustaining agriculture, replenishing water supplies, and influencing the economies of multiple nations. The Indian Ocean, where warm air rises and forms a low-pressure area over the subcontinent, is the source of this monsoon. The southwest's moisture-laden winds sweep across the ocean, accumulating moisture and delivering substantial rainfall to the area.

12 Berar—Berar, historically known as a significant region in central India, has played an important role in Indian history. This region, also known as Vidarbha in ancient texts, was strategically located, serving as a corridor between northern and southern India. Berar's historical significance is underscored by its mention in various ancient and medieval Indian scriptures and records. Throughout its history, Berar has been known for its agricultural productivity, particularly in cotton cultivation, which remains an economic staple. Today, Berar corresponds roughly to the Amravati and Akola divisions of Maharashtra, keeping its historical legacy as a region of cultural and agricultural importance.

13 India's Agricultural Cycle—India's agricultural cycle, which mainly revolves around the monsoon season, is closely linked to the country's climate. The two primary cropping seasons of the cycle are Kharif and Rabi. Crops are sown at the start of the monsoon and harvested at the end of the season, which coincides with the South-West Monsoon (June to September). Rice, corn, sorghum, and pulses are the main crops grown during Kharif. The winter months of October through March are known as the Rabi season. In this season, crops are planted in the fall and harvested in the spring. Rabi crops, including wheat, barley, and peas, are cultivated during this season.

14 Mr. Kamini Kumar Chanda—Mr. Kamini Kumar Chanda was a notable figure during the 1918 famine in India, which coincided with the global influenza pandemic and affected large parts of the country, particularly Gujarat and parts of Maharashtra. As a social reformer and humanitarian, Mr. Chanda played a pivotal role in organizing relief efforts for the affected populations. His work primarily focused on the distribution of food and medical supplies, which were critical because of the compounded impact of famine and disease.

15 Relief Camps—Relief camps became essential for the survival of many affected populations during the 1918 famine that struck India during the global influenza pandemic. The main purpose of these camps was to offer basic medical care, food, and shelter to people who were severely affected by the disease outbreak and food scarcity. The harsh and crowded conditions inside the camps, coupled with the lack of access to clean water and medical supplies, might worsen the spread of influenza.

References

Books

Arnold, D. (1988). *Famine: Social crisis and historical change*. Blackwell.

Arnold, D. (1993a). *Colonizing the body: State medicine and epidemic disease in nineteenth-century India*. University of California Press.

Arnold, D. (2021). Representation and remembrance: The 1918–19 influenza epidemic in India. In G. Beiner (Ed.), *Pandemic re-awakenings: The forgotten and unforgotten 'Spanish' flu of 1918–1919* (pp. 187–C10.P27). Oxford Academic. (Online edition).

Arnold, D. (2022). *Pandemic India: From cholera to Covid-19*. Hurst & Company.

Bhatia, B. M. (1963a). *Famines in India: A study of the aspects of the economic history of India (1860–1965)*. Asia Publishing House.

Bhatia, B. M. (1963b). *The history of Indian famines and development of famine policy (1858–1918)*. Asia Publishing House.

Bhatia, B. M. (2006). Nature and causes of famines in India. In B. Nand (Ed.), *Famines in Colonial India: Some unofficial historical narratives* (pp. 507–533). University of Delhi.

Blair, C. (2006). Indian famines: Their historical, financial and other aspects. In B. Nand (Ed.), *Famines in Colonial India: Some unofficial historical narratives* (pp. 67–157). University of Delhi.

Blyn, G. (1966). *Agricultural trends in India,* 1891–1947*: Output, availability, and productivity*. University of Pennsylvania Press.

Brennan, L. (1984). The development of the Indian famine codes: Personalities, politics, and policies. In B. Currey & G. Hugo (Eds.), *Famine* (pp. 1–26). *The geo journal library* (Vol. 1). Springer. https://doi.org/10.1007/978-94-009-6395-5_6

Brennan, L. (2012). The development of the Indian famine codes: Personalities, politics, and policies. In B. Currey & G. Hugo (Eds.), *Famine as a geographical phenomenon* (pp. 91–111). Springer.

Chakrabarti, P. (2012). *Bacteriology in British India: Laboratory medicine and the tropics*. University of Rochester Press.

Chhun, M. (2015, August 12). *Death and disorder: The 1918–1919 influenza pandemic in British India* (Unpublished doctoral dissertation). Department of History, University of Colorado.

Davis, M. (2001). *Late Victorian holocausts: El Niño famines and the making of the third world*. Verso.

Dyson, T. (Ed.). (1989). *India's historical demography: Studies in famine, disease and society* (Collected Papers on South Asia, No. 8). Curzon Press Limited.

Fagan, B. (1999). *Colonial policies and their impact on food security in British India*. Oxford University Press.

Famine Inquiry Commission. (1918). *Report on Bengal*. Government of India Press.

Famine Inquiry Commission. (1945). *Report on Bengal* (Woodhead Committee Report). Government of India Press.

Felix, J. (2012). *Managing scarcity: The famine codes and colonial governance in British India*. Oxford University Press.

Foodstuffs and Transport Board. (1918, August 2). *Report on relief efforts during the 1918 famine*. Government Printing Office.

Foucault, M. (2008). *The birth of biopolitics: Lectures at the Collège de France, 1978–1979* (G. Burchell, Trans.). Palgrave Macmillan. (Original work published 2004)

Ghosh, K. (1944). *Famines in Bengal: 1770–1943*. National Council of Education.

Government of Bengal. (1913). *The Bengal famine code*. The Bengal Secretariat Book Depot.

Harrison, M. (1994). *Public health in British India: Anglo-Indian preventive medicine 1859–1914*. Cambridge University Press.

Maharatna, A. (1992). *The demography of Indian famines: A historical perspective* [PhD thesis, University of London].

McAlpin, M. B. (1983). *Subject to famine: Food crisis and economic change in Western India, 1860–1920*. Princeton University Press.
Miller, R. (1902–1903). *Famine relief and revenue policies in British India*. Government Press.
Mills, I. D. (1989). Influenza in India during 1918–19. In T. Dyson (Ed.), *India's historical demography: Studies in famine, disease, and society* (pp. 222–226). Curzon Press.
Report of the Indian Famine Commission. (1880). *Part I. Famine relief* (600 pp.). George Edward Eyre and William Spottiswoode.
Report of the Indian Famine Commission. (1898). Government of India Press (pp. 359–363).
Sen, A. (1981). *Poverty and famines: An essay on entitlement and deprivation*. Oxford Academic.
Sen, A. (1983). *Poverty and famines: An essay on entitlement and deprivation*. Oxford University Press.
Simonow, J. (2015). *Responses To famine and displacement in nineteenth and twentieth century India*. ODI. https://www.jstor.org/stable/resrep50682.5
Simonow, J. (2023). *Colonial strategies for famine prevention: Agricultural productivity and infrastructure in British India*. Cambridge University Press.
Srivastava, H. S. (1968). *The history of Indian famines and development of famine policy* (1858–1918). Sri Ram Mehra & Co. Publishers.
Stahl, R. M. (2016). The economics of starvation: Laissez-Faire ideology and famine in colonial India. In T. Thorup (Ed.), *Intellectual history of economic normativities* (pp. 169–184). Palgrave Macmillan.
The Hindu. (2018, September 30). *Agricultural situation: Outlook in Bombay*. https://www.thehindu.com/agricultural-situation-outlook-in-bombay
Tirmizey, K. (2020, May 23). *Pandemics and hunger: Lessons from the 1918 pandemic in India*. India Essay. https://indiaessay.in/pandemics-and-hunger-lessons-from-the-1918-pandemic-in-india/
Turner, M. (1918). *Agricultural disruptions and famine in colonial Bengal*. Harper & Brothers.
White, F. N. (1919). *The influenza pandemic of 1918 in India: The sanitary commissioner with the Government of India*. Government Monotype Press.
Williams, H. (1985). *Famine and relief administration in British India*. Routledge.
Wood, G. (1918). *Famine codes: Their principles and their results*. Macmillan.

Articles

Arnold, D. (1979). Looting, grain riots and government policy in South India 1918. *Past & Present*, *84*, 111–145.
Arnold, D. (1993b). Social crisis and epidemic disease in the famines of nineteenth century India. *Social History of Medicine*, *6*(3), 385–404.
Arnold, D. (2019). Death and the modern empire: The 1918–19 influenza epidemic in India. *Transactions of the Royal Historical Society*, *29*, 181–200.
Bagchi, A. K. (2014). Indian economy and society during world war one. *Social Scientist*, *42*(7/8), 5–27.
Brainerd, E., & Siegler, M. V. (2003). The economic effects of the 1918 influenza epidemic. *CEPR Discussion Papers*, *3791*, 1–46.
Brennan, L., Heathcote, L., & Lucas, A. (1984). The causation of famine: A comparative analysis of Lombok and Bengal, 1891–1974. *South Asia*, *7*(1), 1–26.
Chhun, M. (2019–2020). A good winter rain will put everything right: The British Government in India's Response to the 1918 influenza pandemic and famine. *Journal of Pandemics in Historical Perspective*, *19*, 1–11.
Chhun, M. (2020, April 30). How the 1918 flu pandemic killed 12 million Indians. *Madras Courier*.https://madrascourier.com/insight/how-the-1918-flu-pandemic-killed-12-million-indians/

Greenough, P. R. (1980). Indian famines and peasant victims: The case of Bengal in 1943–44. *Modern Asian Studies*, *14*(2), 205–235.
Haggis, J., Jarrett, S., Taylor, D., & Mayer, P. (1986). By the teeth: A critical examination of James Scott's the moral economy of the peasant. *World Development*, *14*(12), 1435–1455.
Kalpagam, U. (2002). Colonial governmentality and the public sphere in India. *Journal of Historical Sociology*, *15*(1), 35–58.
Kaur, S. (2022). Agrarian crisis in India: Causes and consequences. *Apeejay Journal of Management & Technology*, *17*(1), 24–42.
Kumar, N. (2016). Economic impact of British colonial rule on Indian agriculture: A review. *International Research Journal of Social Sciences*, *5*(2), 56–58.
Kumar, R. (2018). An overview of land revenue systems of British India. *Research Review International Journal of Multidisciplinary*, *3*(6), 518–520.
Matthews, D. H. (2008). Inaccurate conceptions: Disputed measures of nutritional needs and famine deaths in Colonial India. *Modern Asian Studies*, *42*(6), 1189–1212.
Mills, I. D. (1986). The 1918–1919 influenza pandemic—The Indian experience. *Indian Economic and Social History Review*, *23*(1), 1–40.
Mishra, V., Tiwari, A. D., Aadhar, S., Shah, R., Xiao, M., Pai, D. S., & Lettenmaier, D. (2019). Drought and famine in India, 1870–2016. *Geophysical Research Letters*, *46*(4), 2075–2083.
Ojo, O. B. (2020). Socio-economic impacts of 1918–19 influenza epidemic in Punjab. *Journal of Asian and African Studies*, *55*(7), 1023–1032.
Padel, F. (2012). Review: Structural violence and the Bengal famine of 1943. *Economic and Political Weekly*, *47*(44), 26–28.
Passmore, R. (1951). Famine in India: An historical survey. *The Lancet*, *258*(6677), 303–307.
Roy, T. (2002). Economic history and modern India: Redefining the link. *The Journal of Economic Perspectives*, *16*(3), 109–130.
Sahu, A. C. (1978). Export of food grains, a potent cause of famines in India between 1860 and 1900. *Proceedings of the Indian History Congress*, *39*(II), 808–815.
Sen, A. (1977). The making of a disaster: A note on the Bengal samine. *Cambridge Journal of Economics*, *1*(1), 33–54.
Srivastava, R. P. (1985). Famine, disease, and the social order in early modern India. *Indian Economic & Social History Review*, *22*(2), 139–165.
Tabor, M. H. (1910). Famine relief in India. *Charity Organization Review*, New Series, *27*(162), 295–302.
Tambolkar, S., Pustake, M., Giri, P., & Tambolkar, I. (2022). Comparison of public health measures taken during Spanish Flu and COVID-19 pandemics: A narrative review. *Journal of Family Medicine and Primary Care*, *11*(5), 642–647.
Taylor, W. (1873). Famines in India: Their remedy and prevention. *East India Association*, *7*, 143–182.
Tiwari, K. A., & Sharma, S. R. (2023). Impact of British colonial rule on Indian peasantry. *Indian Journal of Social Studies and Humanities*, *1*(14), 25–31.

Archival Sources

Books and Reports

Bengal Famine Report 1918. (1918). Government of India.
Famine Inquiry Commission. (1945). *Report on Bengal (Woodhead Committee Report).*
Report of the Indian Famine Commission. (1901). *Appendix I to V, evidence of witness.* Calcutta.
Report of the Indian Famine Commission. (1918). pp. 359–63.
Resolution on the administration of famine relief in the United Provinces of Agra and Oudh during the years 1907 and 1908. (1918). Government Press, United Provinces.

Government Documents

Campbell, C. (1918, August 30). Campbell to Secretary, Rev. (Spl.). T.N.A., G.O. 455, Rev. (Spl.) (Conf.), 30 September 1918.
Cardew, Note. (1918, September 15). T.N.A., G.O. 593, Rev. (Spl.) (Conf.), 13 October 1918.
Famine Proceedings 1874–1919. (1874–1919). Famine was a branch of the Revenue, Agriculture, and Commerce (Agriculture and Horticulture) from 1874 to 1879; from 1880 to June 1881, it was in the Home, Revenue, and Agriculture Department from July 1881 to 1919. It was a part of the Revenue and Agriculture Department.
Famine Programmes. (1902, November). Nos. 10 to 22.
Famine Programmes. (1902, November). No. 23.
Famine Programmes. (1902, November). No. 113.
Famine Programmes. (1903, May). No. 1.
Famine Programmes. (1903, May). Nos. 1, 2, 3, and 4.
Famine Programmes. (1903, May). No. 4.
Famine Programmes. (1903, September). No. 5, Circular No. 21-96-3 from J. O. Miller, Secretary to the Govt. of India to local Governments and Administration, Dept. of Revenue and Agriculture, Famine, Simla, 23 September 1903; F.C. 1901, Report para 216.
Famine Programmes. (1905, March). No. 13.
Famine Programmes. (1905, November). No. 1.
Famine Programmes. (1906, January). Nos. 4 to 7.
Famine Programmes. (1918, March). Nos. 1 to 3.
Proceedings of the Govt. of Bengal. (1918, December). Municipal Dept. Sanitation Branch, File No: S Q-5 and S Q–2.
Proceedings of the Govt. of India. (1919, November). Home Department, Nos. 300–305.
Resolution Govt. of India Dept. of Revenue and Agriculture (Famine) No. 12-43-30, dated 26th August 1901; Famine Progs. No. 23, November 1902; Dispatch No. 73 of 1902 from the Govt. of India, dated 30th October 1902; Famine Programmes. No. 1, May 1903.
Wood, R. B. (1918, September 15). Director of Civil Supplies to Secretary, Rev. (Special). T.N.A., G.O. 841, Rev. (Spl.), 5 December 1918.

Newspapers

From the Archives June 26, 1918. (2018, June 26). Curious fever epidemic in Bombay. *The Hindu*.
Lokopakari. (1918, September 23). In Native Newspaper Reports; *Indian Patriot*, 10 September 1918, cutting in T.N.A., G.O. 922, Public (Conf.), 8 October 1918.
The famine and the flu. (1918, September 19). *The Hindu*, p. 5.
The Hindu. (1918, September 4). p. 5.
Turner, J. A. (1918, September 28). Influenza pandemic: Health officer's appeal. *Times of India*.

4 Diseases, Medicine, and Colonialism

Influenza and the Politics of Imperialism

The Influenza Crisis: A Turning Point in Colonial Medicine and Nationalist Movements

The intersection of disease, medicine, and colonialism is intricate, with infectious diseases often playing a significant role in colonial expansion and maintenance. The 1918–20 Influenza Pandemic exemplifies how epidemics[1] can significantly influence imperial rule and nationalist resistance (Tumbe, 2020, pp. 127–175). The present chapter examines the Indian subcontinent during British colonial administration, focusing on the Indian Medical Service's (IMS) role in containing the devastating influenza pandemic within India's diverse population, highlighting the complex interplay between imperial control and public health (Rai, 2018, pp. 827–830).

The influenza outbreak highlighted power dynamics in colonial societies. Colonial authorities used public health measures to reinforce imperial legitimacy, while nationalist leaders criticized the colonial medical system and demanded self-governance (Arnold, 2022, pp. 187–198). The chapter also explored the commercial exploitation of public health anxieties during the pandemic (Bayly, 1975, p. 11). Entrepreneurs exploited fear and uncertainty by marketing "cures", highlighting the conflict between public welfare and private enterprise's profit motives amid a global health crisis (Beiner, 2021, pp. 45–55).

The Influenza Pandemic of 1918–20 was a significant event in the history of disease, medicine, and imperialism, highlighting the interplay between colonial power, nationalist resistance, and international health governance. The Indian subcontinent's experiences under British rule exemplify this complex interplay (Kupperberg, 2008, pp. 12–23).

Disease, Medicine, and Imperialism

David Arnold, in his work "Colonizing the Body: State Medicine and Epidemic Disease in Nineteenth-Century India," asserts that the medical history of India is deeply intertwined with the narrative of British colonialism. He describes medicine as a battleground where the authority and effectiveness of western science were both proclaimed and contested.

DOI: 10.4324/9781003656647-5

> *It is crucial to recognize that colonialism imposed not only political control but also sought to regulate the health and bodies of the colonized populations. In this context, medicine served as both an instrument of imperial power and a means for the colonized to resist and challenge that authority.*
> (Arnold, 1993, pp. 7, 9)

The tone of these narratives has helped to shape the current discourse courteously. These narratives portray the interplay of disease, medicine, and imperialism, which took centre stage during the influenza pandemic in India. Imperialism played a significant role in both the dissemination of the disease and the response to it (Arnold, 1988, pp. 1–26). European colonial powers, primarily European nations, established empires in Africa, Asia, and the Americas, acquiring unparalleled global control by the late 19th century. This included extensive settlement expansion, global trade, and transportation routes, and European authority over non-European territories (Kohn, 2007, pp. 214–216). This dominance significantly impacted the history of disease, its dissemination, and global communities' ability to withstand western power and influence (Hays, 2009, pp. 179–213). Colonial empires, like other diseases, not only facilitated the global spread of the influenza (respiratory) virus[2] but also influenced how different regions experienced and managed the pandemic (Crosby, 2003, pp. 17–37). Colonial healthcare systems were often inadequate, catering more to European settlers' needs than local populations, a disparity highlighted during the pandemic because of inadequate supplies, personnel, and infrastructure (Harrison, 1994, pp. 75–102).

The Spanish Influenza outbreak in India in 1918–19 was influenced by the interplay of disease, medicine, and imperialism. The British colonial administration's policies and priorities shaped the distribution of medical resources, accessibility of healthcare services, and overall pandemic management, highlighting the unique challenges faced by India during this time (Arnold, 1993a, pp. 240–290). Imperialism significantly impacted disease transmission and control in India during the Spanish Influenza outbreak because of the British colonial governance system prioritizing colonial rulers' needs (Chakrabarti, 2013, pp. 101–122). This unequal power dynamic influenced the allocation of resources for healthcare and disease control, with a focus on maintaining the health of the British officials and military personnel rather than the general Indian populace (Byerly, 2010, pp. 82, 85–87). Imperial neglect and British policies in India exposed the population to influenza virus spread, resulting in uneven distribution of medical resources during the pandemic (Harrison, 1994, pp. 202–227). Hospitals and healthcare facilities in urban centres, where British officials lived, received better funding and support compared to rural areas where most of the Indian population lived (Kumar, 1994, p. 145). The Spanish Influenza's impact in rural India was exacerbated by unequal healthcare access, highlighting the underlying inequalities perpetuated by imperialism in India (Arnold, 2019, pp. 182–185).

Medicine, as a tool of imperialism, played a dual role during the Spanish Influenza outbreak in India. On one hand, western medical knowledge and practices were introduced by the British colonial administration, leading to advancements in healthcare and disease management (Arnold, 2000, pp. 9–19). British authorities established medical colleges, training programmes, and hospitals in India, promoting modern medical practices. Western medicine was crucial in diagnosing and treating influenza cases, providing relief. However, the Eurocentric approach[3] promoted by the British administration had limitations during the Spanish Influenza outbreak, despite that this approach very often disregarded traditional Indian healing practices[4] and indigenous knowledge systems[5] (Bhattacharya, 2006, pp. 105–163). The exclusion of indigenous communities from pandemic response efforts because of marginalization of local medical traditions and imposing western practices reflected imperial power dynamics (Chakrabarti, 2012, pp. 136–137).

India's dependency on western medicine during the Spanish Influenza outbreak underscored its dependence on imported supplies, exacerbated by disruptions in global supply chains because of World War I (Mills, 2014, p. 57). India's reliance on imported medical supplies exposed the vulnerabilities of the country's healthcare system to external forces, further underscoring the impact of imperialism on disease management during the pandemic (Harrison, 2012, pp. 80, 247). The Spanish Influenza outbreak in India in 1918–19 highlighted the complex relationship between disease, medicine, and imperialism. British colonial rule influenced healthcare systems, response strategies, and the pandemic trajectory. Unequal medical resource distribution, western medical practices, and dependency on imported supplies were manifestations of imperialism's impact on disease control (Amrith, 2006, p. 43). The Spanish Influenza outbreak in colonial India underscores the need for fair and culturally sensitive disease management and healthcare delivery, influenced by disease, medicine, and imperialism (Harrison, 2010, pp. 189–190). The Spanish Influenza outbreak in India in 1918–19 highlighted the need for systemic inequalities and restructuring healthcare systems to ensure fair access to medical resources and culturally sensitive care. The legacy of imperialism in healthcare policies caused decolonizing approaches, prioritizing local knowledge and community engagement, and building resilient, responsive healthcare systems for diverse populations (Amrith, 2006, pp. 72–98). The Spanish Influenza outbreak in India underscored the need for integrating indigenous healing practices and knowledge systems into public health strategies to promote health and well-being (Mukharji, 2016, pp. 1–35). During the Spanish Influenza pandemic, local healers and traditional medicine practitioners provided support to communities without formal healthcare, integrating traditional practices with modern methods for improved health outcomes (Sen, 2005, pp. 42–45). India's dependency on western medicine during the Spanish Influenza outbreak underscored its dependence on imported supplies, exacerbated by disruptions in global supply chains because of World War I (Mills, 2014, p. 57). India's reliance on imported medical supplies exposed the vulnerabilities of the country's healthcare system to external forces, further underscoring the impact of imperialism on disease management during the pandemic (Harrison, 2012, pp. 80, 247).

The Spanish Influenza outbreak underscored the need for robust public health infrastructure and healthcare system strengthening, while India's healthcare system's vulnerabilities during the 1918–19 pandemic exposed its vulnerabilities

(Johnson & Mueller, 2002, pp. 105, 107–110). Resilient healthcare systems prioritize preventive care, early detection, and rapid response to mitigate disease outbreaks and safeguard population health. The Spanish Influenza pandemic in India underscored global health interconnectedness and international cooperation in addressing transnational health challenges (Taubenberger & Morens, 2006, pp. 15–22). The rapid spread of the influenza virus across borders during the 1918–19 pandemic highlighted the need for coordinated efforts among countries to prevent, detect, and respond to infectious diseases (Barry, 2004, p. 53). Collaborative initiatives, such as information sharing, resource mobilization, and joint research efforts, can help strengthen global health security and enhance the capacity of countries to effectively manage pandemics and health emergencies (Crosby, 2003, pp. 295–311).

The Spanish Influenza outbreak in India from 1918 to 1919 highlighted the significant impact of disease, medicine, and imperialism on public health and healthcare systems. British colonial rule influenced sociopolitical structures, healthcare policies, and response mechanisms, providing insights into public health governance, healthcare delivery, and community resilience during health crises (Arnold, 1988b, pp. 1–27). The 1918–19 influenza outbreak in India underscores the impact of disease, medicine, and imperialism on public health systems. It underscores the need for a comprehensive strategy to address health inequalities, promote social fairness, and improve health equality for all groups. Analyzing imperialism's influence on healthcare strategies can help establish more diverse, culturally aware public health structures (Elbe, 2012, pp. 56–58).

Resistance and Distrust: Indigenous Reactions to Colonial Medical Authority During the 1918 Influenza Pandemic in Bengal

During the Spanish Influenza outbreak of 1918–19 in colonial Bengal, conflicts emerged between local stakeholders—including indigenous physicians, nationalists, and vernacular media—and the colonial medical authorities. The response of the British colonial administration to the pandemic faced significant criticism for being insufficient, culturally insensitive, and politically driven. Local practitioners, many of whom were educated in traditional systems such as Ayurveda and Unani, alongside those holding western medical qualifications, frequently challenged the standardized colonial medical approaches that disregarded local health beliefs, spiritual healing methods, and environmental factors. Numerous such practitioners articulated their critiques in medical journals and popular newspapers, emphasizing the shortcomings of the Indian Medical Service (IMS) in meeting the distinct needs of Bengal's rural and urban impoverished populations. Bengali doctors, including Dr. Nilratan Sircar and others connected to nationalist movements, openly denounced the indifference of the colonial government and began promoting self-reliance through traditional remedies, home-based care, and community relief efforts (Mukherjee, 2017a, p. 91).

Nationalist leaders and organizations, particularly those associated with the Indian National Congress and local Swadeshi movements, perceived colonial health initiatives as a means of extending imperial dominance. They contended that British officials prioritized the health of European elites and military installations over that of the indigenous population. This viewpoint was exacerbated by the unequal distribution of quinine, the rapid burial of Indian corpses without appropriate ceremonies, and the scarcity of accessible medical services in rural areas such as Dacca, Pabna, and Rangpur. As a result, there was a notable increase in grassroots opposition to colonial health initiatives, including refusals to accept treatment from government-operated dispensaries. The populace, particularly in remote villages, frequently rejected government-issued medications, suspecting them to be experimental or ineffective mixtures. A profound political mistrust prompted many individuals to seek assistance from local healers, traditional medicine, and religious institutions rather than embracing western medical practices (Harrison, 1994, p. 274).

Local vernaculars such as the *Amrita Bazar Patrika* and *The Bengalee* played a crucial role in amplifying public dissatisfaction. These newspapers criticized the colonial government's negligence and highlighted distressing images of neglected corpses, inadequately equipped hospitals, and untrained caregivers. They also praised local relief initiatives, frequently underscoring nationalist ideals like self-sufficiency and indigenous expertise. Some editorials even charged the government with exploiting the pandemic to curtail civil liberties and postpone reforms. The media emerged as a powerful instrument for shaping public sentiment, not only to condemn the colonial administration but also to promote solidarity and mutual assistance within Bengali society. As a whole, it can be said that the influenza pandemic in Bengal represented a significant convergence of health, politics, and resistance (Mukherjee, 2017b, pp. 134–138). Indigenous healthcare practitioners, nationalist leaders, and vernacular media collectively forged a robust narrative that questioned the authority and legitimacy of colonial medical efforts. Public refusals of treatment, stemming from political scepticism and cultural discord, highlighted the widespread distrust of imperial institutions during one of the most catastrophic public health crises in Indian history.

Influenza Pandemic and the Indian Medical Service (IMS)

> *Nandini Bhattacharya, in her work "Contagion and Enclaves: Tropical Medicine in Colonial India," emphasizes the impact of the Indian Medical Service (IMS) during the influenza pandemic. She notes that "The 1918 influenza pandemic exposed the significant shortcomings of the colonial medical system in India. The Indian Medical Service, inundated with a high volume of cases and deaths, found it challenging to deliver adequate help, underscoring the profound inequalities in healthcare between the colonial authorities and the Indian population."*
>
> (Bhattacharya, 2012, p. 145)

The narrative's tenor has significantly contributed to shape the current discourse positively. This highly relevant narrative makes the present researcher to think that it is absolutely necessary to bring the historical context of the Indian Medical Service right at the beginning of the current discourse. The author focuses on the social necessity and reasons behind the Indianization of the Indian Medical Service (IMS) during the 1918–19 Spanish Influenza pandemic. The IMS failed to provide adequate services to the Indian populace, particularly the rural population, despite the necessity for medical care. Understanding the factors that impacted the IMS system is crucial to comprehending its failure during such a devastating pandemic.

The Indian Medical Service (IMS) has been in operation since the early days of British colonial rule, initially providing medical services in Bengal, Madras, and Bombay. During the early decades of the 19th century, as the English East India Company[6] combined its command over these presidencies, the requirement for organized clinical consideration for its soldiers and authorities became clear (Kumar, 1998, p. 93). The earliest of the clinical benefits laid out in the English administrations in India was the Madras Medical Service,[7] which was established in 1763. This was trailed by the Bengal Medical Service[8] in 1764 and the Bombay Medical Service[9] in 1785 (Arnold, 1993b, p. 35). Initially concentrating on the well-being of British soldiers, military medical services subsequently broadened their scope to encompass civilian healthcare. However, challenges like tropical diseases, limited medical knowledge, and harsh Indian climate hindered the administration of clinical benefits (Kumar, 2006, p. 47).

The administrations initially had few specialists and partner specialists who were often under-resourced. As the colonial population and local Indian communities grew, the presidency expanded its medical services to civilian healthcare. By the mid-19th century, these services had advanced significantly, including emergency clinics, dispensaries, and participation in health initiatives like smallpox immunization campaigns. Medical education also became a focus, with the establishment of a Medical College in Calcutta, Madras, and Bombay (Harrison, 2006, p. 175). European institutions educated European doctors and started teaching Indian doctors, leading to the formation of the Indian Medical Service (IMS) in 1896. The IMS incorporated highly qualified specialists from England, many of whom were alumni of prestigious institutions like the Royal College of Surgeons. These officers worked in both military and civilian sectors, contributing to the establishment of clinics, medical colleges, and general health drives. The IMS also contributed to clinical exploration and the advancement of medical science in India, particularly in the treatment of tropical diseases prevalent in the region (Oberoi, 2015, pp. 61–74). The Indian Medical Service (IMS) was criticized for being an instrument of colonial control, often aligning with British interests rather than the Indian population's needs. Indian medical professionals were often excluded from the IMS's hierarchy, limiting their advancement opportunities. Despite this, the IMS laid the groundwork for India's current medical establishments and practices, impacting Indian medical care even after 1947's autonomy. India's healthcare system is built on the foundation of IMS's medical colleges, hospitals, and public health initiatives, contributing to the country's ongoing efforts to improve public health and medical education (Crawford, 1914, pp. 235–244).

During the Spanish Influenza, the Indian Medical Service (IMS) faced challenges in colonial Bengal, particularly because of the global health crisis, which devastated populations worldwide (Chandavarkar, 1992, pp. 125–149). The IMS, a key part of British colonial administration, played a pivotal role in response efforts, using medical interventions and public health strategies, facing limitations, and influencing sociopolitical implications (Mills, 2004, pp. 1–15). The IMS, responsible for diagnosing and treating influenza cases, faced overwhelming medical services during the pandemic. Hospitals and dispensaries were filled, and makeshift arrangements were made to accommodate the overflow of patients. British and Indian doctors, along with many other practitioners, worked tirelessly to manage the influx (Arnold, 2019, pp. 185–189). The researchers focused on treating symptoms and understanding the virus's nature, as standard treatment protocols were palliative, focusing on alleviating fever, cough, and pain because of the lack of antiviral drugs (Johnson & Mueller, 2002, pp. 111–113).

Besides direct medical care, the IMS implemented several public health measures to curb the spread of the disease. Quarantine[10] and isolation were common practices, although their effectiveness was limited by the dense and often impoverished living conditions in Bengal. IMS propaganda effectively targeted urban areas, but neglected rural populations, leading to fatal disease severity and horror because of lack of awareness (Humphries, 2013, pp. 58–109). Public health campaigns aimed to educate the population about hygiene practices, which were limited by literacy rates and communication barriers, while the IMS neglected to provide clean water and sanitation facilities, crucial for preventing secondary infections (Crosby, 2003, p. 57). The Indian Medical Service (IMS) played a crucial role in data collection and epidemiology during the pandemic. However, the lack of proper record-keeping and maintenance of detailed records hindered the monitoring of the outbreak's trajectory and resource allocation. The IMS's efforts were part of the colonial administration's attempt to maintain control during a crisis. The pandemic scale and healthcare infrastructure limitations often compromised the reliability of this data. The IMS faced a critical challenge in the scarcity of medical personnel and supplies, especially in Bengal (Killingray & Phillips, 2003, p. 85). The IMS faced shortages of drugs, medical equipment, and basic supplies because of World War I, which strained resources and diverted attention to the war effort. This dual burden led to difficult decisions about resource allocation and care prioritization (Arnold, 2019, pp. 185–188).

In such a vacillating state, the Indian Medical Service (IMS) disproportionately concentrated its efforts on protecting the health of British officials, military personnel, and essential economic hubs, often neglecting the public health needs of rural and indigenous communities throughout colonial Bengal. As an entity of the colonial system, the IMS prioritized the safeguarding of imperial interests—particularly the maintenance of administrative functions, the security of European settlements, and the operational integrity of ports, railways, and plantations crucial to the colonial economy. This selective allocation of resources resulted in significant areas of Bengal, especially districts such as Mymensingh, Bogra, and Faridpur, experiencing a severe shortage of medical care, medications, and burial facilities. This strategy mirrored the overarching racial and class prejudices inherent in colonial public health policies, where the lives of Europeans and imperial profits were deemed more valuable than those of the colonized populace. The limited hospitals and trained medical staff were primarily situated in urban areas like Calcutta and military bases, leaving rural regions reliant on untrained volunteers or local practitioners. The actions and inactions of the IMS fostered widespread discontent and faced considerable criticism from both nationalist groups and the vernacular media of the era (Harrison, 1994, pp. 214–218).

For such inexplicable biased acts, the Indian Medical Service (IMS) faced criticism for its response to the Spanish Influenza because of disparities in healthcare access and quality. The colonial healthcare system was designed to benefit European and affluent Indian communities, who enjoyed superior facilities and resources. The pandemic highlighted these inequalities, leading to increased dissatisfaction and resentment among the Indian population. The IMS's efforts were criticized for their inadequate care provision (Chakrabarti, 2014, pp. 101–122). The IMS faced logistical and infrastructural challenges in Bengal because of its dense population and inadequate transportation networks, causing difficulties in medical service delivery and remote areas. The pandemic highlighted the need for a robust, decentralized public health system to address these limitations (Harrison, 1996, pp. 438–443).

The sociopolitical context of colonial Bengal influenced the IMS's effectiveness, as nationalist sentiments and opposition to British rule increased. The pandemic fueled anti-colonial sentiments, with Indian leaders criticizing the British government for inadequate protection and welfare neglect. This led to political mobilization and nationalist movements, highlighting the need for improved healthcare and protection (Chatterjee, 1993, pp. 158–172).

The IMS and colonial administration addressed a growing health crisis by increasing medical personnel supply through mobilizing medical students and retired professionals. However, sub-assistant medical practitioners were sent instead of doctors, leaving people in limbo and leading British doctors to flee to the mountains (Harrison, 1994, pp. 166–202). The IMS collaborated with local health practitioners and traditional healers to expand their reach, but these efforts were often too late because of the pandemic's already devastating effects (Guha, 2001, pp. 141–142). The IMS's role during the Spanish Influenza in colonial Bengal was significant, demonstrating public health commitment and a coordinated medical response (Guha, 2012, pp. 31–58). However, their failures exposed the inequalities of the colonial healthcare system. The pandemic highlighted the need for a more inclusive, fair approach to healthcare, addressing the needs of all population segments (Pati, 2019, pp. 50–56). During the Spanish Influenza pandemic in colonial Bengal, the Indian Medical Service (IMS) struggled to provide adequate medical care, public health interventions, data collection, and resource management. Systemic limitations and sociopolitical challenges undermined their efforts, testing their resilience and revealing the inadequacies of the colonial healthcare system. This experience highlighted the importance of fair and effective public health systems, especially during crises, and fueled India's struggle for independence (Chakrabarti, 2020, pp. 83, 95–99).

During the Spanish Influenza pandemic of 1918–19, the Indian Medical Service (IMS) played a crucial yet challenged role across various districts of colonial Bengal. In the districts of 24 Parganas, Nadia, Murshidabad (under the Presidency Division), Burdwan, Birbhum, Bankura, Midnapur, Hooghly, Howrah (under the Burdwan Division), Dinajpur, Jalpaiguri, Darjeeling, and Malda, the IMS undertook a range of activities aimed at managing and mitigating the impact of the pandemic. These activities included medical care, public health interventions, data collection, and logistic coordination, though they were often hampered by systemic constraints and sociopolitical issues. In the densely populated district of 24 Parganas, the IMS focused on establishing temporary clinics and expanding existing hospital facilities to cope with the overwhelming number of influenza cases. Makeshift clinics were established in schools and community centres to provide symptomatic relief for patients with influenza. Medical staff worked tirelessly to disseminate public health information about hygiene and sanitation, despite communication barriers and widespread illiteracy, to prevent the disease's spread (Arnold, 2004, pp. 49–57).

Nadia and Murshidabad, being rural districts with less developed healthcare infrastructure, posed significant challenges for the IMS. The IMS faced a shortage of medical supplies and overwhelmed dispensaries and hospitals. They mobilized local health practitioners and traditional healers to reach remote villages and conducted outreach programmes to educate the rural population on quarantine and isolation (Ramanna, 2002, pp. 8–48). In the Burdwan Division, comprising districts such as Burdwan, Birbhum, Bankura, Midnapur, Hooghly, and Howrah, the IMS faced similar challenges. Burdwan, despite being an urbanized district, possessed a greater number of medical resources, but there was a lack of timely supply of essential medical supplies. IMS established additional care centres and coordinated with local authorities to manage disease spread. Birbhum and Bankura, with rural settings, focused on outreach and education. Midnapur required tailored public health messages (Chandra & Eva, 2014, p. 510). Howrah and Hooghly, being industrial and densely populated districts, experienced rapid transmission of the virus. The IMS partnered with local industrialists to establish infirmaries and conduct health education campaigns in congested districts, emphasizing cleanliness and preventing secondary infections, despite the challenging isolation and sanitation tasks.

In the northern districts of Dinajpur, Jalpaiguri, Darjeeling, and Malda, the IMS's efforts were complicated by geographical and infrastructural constraints. The IMS used mobile medical units to reach remote areas in Darjeeling, Jalpaiguri, and Dinajpur, collaborating with tea estate managements to provide care for labour populations. In Malda, the focus was on preventing disease spread through small towns and villages through extensive travel and outreach efforts (Klein, 1988, pp. 639–645). The IMS provided direct medical care, public health interventions, and logistical coordination in districts to manage the pandemic's impact. However, because of the crisis's scale, limited resources, and infrastructural challenges, their response was often inadequate, highlighting the need for a stronger public health system.

During the Spanish Influenza pandemic of 1918–19, the Indian Medical Service (IMS) played a pivotal role in combating the widespread health crisis across various districts in the then Bengal, including Khulna, Rajshahi, Rangpur, Bogra, Pabna, Dacca, Mymensingh, Faridpur, Bakargunj, Chittagong, Noakhali, and Tippera. The IMS's efforts in these regions encompassed direct medical care, public health interventions, and logistical coordination, albeit under severe constraints posed by limited resources, infrastructural challenges, and the sociopolitical context of colonial rule. The IMS in Khulna faced a rapidly spreading epidemic in an urban and rural district. Overcrowded medical facilities led to temporary clinics and care centres. The IMS provided symptomatic relief, focusing on fever and cough relief. Public health campaigns were educated the population on hygiene practices, but limited by communication barriers and poverty. The Indian Medical Service (IMS) has mobilized local health practitioners and traditional healers to reach remote villages in rural districts like Rajshahi, Rangpur, and Bogra, focusing on quarantine and isolation measures to curb virus spread. However, implementing these measures in these communities, where people live in close quarters and have limited access to clean water and sanitation facilities, remains challenging (The Statesman, 1918, p. 6). The IMS in Pabna and Dacca used existing hospitals and dispensaries to handle overflow patients, while also coordinating with local authorities to enforce public health measures like quarantine and social distancing, despite challenges such as high population density and inadequate enforcement mechanisms. The IMS has deployed mobile medical units to Mymensingh and Faridpur, addressing healthcare needs in rural areas and educating the population on preventive measures, focusing on secondary infections because of poor sanitation and water access (The Times of India, 1918, p. 4). The IMS in Bakargunj faced logistical challenges because of the district's infrastructural limitations. Despite collaboration with local authorities and community leaders, efforts to distribute medical supplies and establish temporary care centres were hindered by inadequate infrastructure.

The IMS in Chittagong focused on managing the pandemic through organized public health campaigns and medical interventions. The district's infrastructure enabled the establishment of isolation wards in hospitals and temporary facilities for influenza treatment, while coordinating with local industries for infirmaries (The Calcutta Gazette, 1918, p. 12). The IMS in Noakhali and Tippera faced challenges because of rural settings, requiring temporary clinics, care centres, and community networks to spread public health messages, while also overcoming logistical barriers to deliver medical supplies and personnel (Amrita Bazar Patrika, 1918, p. 7). Overall, the Indian Medical Service's (IMS) response to the Spanish Influenza pandemic in colonial Bengal was inadequate because of the crisis's scale, limited resources, and infrastructural challenges. The pandemic exposed deep-seated inequalities and infrastructural deficits in the colonial healthcare system, underscoring the need for more robust public health infrastructure and greater resource allocation in future health crises. The pandemic was one of the deadliest in history, and the IMS faced significant challenges in providing adequate care and containment. This perceived negligence and inadequate response led to widespread public discontent and various reactions among the people of Bengal.

One of the primary reactions was that the Indian population experienced anger and frustration because of the IMS's inability to meet the immense healthcare demands, leading to overcrowding of hospitals and clinics. This perception of the colonial government prioritizing European and elite Indian communities over the general population further fueled public resentment, highlighting the deep-seated inequalities in the colonial system (The Times of India, 1918, p. 5). Rural areas in Nadia, Murshidabad, and Bankura faced dire healthcare conditions because of minimal infrastructure. Villagers relied on traditional healers and home remedies, leading to high mortality rates and a sense of abandonment. Reports of villages being destroyed without medical intervention fueled a growing sense of betrayal and neglect by colonial authorities (Amrita Bazar Patrika, 1918, p. 7). Urban centres like Calcutta experienced significant unrest because of the influenza, particularly affecting the poor living in densely populated and unsanitary conditions. The IMS's inability to provide effective care and rapid virus spread led to widespread fear and panic. Public gatherings, protests, and demonstrations grew as people demanded better healthcare and decisive action from authorities (The Statesman, 1918, p. 6).

Nationalist leaders, including Mahatma Gandhi and Rabindranath Tagore, used widespread discontent to fuel the anti-colonial movement. They criticized the British government's inadequate response to the pandemic, arguing that the neglect of the Indian Medical Service (IMS) symbolized broader colonial exploitation and mismanagement of India. The pandemic became a powerful symbol of colonial oppression and fueled independence movement support (Arnold, 2019, pp. 197–200). Local newspapers and publications significantly influenced public opinion by reporting on the IMS's shortcomings and the colonial government's response, often highlighting personal stories of loss and suffering. This media coverage spread awareness, united societal criticism, and served as a platform for grievances and accountability (Gupta, 2007, pp. 266–271). Community organizations and social groups filled the gap left by the IMS by organizing relief efforts, providing basic medical care, distributing food, and educating people about hygiene practices. These grassroots efforts highlighted the failures of the official healthcare system and showed the resilience and solidarity of the Indian people during the crisis. Religious and cultural leaders also played a significant role in public reaction, organizing community responses and offering solace to those affected by the pandemic. Temples, mosques, and churches became centres of support, often criticizing colonial authorities for neglect and indifference (Kudaisya, 2016, pp. 48–53).

In conclusion, the shortcomings of the Indian Medical Service during the Spanish Influenza pandemic in colonial Bengal from 1918 to 1919 incited widespread anger and frustration among the populace, underscoring the disparities and inefficiencies inherent in the colonial healthcare system. This led to nationalist sentiment and strengthened the anti-colonial movement. The pandemic exposed the Indian populace's vulnerabilities and underscored the need for a fairer healthcare system, contributing to India's independence struggle.

Colonial Supremacy and the Interplay Between Disease and Vaccination During Spanish Influenza

Vaccination[11] is a straightforward, secure, and efficient method of safeguarding against harmful diseases before encountering them. Vaccines are a natural defense mechanism that helps to develop resistance to specific infections and enhance the immune system. They contain inactivated or weakened forms of germs, such as viruses or bacteria, and do not cause the disease or its complications. Vaccines are administered through injections, orally, or sprayed into the nose. They lower the risk of contracting a disease by collaborating with the body's natural defenses. Upon receiving a vaccine, the immune system reacts by identifying the invading germ and producing antibodies, which are proteins naturally generated by the immune system to combat disease. This makes vaccines a safe and intelligent approach to triggering an immune response without causing illness. Vaccines are highly effective, as they prevent us from falling ill in the first place and protect us at various stages of life. It is crucial to ensure that all vaccines are kept up to date to avoid severe illness (WHO, 2024, p. 1).

The Spanish Influenza pandemic of 1918–19 in India was a significant event that led to the colonial administration recognizing the need for vaccination programmes. The pandemic had a devastating impact on the Indian population, resulting in the loss of 10–20 million lives, posing a significant threat to the colonial government's ability to maintain order and stability. The colonial authorities were also concerned about the potential economic and political consequences of the pandemic, as a weakened workforce could negatively impact industrial output, tax collection, and trade, which were vital for the colonial structure and administrative system. The government's response to the health crisis could lead to public unrest and civil disobedience. The colonial rulers understood that managing the pandemic was not only a medical necessity but also crucial for maintaining their political and economic supremacy (Chandra, 2008, pp. 387–395).

The colonial regime started extensive vaccination drives, using administrative resources, medical facilities, and coercive authority to distribute and administer the limited flu vaccine, despite logistical issues, public doubt, and resistance, as a concentrated effort to protect their interests and maintain population control (Killingray & Phillips, 2003, pp. 239–241). The 1918 Spanish Influenza pandemic, causing around 50 million deaths globally, was largely because of a lack of clarity about its causative agent, leading to confusion and scientific uncertainty. Misconceptions, such as the belief that the virus was caused by a bacterial infection (Kolata, 1999, pp. 3–34), significantly impacted public health measures, treatment strategies, and scientific investigations during and after the pandemic (Arnold, 1987, pp. 173–178).

Early Theories and Misconceptions

The early 1900s saw significant growth in microbiology, with pathogenic bacteria being identified as key to medical science. Scientists like Robert Koch and Louis Pasteur made significant discoveries, providing a framework for understanding infectious diseases. However, this led to the misattribution of the Spanish Flu to bacterial origins. In 1892, German physician Richard Pfeiffer[12] discovered Haemophilus influenzae,[13] believed to be the causative agent of influenza. During the 1918 pandemic, patients were frequently infected with Haemophilus influenzae,[15] solidifying the belief that this bacterium was the cause of the Spanish Flu. The prevailing bacteriological perspective and secondary bacterial infections in influenza patients further perpetuated this misunderstanding (Morens et al., 2009, pp. 225–227).

The Role of Secondary Bacterial Infections

The Spanish Flu's association with bacteria is largely because of the prevalence of secondary bacterial infections among influenza patients. Influenza viruses cause significant damage to respiratory epithelium,[14] making it susceptible to colonization by bacterial pathogens. Many infected individuals later develop pneumonia, often leading to death. The bacteria commonly involved in these secondary infections included *Streptococcus pneumoniae, Staphylococcus aureus,* and *H. influenzae* (Brundage & Shanks, 2008, pp. 1193–1195).

Secondary bacterial infections often overshadowed viral symptoms, leading to autopsies revealing bacterial pneumonia as the immediate cause of death. This confusion was exacerbated by the lack of diagnostic tools to differentiate between primary viral infections and secondary bacterial complications. Here, one news may be mentioned regarding the controversy about bacteria or a virus—*The Statesman, on October 18, 1918, page 5, featured an article titled "Influenza Epidemic: A Bacterial Infection?". This piece examined the dominant theories regarding the origins of the influenza pandemic and emphasized the continuing discussion among medical professionals concerning whether the illness was caused by bacteria or a virus.*

The text highlights the ongoing debate in the medical community about the origin of the pandemic, highlighting the limited understanding of the disease and the challenges faced in identifying its cause, which impacted the development of effective treatments and public health strategies.

Diagnostic Limitations and Technological Constraints

During the 1918 pandemic, basic diagnostic techniques did not detect viruses. Bacterial culture methods and microscopic examination were effective for bacteria, but not viruses. The understanding of viruses as distinct pathogens was relatively new, with the first tobacco mosaic virus[15] discovered in 1898. Electron microscopy allowed for virus visualization in the 1930s, but limited influenza detection (Taubenberger & Morens, 2006, pp. 15–18).

Scientific Research and Shifting Paradigms

In 1901, American bacteriologist William H. Park proposed a filterable agent as the cause of influenza, despite the belief it could be a virus. In the 1930s, British researchers successfully isolated the influenza A virus in ferrets, revolutionizing diagnosis, treatment, and prevention strategies (Smith et al., 1933, pp. 66–67).

Colonial Administration Responses

> *In the Bengalee local newspaper on July 17, 1918, page 2, H. M. Crake, the Health Officer for the Corporation of Calcutta, published an article titled "Rational Method of Preventing Infection." The article stated that during influenza epidemics, secretions from the nose, throat, and respiratory tract are typically highly infectious. Since the disease's germs are seldom detected in the bloodstream, it suggests that influenza is primarily a localized infection, with general symptoms arising from toxins released by the bacilli. It is a reasonable hypothesis that, most times, the bacilli are confined to the upper respiratory tract—specifically, the nose and throat—during the initial stages of infection. If this hypothesis holds true, eliminating the local infection before it can spread should prevent an outbreak. The most logical method of prevention appears to be the disinfection of the nose and throat using an antiseptic nasal douche. Recent studies have showed that a saturated aqueous solution of thymol is the most effective mouthwash available.*

Colonial administrations implemented public health measures and treatment protocols based on the belief that the Spanish Flu was caused by bacteria. They used bacterial vaccines to protect against H. influenzae and other bacteria, but they were ineffective against the influenza virus itself (Crosby, 2003, pp. 17–37). Limited healthcare infrastructure and resource constraints hinder pandemic response, while bacterial vaccines and antibiotics provide relief, and public health campaigns focus on hygiene and sanitation (Tomkins, 1992b, pp. 440–445). The 1918 Spanish Influenza pandemic highlighted the challenges of understanding and combating infectious diseases, highlighting the limitations of scientific knowledge and the influence of prevailing paradigms on public health responses. Despite the loss of life, advancements in virology and public health practices have improved our ability to respond to future pandemics, emphasizing the importance of continuous scientific inquiry and international collaboration. *The Statesman* March 4, pg.9, 1919 published a news titled, "Influenza in India–Sanitary Commissioner's Report" which has been highlighted earlier.

The 1918 Spanish Influenza pandemic prompted colonial scientists to focus on bacterial vaccines, with pathological laboratories in British-ruled India working diligently to create vaccines. Institutions like the Central Research Institute in Kasauli and the Haffkine Institute in Bombay were key hubs for bacteriological studies and vaccine manufacturing (Arnold, 1989, pp. 125–129).

Central Research Institute (Kasauli)

The Central Research Institute (CRI) in Kasauli, founded in 1905, was a leading research facility focused on vaccine development. During the Spanish Influenza pandemic, the institute developed a bacterial vaccine targeting Haemophilus influenzae and other bacteria. Led by Dr. S. R. Christophers, the institute successfully produced a vaccine that offered a defense against secondary bacterial infections, a common cause of death in influenza patients. This approach, comprising inactivated preparations of H. influenzae, Streptococcus pneumoniae, and other bacterial pathogens, significantly reduced mortality rates (Kumar, 2012, pp. 435–439).

Haffkine Institute (Bombay)

The Haffkine Institute in Bombay, founded in 1899 by bacteriologist Waldemar Haffkine, played a crucial role in vaccine production during the Spanish Flu pandemic. Led by Dr. T. F. Hughes, the institute developed a bacterial vaccine containing strains like H. influenzae and Streptococcus pneumoniae, which were believed to contribute to severe pneumonia in influenza patients. This strategy aimed to minimize the pandemic's impact by reducing secondary bacterial infections (Kurian, 2007, p. 63).

The local newspaper, *The Englishman*, released an article entitled "*Influenza in Tea Gardens: Beneficial Inoculation*" on April 23, 1919 (p. 9), which is crucial to emphasize in this context—

> *The published news illustrates the shortcomings of the colonial public health response to the 1918 influenza pandemic in the tea gardens of Assam. Although the response seemed proactive—evidenced by inoculation campaigns and partnerships with institutions like the Pasteur Institute—the underlying goal was economic preservation rather than genuine humanitarian concern. The coolie labor force was treated as interchangeable components rather than as individuals, with health initiatives aimed at sustaining productivity instead of promoting well-being.*
>
> *The texts underscore a system plagued by inadequate resources, where overburdened personnel and insufficient infrastructure struggled to meet overwhelming demand. Inoculation efforts were advocated despite questionable effectiveness, relying more on anecdotal reports than on scientific evidence. Appeals for government help and integrating vaccinations for various diseases reveal a reactive and poorly coordinated approach. Ultimately, these documents highlight a colonial medical framework that prioritized industrial interests over the preservation of life, exposing significant ethical and logistical deficiencies.*

Challenges and Impact

The production of bacterial vaccines in India during the Spanish Influenza pandemic was a significant challenge because of limited understanding of the disease's cause and inadequate diagnostic tools. The vaccines were based on the mistaken assumption that bacteria were the primary cause, which led to the development of vaccines that were ineffective in preventing the virus. However, the Central

Research Institute in Kasauli and the Haffkine Institute in Bombay made significant contributions to vaccine production, distributing and administering vaccines that might reduce mortality rates by preventing secondary bacterial infections. Their work underscored the importance of understanding disease aetiology, scientific adaptability, and vaccination's role in public health. Their work continues to guide contemporary infectious disease outbreak responses, emphasizing the need for rigorous scientific investigation, evidence-based policymaking, and international collaboration (Davis, 2005, pp. 69–81).

Colonial Mindset and the Response of Indian Medical Professionals

British physicians endeavoured to create a vaccine aimed at curbing the spread of influenza; however, their attempts were thwarted by the elusive nature of the disease's cause. Lt. Col. Mac Taggart proposed a vaccine composed of inactivated influenza bacilli, pneumococci, and streptococci, yet this suggestion lacked any experimental validation. The Indian Medical Service (IMS) made substantial investments in vaccination initiatives, but these efforts did not yield success. Sanitary Commissioner Norman White voiced his exasperation regarding the public's misconceptions about the vaccine development process, noting that only 300000 doses would be reserved for potential future outbreaks, leaving the rest exposed to natural factors (Foley, 2005, pp. 200–207). In India, the British medical authority MacTaggart expressed a tempered sense of hope regarding the bacteriology of the illness, asserting that a precise understanding of its nature is essential for effective intervention. He highlighted the divergent perspectives within the British medical community in India, which grappled with the dual challenges of addressing the ongoing pandemic and preventing future epidemics, with the former being viewed as a critical element in lowering mortality rates (Arnold, 2010, pp. 430–433; Chhun, 2015, p. 143).

Despite prevailing scepticism, the government produced a flu vaccine that was made accessible to civil surgeons, health officers, and private practitioners upon request. The United Provinces Medical Manual outlined protocols for the vaccine's storage and administration, while also acknowledging the absence of conclusive evidence regarding its effectiveness as a preventive or therapeutic measure. This situation prompts inquiries into the potential for willful ignorance and desperation within western medicine, as vaccines were developed despite uncertain efficacy in response to the urgent demand for action (Bashford, 2006, p. 74).

In 1919, Major White's theory suggesting that individuals who had previously experienced influenza waves developed natural immunity was met with scepticism, underscoring the medical community's uncertainty and inability to effectively address the outbreak (Worboys, 2000, p. 35). Debendranath Sen identified a mucoid substance in the recesses of the nasal cavity that contained the same Pfeiffer's Bacillus, which opened new avenues for research aimed at combating the disease, as noted in a letter to the Indian Medical Gazette (Sen, 1919, p. 387). The medical community's understanding of influenza treatment was constrained by their limited knowledge. Captain Cecil Webb Johnson, a member of the Royal

Army Medical Corps, contributed a letter to the Indian Medical Gazette that proposed some contentious treatment methods (Whitehead, 1999, p. 41). In his correspondence, Webb Johnson stressed the necessity of refraining from food intake until the fever had resolved and cautioned against excessive nourishment. He also recommended the judicious use of alcohol, likening it to a whip or spur that could influence the outcome of a race. Johnson highlighted the importance of safeguarding the heart and lungs from the onset of the illness. Despite scepticism expressed in medical journals, the Indian Medical Service formed collaborations with voluntary organizations to staff dispensaries and temporary hospitals, leaving rural populations to manage on their own (Harrison, 2004, pp. 8–38).

The Indian flu encountered a paradox stemming from geographical constraints, as the virus proliferated swiftly in densely populated urban centres with efficient systems, while it proved more lethal in rural regions because of a lack of organized relief initiatives. Disparities in wealth and poverty played a significant role in the pandemic's impact. Although the urban poor had access to relief centres, their distrust of the government hindered effective help, whereas the rural poor experienced significant neglect. The Indian Medical Mission was inadequately equipped to address the crisis, and S.S. Vyas, a sub-assistant surgeon in Indore, emphasized the collaborative efforts of the medical community, which included a group of approximately 15 doctors who volunteered to establish medical depots for the distribution of free medicines (Vyas, 1919, p. 457).

Common Peoples' Perception and Misconception

Throughout the pandemic, the medical community faced challenges in comprehending the characteristics of influenza, which prompted the colonial administration to focus on the development of bacterial vaccines to manage the disease and reduce death rates. This approach, however, neglected the viral component of the infection, leading to feelings of disappointment and resentment among the affected populations. The vaccination campaigns started by the Bengal administration were based on the incorrect belief that the disease had a bacterial origin, targeting bacterial pathogens associated with secondary infections in those suffering from influenza. While these vaccines were effective in reducing bacterial complications, they did not tackle the underlying viral infection, resulting in continued high rates of illness and mortality (Arnold, 1993a, p. 61).

Public Protests and Reactions

During the influenza pandemic of 1918–19 in colonial Bengal, local newspapers voiced their discontent regarding the colonial government's failure to produce and distribute an effective vaccine. *The Amrita Bazar Patrika*, a leading Bengali local vernacular, condemned the colonial administration for its inadequate response to the health crisis, accentuating the severe consequences of the outbreak on the local community and the pressing need for medical solutions, including vaccines. Likewise, *The Bengalee*, another significant newspaper, conveyed its dissatisfaction with the government's handling of the pandemic in an article dated December 7, 1918. This publication criticized the government's lack of preparedness for a health emergency and its inability to mobilize resources for vaccine development and distribution, drawing attention to the suffering endured by the populace and calling for more decisive actions to address the disease (Kleinman & Watson, 1990, pp. 864–868). The government has been blamed for the shortage in medical care during the pandemic, with efforts to extend allopathic treatment described as inadequate. Alternative treatments were also lacking, and hospitals were closed because of lack of medical personnel. Despite this, the public held the government accountable, emphasizing the importance of not stagnating in efforts to save lives and ease suffering. The article highlights the nation's struggle with widespread death and limited healthcare access, with rural Bengal reaching its peak. The government appears to be at a standstill, highlighting the need for continued efforts to save lives and ease suffering (Killingray & Phillips, 2003, p. 89).

The increasing fatalities and unchecked outbreak in Bengal led to locals protesting against colonial medical procedures, citing the colonial government's inadequacy and the ineffectiveness of vaccinations. Historical records show gatherings and protests were organized to show discontent with the epidemic management, particularly the lack of openness and neglect of indigenous health customs. The colonial administration's attempts to enforce vaccination, sometimes using force, further aggravated the situation, leading to a lack of trust and resentment. In rural regions, resistance to vaccination was even more pronounced, with many communities rejecting vaccines and opting for local healers and remedies.

Calcutta's local newspapers and leaders criticized the colonial government's handling of the pandemic, questioning the scientific rationale behind vaccination campaigns. Public gatherings became platforms for expressing grievances, leading to civil disobedience and widespread frustration among the population. The failure of vaccination programmes and high mortality rates resulted in public protests and dissent in various districts of Bengal, including 24 Parganas, Nadia, Murshidabad, Burdwan, Birbhum, Bankura, Midnapore, Hooghly, Howrah, Dinajpur, Jalpaiguri, Darjeeling, and Malda. Similar reactions were observed in other districts of colonial Bengal such as Khulna, Rajshahi, Rangpur, Bogra, Pabna, Dacca, Mymensingh, Faridpur, Bakargunj, Chittagong, Noakhali, and Tippera. Disillusioned by the colonial administration's inability to control the disease and the inefficacy of the vaccines, people in these areas organized public meetings and demonstrations to express their discontent. The protests were fueled by the clear failure of the vaccines and the perceived negligence of the colonial health authorities. During the Spanish Influenza pandemic, both urban and rural communities resisted vaccination, favouring traditional medicine and local health practices. This dissent highlighted distrust of colonial administration and the need for transparent public health measures. The pandemic emphasized the importance of local expertise and public confidence in health interventions.

In 1918–19, physicians and researchers had limited knowledge of viruses and the immediate causes of death during the pandemic. They understood viruses as causative factors for disease and death, with bacterial secondary infections being the primary cause of influenza deaths. However, they could not pinpoint a specific bacterium as the cause of death. Vaccine makers used a cautious approach, considering multiple serotypes of Pneumococcus, which may have impacted vaccination effectiveness (Bristow, 2012, pp. 14–20). During 1918–19, the effectiveness of the Spanish Influenza vaccine was debated, with some arguing that bacterial vaccines were ineffective because of a lack of understanding of the virus as the causative agent and others criticizing vaccine outcomes for not meeting modern medical trial evaluation standards. However, the medical and technological contexts of the time were different, and health authorities and experts were not naïve about pharmaceutical interventions for influenza or mortality causes. Despite its use, the Spanish Influenza vaccine could not claim complete success.

Medical Advertisements During Influenza Pandemic—An Attempt for Commercializing Public Health

In 1918, the influenza pandemic prompted businesses to exploit the public's fear and need for medical solutions. Advertisements for fever pills, nasal sprays, and anti-influenza cigarettes targeted a population desperate for relief. Local and international companies competed for consumer trust by making unverified claims about their products' effectiveness. This commercialization of public health revealed the conflict between profit-driven motives and genuine medical necessities, reflecting the broader exploitation and opportunism in the colonial economy. The proliferation of such advertisements not only highlighted the deficiencies in official medical responses but also significantly influenced public perceptions and behaviours during one of the deadliest pandemics in history (Tomkins, 1992a, pp. 435–439).

During the 1918–19 Spanish Influenza pandemic, colonial governments and commercial entities used medical advertisements to deceive the public, promoting ineffective cures and preventive measures, such as "Influenza Cure Tablets", and sensationalist advertising by pharmaceutical companies, often using dubious testimonials and pseudo-scientific jargon (Honigsbaum, 2009, p. 151). Misinformation during the Spanish Influenza outbreak led to public health crises by diverting attention from effective measures like quarantine, hygiene, and social distancing. Colonial governments failed to regulate these ads effectively, undermining public trust in medical authorities and the government. Profit-driven agendas and false information significantly impacted the epidemic's trajectory, preying on public fears and impeding authentic disease control measures. This exploitation underscores the importance of ethical guidelines and truthful information in public health messaging (Bristow, 2012, p. 35).

Throughout the Spanish Influenza pandemic, pharmaceutical companies specializing in both Ayurvedic and Western medicines used medical advertisements as a key tactic to take advantage of the widespread fear and urgency. These ads enabled companies to quickly reach a large audience, offering fast and simple solutions to those affected. During the Spanish Influenza pandemic, pharmaceutical companies used medical advertisements to reach a large audience and offer quick solutions. They used sensational language, testimonials, and pseudo-scientific assertions to instil urgency and trustworthiness in their products. Ayurvedic practitioners showcased traditional medicine effectiveness, while western companies highlighted scientific advancements. This strategy helped boost sales and establish a strong market presence amid the global health emergency (Arnold, 2019, pp. 185–189).

Figure 4.1, the schematic diagram, depicts the intricate network of influences and strategies used during the Spanish Flu pandemic of 1918, highlighting the interplay between colonial power, public health, and commercial interests. It reveals how colonial influence influenced public health practices and promoted western medical products. The pandemic also served as a battleground for market share and cultural influence, with local companies like Bengal Chemical and Pharmaceutical Works Ltd. competing with British companies to maximize profits. The diagram also highlights the use of persuasive marketing techniques, including misleading claims and media endorsements, to target audiences and promote products. This network reveals the 1918 influenza pandemic in colonial Bengal as a complex event that affected almost every aspect of society. It highlights the interaction

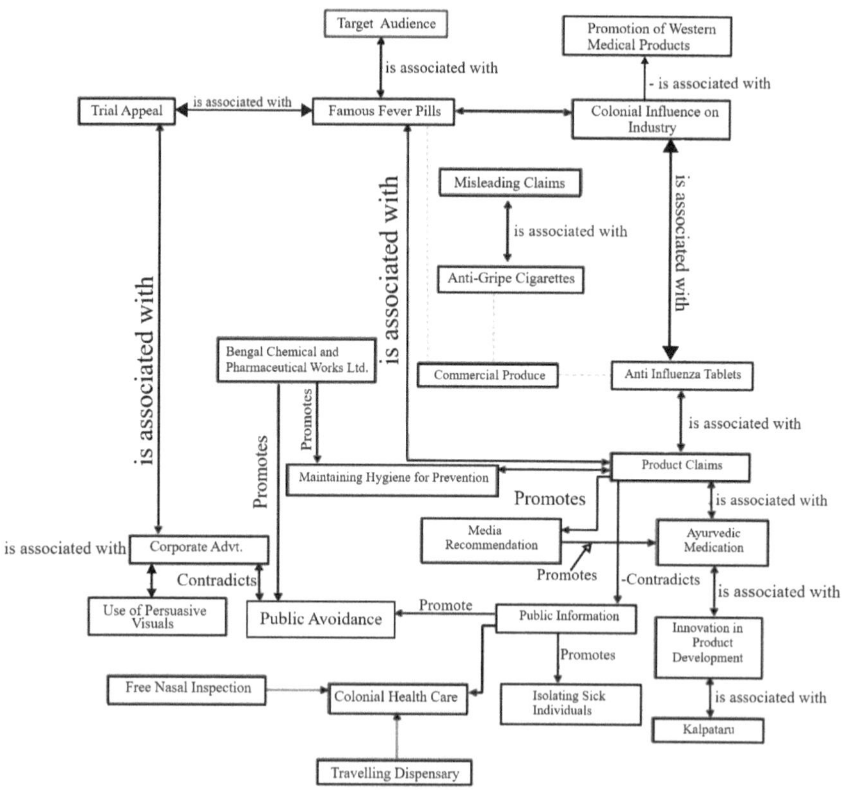

Figure 4.1 Schematic Diagram Showing Complex Network of Influences for Commercialization of Medical Advertisements

between colonial power structures, emerging local industries, traditional practices, and modern medical approaches.

The pandemic appears to have been a catalyst for innovation and change, exposing and potentially exaggerating existing social and political tensions. This multi-level response to the crisis likely had long-lasting effects on the Indian healthcare system, the pharmaceutical industry, and the public's relationship with both the colonial authorities and the medical establishment. The network has been divided into several dimensions to further investigate the actual scenario.

Famous Fever Pills: The prominence of "Famous Fever Pills" in the network suggests these medications played a crucial role during the pandemic. This reflects a reliance on symptomatic treatment, as specific antiviral medicine did not exist. It is possible that these pills became a symbol of the medical response to the pandemic, representing both hope for relief and the limitations of medical knowledge. It also reflects the desperate search for effective treatments during the pandemic. They may have been promoted heavily by both colonial authorities and local manufacturers, possibly leading to debates about their efficacy and accessibility. Figures 4.2 and 4.3 show how these medical advertisements targeted their marketing to capture the stereotype of people and make them believe in medications which in reality offered no rescue.

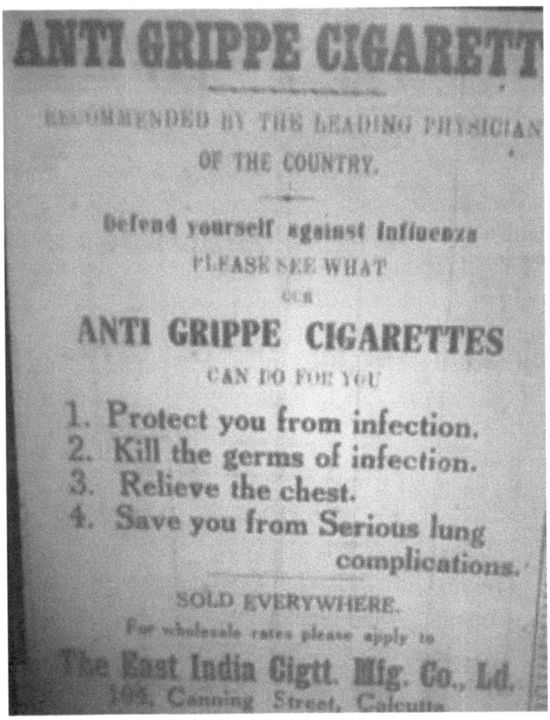

Figure 4.2 Advertisement Propagating About Anti-Grippe Cigarettes for Saving Oneself

Source: The Bengalee, 1918, November 7, p. 6

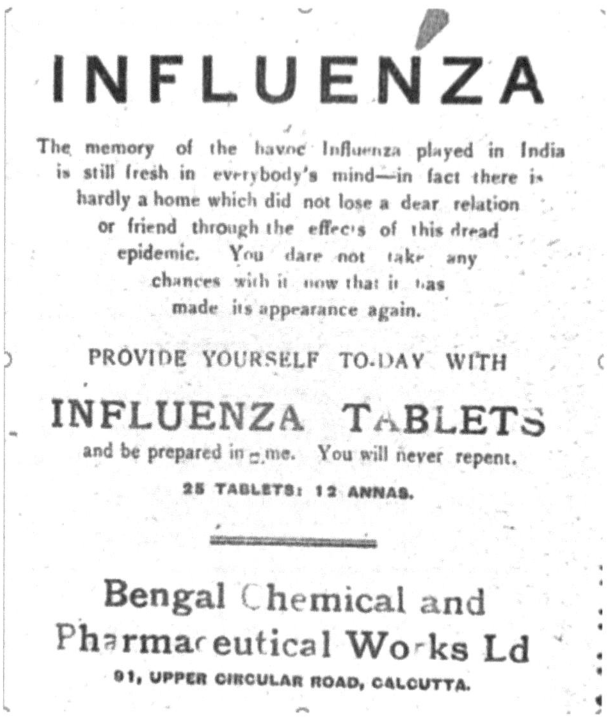

Figure 4.3 Advertisement of Influenza Medicine
Source: The Statesman, January 5, 1919, p. 10

Colonial Context: The diagram reveals the complex power dynamics during the pandemic, with British colonial interests shaping the response. The promotion of western medical products and industry influence may have created internal tensions with traditional Indian medical practices and local healthcare systems, potentially marginalizing indigenous knowledge and treatments.

Pharmaceutical Industry: Bengal Chemical and Pharmaceutical Works Ltd. is a key player in local pharmaceutical manufacturing, playing a multifaceted role in hygiene promotion and product claims. The industry experienced rapid growth and transformation during the pandemic, laying the groundwork for future developments in Bengal's medical sector. The pandemic presented an opportunity for modernization and expansion of local pharmaceutical capabilities, while also highlighting tensions between profit motives and public health needs.

Public Health Measures: The public health strategies mentioned, including public avoidance, isolating ill individuals, and free nasal injections, represent a multi-pronged approach to combat the pandemic, likely a mix of colonial policies and local adaptations, potentially facing challenges because of cultural differences, resource limitations, and potential resistance from the local population.

Traditional Medicine: The presence of Ayurvedic medication in India's medical network shows the resilience of traditional practices, even under colonial rule. The pandemic may have sparked debates about the efficiency of different medical systems, potentially influencing long-term attitudes towards the contrast between traditional and western medicine.

Questionable Practices: Misleading claims in health products like anti-grippe cigarettes and anti-influenza tablets reveal the darker side of medical marketing and challenges in regulating claims during pandemics. This highlights desperation and confusion, leading people to try unproven or harmful remedies.

Healthcare Delivery: The mention of travelling dispensaries alongside colonial healthcare suggests a diverse and potentially improvised system, possibly aiming to reach remote or underserved populations during the crisis, highlighting the challenges of providing widespread healthcare in a diverse colony.

Target Audience: Target audience node suggests strategic pandemic management, possibly involving tailored interventions for different demographics, reflecting an early understanding of public health needs, but raising equity concerns in colonial healthcare delivery (Sharma, 2009, pp. 213–217).

The 1918 influenza pandemic significantly impacted colonial Bengal's society, healthcare, and industry. Medical advertisements represented hope and limitations of medical knowledge, while the colonial context highlighted power dynamics and marginalization of traditional Indian practices. The Bengal Chemical and Pharmaceutical Works Ltd. played a crucial role in public health education and blending colonial policies with local adaptations. Ayurvedic medicine emphasized the resilience of traditional practices. The pandemic exposed exploitation and facilitated innovation in healthcare delivery, exposing and amplifying existing social and political tensions (Pillai, 1974, p. 29).

Complex Interplay Between Colonial Power, Nationalist Responses, and Global Health Governance During Influenza Pandemic

During the 1918–19 influenza pandemic in India, which occurred during British colonial rule, the intricate relationship between imperial power, nationalist movements, and global health initiatives was brought to light. The virus spread rapidly in densely populated cities and villages, but the colonial administration faced challenges in responding because of limited resources and a focus on maintaining order. Indian nationalist leaders, inspired by the suffering of their people, condemned the government's inaction and organized relief efforts independently from colonial authorities. Meanwhile, international health organizations such as the League of Nations struggled to coordinate a global response, hindered by conflicting national interests and the aftermath of World War I. This complex interplay between colonial rule, nationalist movements, and the constraints of early global governance significantly influenced the impact of the influenza pandemic in India, providing valuable historical insights for navigating the intersection of public health, politics, and power (Bhatia, 2001, p. 58).

Nationalist Protests in the Wake of the Combined Onslaught of Spanish Influenza and Famine After World War I

After World War I, India faced many challenges, fueling the nationalist movement. Indian nationalists hoped for greater political autonomy and self-governance from

British support. However, expectations were unfulfilled, leading to frustration and calls for independence. The Spanish Influenza pandemic of 1918–19 further exacerbated the situation, resulting in millions of deaths and economic hardships. This eroded public confidence in the British administration's ability to effectively govern and protect the population, further affecting the country's resources and infrastructure (DeWitt, 1978, pp. 185–189).

In the crisis, Indian nationalist leaders like Mahatma Gandhi mobilized the masses for self-rule, leading to the Indian National Congress intensifying its calls for "Swaraj" (self-rule) and civil disobedience campaigns. The end of World War I marked a significant turning point in India–British relations, with Indian soldiers making significant sacrifices and contributing to the Allied victory. Indian nationalists hoped for greater political autonomy and self-governance, but the British government failed to fulfil these expectations (Erikson, 1970, pp. 19–33). The Government of India Act of 1919, also known as the Montagu–Chelmsford Reforms,[16] was viewed as a disappointment by the Indian nationalist movement. While the act introduced some aspects of self-governance, such as the expansion of legislative councils and the establishment of provincial autonomy, it fell short of the demands for increased political representation and decision-making power (Collected Works of Mahatma Gandhi,[17] 1919, p. 169). The act maintained British control over key governance areas, fueling nationalist leaders' resentment. India also suffered the devastating impact of the Spanish Influenza pandemic, which emerged in 1918 and spread worldwide, resulting in 10–20 million deaths, particularly on the Indian subcontinent (Arnold, 2021, p. 98).

The Spanish Flu caused significant loss of life and economic disruption in India, affecting the healthcare system and infrastructure. The outbreak also led to a famine in certain parts of the country, resulting in widespread food shortages and starvation. The Bengal region, particularly, experienced a severe famine, resulting in about 3 million deaths. This event further diminished public confidence in the British administration's ability to govern and protect the population. The pandemic, agricultural disruption, and poor monsoon season further exacerbated the situation (Gandhi, 2024, p. xvi). The devastating consequences of the Spanish Flu and the famine, along with the political disillusionment following the war's end, created a volatile and explosive environment in India. Considering the immense crisis, Indian nationalist leaders mobilized the masses and directed their discontent towards a more assertive and organized movement for self-rule.

Following World War I, Mahatma Gandhi, Bal Gangadhar Tilak,[18] and Annie Besant[19] addressed the Spanish Influenza pandemic and famine in India through political activism and humanitarian efforts. The pandemic and famine exposed the shortcomings of British colonial governance. Gandhi advocated for self-governance, emphasizing self-sufficiency, local autonomy, and community well-being. He organized relief initiatives, mobilized volunteers, and promoted traditional Ayurvedic treatments and sanitation practices, strengthening his connection with the common people and his dedication to Swaraj (Sarkar, 1989, pp. 195–204). Bal Gangadhar Tilak, a leader in the Indian independence movement, used the pandemic to advocate for self-rule and criticize British authorities for inadequate healthcare and help. Annie Besant, a prominent figure in the Theosophical Society[20] and Indian Home Rule Movement,[21] emphasized the need for a government led by Indians to effectively address the populace's needs. These leaders fueled public sentiment against British governance, turning the despondency from influenza and famine into a renewed call for independence, ultimately driving transformation and reshaping the crisis into a powerful catalyst for change (Bose, 2006, pp. 148–160). The aftermath of World War I, the Spanish Flu, and the famine in India led to a volatile and explosive environment, marking a turning point in the country's journey towards independence. The Indian people, guided by nationalist leaders, became united and resolute in their quest to break free from colonial rule. The reactions to these events were diverse, reflecting the country's political and social environment. Nationalist leaders experienced disappointment because of the British government's failure to fulfil wartime promises, fueling a renewed sense of urgency in their pursuit of self-governance. The pandemic and famine also intensified the suffering of the Indian people and eroded their confidence in the colonial administration's ability to govern and protect them effectively (Jalal, 2001, pp. 290–297).

The Indian nationalist movement acquired momentum and mobilized the masses through radical forms of resistance, such as the Non-Cooperation Movement[22] and the Quit India Movement.[23] These movements aimed to challenge British rule and compel colonial authorities to meet their demands. The country's independence in 1947 resulted from the success of these movements and increasing international pressure on the British Empire after World War II. Despite facing sacrifices and challenges, the Indian people showed resilience and determination to shape their destiny as a sovereign nation (Guha, 2007, pp. xvi–xvii).

Nationalist Protest Against Rowlatt Act and Jallianwala Bagh Massacre

In 1918–19, India experienced significant unrest, fueled by the Spanish Influenza pandemic. The Rowlatt Act[24] and Jallianwala Bagh Massacre[25] were key events in igniting nationalist sentiments against British colonial rule. The Rowlatt Act, implemented in 1919, allowed the British government to detain suspected sedition without trial, leading to widespread condemnation and protests. Mahatma Gandhi transitioned from relief efforts to leading a non-violent resistance movement against the Act. His call for a nationwide strike on April 6, 1919 demonstrated the growing unity and determination of the Indian populace (Donald, 1971, p. 198). The Jallianwala Bagh Massacre on April 13, 1919 was a brutal incident in Amritsar, India, where British troops killed hundreds of unarmed people. The incident exposed the harsh reality of British colonial rule and sparked anti-colonial sentiments. Leaders from various regions and communities denounced the massacre, turning it into a focal point for the Indian independence movement. The unity displayed by Indians in response to the violence overshadowed religious and regional differences, strengthening their determination to fight for freedom (Kim, 2019, pp. 200–250). The Spanish Influenza pandemic worsened the suffering of the

Indian population during the colonial war, resulting in millions of deaths and worsening economic challenges. The Rowlatt Act, Jallianwala Bagh Massacre, and the pandemic created a volatile environment of discontent and resentment, leading to a surge in nationalist sentiment. This period marked a pivotal moment in the Indian independence movement, as the populace rallied with renewed determination and solidarity towards self-rule, disillusioned by the British response to their suffering (Brown, 1994, pp. 71–85).

Nationalist Response to the Global Health Governance

During the Spanish Influenza pandemic in Bengal, British colonial officials frequently depicted the crisis in their official communications and medical reports as stemming from India's climatic conditions, inadequate hygiene, and a perceived indigenous "fatalism", rather than acknowledging it as a failure of colonial governance. They characterized the outbreak as an unfortunate yet natural calamity, stressing the infrastructural limitations of a vast and "underdeveloped" region, while minimizing the extent of mortality to preserve imperial morale and evade criticism from audiences in Britain or other colonies. Reports dispatched to London often emphasized the alleged ignorance of the local population and their resistance to modern medical practices as significant obstacles to effective intervention, thereby subtly exonerating colonial authorities from direct accountability (Arnold, 2020, pp. 278–280).

In reaction, Indian nationalists vehemently condemned this narrative, charging the British with severe negligence, racial prejudice, and exploitative governance. Publications such as the *Amrita Bazar Patrika* and various nationalist leaders contended that the staggering death toll was not simply a natural disaster but rather a direct consequence of colonial mismanagement and resource exploitation. They highlighted the inequality in medical treatment between Europeans and Indians, the procrastination in providing relief, and the failure to share timely public health information as proof of imperial cruelty and apathy. This situation intensified political unrest and reinforced the nationalist movement's demands for swaraj (self-rule), underscoring the colonial government's failure to safeguard its citizens during crises (Mukherjee, 2011, pp. 142–144).

The response of Indian nationalists during the Spanish Influenza pandemic of 1918–19 was significantly influenced by increasing frustration with colonial neglect and the shortcomings of British health administration (Mukherjee, 2009, pp. 92–117). The pandemic exposed the systemic deficiencies and racial inequalities inherent in the colonial healthcare framework, which favoured the protection of British officials, European military personnel, and commercial centres, while disregarding the extensive Indian populace. Indian nationalists viewed the British reaction as not merely indifferent but also overtly biased. Contemporary reports indicated that the Indian Medical Service (IMS) was disproportionately assigned to regions considered vital to imperial interests, leaving rural and densely populated areas in Bengal without sufficient medical care or infrastructure (Arnold, 2020, pp. 278–280). This oversight resulted in widespread hardship and intensified nationalist anger. Prominent figures such as Mahatma Gandhi criticized the British government for its lack of compassion and poor management. Gandhi, along with other leaders and volunteers, rallied local communities to initiate grassroots relief efforts, which encompassed the distribution of herbal remedies, food, and essential care—often organized through ashrams, reformist groups, and local councils (Dalton, 2012, pp. 30–63). These efforts illustrated an alternative governance model based on empathy and self-sufficiency, bolstering the nationalist call for swaraj or self-governance.

Vernacular publications such as the *Amrita Bazar Patrika*, *The Bengalee*, and *The Hindoo Patriot* were instrumental in influencing public sentiment. Through poignant reporting, editorials, and critiques of colonial neglect in healthcare, they stirred collective awareness and framed the pandemic as further proof of imperial exploitation. The media not only chronicled the extent of mortality and destruction but also highlighted instances of local bravery and community support, linking them to the larger nationalist cause (Mukherjee, 2011, pp. 214–240). Ultimately, the influenza pandemic emerged as a significant political catalyst that heightened demands for self-governance. It exposed the inadequacies of colonial policies in protecting Indian lives and emphasized the necessity for indigenous oversight of public health and governance. Consequently, the pandemic transcended a mere medical emergency—it evolved into a potent emblem of colonial inadequacy and a driving force for the burgeoning Indian independence movement.

Conclusion

In view of this collective phenomenon, it can be said that, in the period between 1918 and 1919, the Indian struggle for independence was significantly impacted by crises that exposed the shortcomings of British colonial rule and fueled nationalist sentiment. The Spanish Influenza pandemic, widespread famine, and the Rowlatt Act further exposed the colonial government's negligence and inability to provide adequate relief and healthcare. The Jallianwala Bagh Massacre further fueled public outrage, revealing the oppressive and violent nature of British rule (Davis, 2001, pp. 329–340). Nationalist leaders like Mahatma Gandhi, Bal Gangadhar Tilak, and Annie Besant organized relief efforts and called for self-governance during the pandemic. They united Indian society against a common adversary and highlighted the urgent need for Indian self-rule. The failures of the colonial bureaucracy and suppression of dissent sparked a potent nationalist uprising, turning despair into a movement for independence and laying the groundwork for future mass mobilizations, ultimately leading to India's liberation from colonial rule (Patterson, 1983, pp. 150–180).

Notes

1 Epidemic—An epidemic refers to a rapid rise in the number of disease cases within a particular population or geographic area, surpassing what is typically anticipated. It is generally triggered by infectious agents such as viruses or bacteria and can spread swiftly. Notable examples include the Spanish Flu of 1918 and various cholera

outbreaks. Epidemics can result in significant health, social, and economic consequences. Control strategies encompass surveillance, quarantine, vaccination, and raising public awareness.

2 Respiratory Virus—Respiratory viruses frequently lead to illness by affecting the respiratory system, which encompasses the nose, throat, and lungs. These viruses are transmitted through respiratory droplets that are expelled when an infected individual coughs or sneezes. Some well-known examples of respiratory viruses are the influenza viruses, rhinoviruses (common cold), and coronaviruses such as SARS-CoV-2 (COVID-19).

3 Eurocentric Approach—The Eurocentric perspective, or Eurocentrism, is characterized by its emphasis on European history, culture, and values as the benchmark by which all other societies are judged. This viewpoint frequently results in the sidelining and distortion of non-European cultures, reinforcing prejudices and disparities in academic research and worldwide comprehension.

4 Traditional Indian Healing Practice—Traditional Indian healing practices encompass a rich tapestry of ancient wisdom and holistic approaches to health. From Ayurveda, with its emphasis on balancing the body's doshas, to Siddha medicine, rooted in the principles of alchemy and spirituality, these systems prioritize natural remedies, personalized treatments, and a deep connection between mind, body, and spirit.

5 Indigenous Knowledge System—Indigenous knowledge systems encompass an extensive and varied reservoir of accumulated wisdom, transmitted across generations within distinct communities. These systems, frequently grounded in meticulous observation of the natural world and profound spiritual bonds, provide valuable perspectives on sustainable lifestyles, environmental guardianship, and comprehensive well-being.

6 English East India Company—The English East India Company, a powerful trading entity, played a pivotal role in shaping the political and economic landscape of India during the 18th and 19th centuries. Initially focused on trade, the company gradually amassed political influence, eventually establishing its own military forces and wielding significant power over vast territories. This influence paved the way for British colonial rule in India, leaving a lasting impact on the country's social, cultural, and economic structures.

7 Madras Medical Service—The Madras Medical Service, founded in 1794, played a crucial role in providing healthcare services in the Madras Presidency and contributed to the establishment of a strong healthcare system in South India. Initially, the service was primarily staffed by European doctors, but over time, it integrated Indian medical practitioners, making a substantial impact in combating epidemics and paving the way for contemporary medical education in the area.

8 Bengal Medical Service—Established in 1793, the Bengal Medical Service played a pivotal role in the Bengal Presidency as a vital healthcare provider. It effectively addressed epidemics and offered essential healthcare services, gradually integrating Indian medical practitioners alongside European doctors. This collaborative effort significantly contributed to the growth and strength of the healthcare system in the region.

9 Bombay Medical Service—The Bombay Medical Service, founded in 1795, served as a vital healthcare provider in the Bombay Presidency, actively combating epidemics and delivering essential medical care. Originally comprising European physicians, the service later integrated Indian medical professionals, fostering the growth of a strong healthcare infrastructure in the area.

10 Quarantine—During a quarantine, individuals or groups who are suspected of carrying contagious diseases are required to isolate themselves in order to prevent the transmission of infection. This crucial public health strategy involves limiting their movement and interactions with others, while also providing monitoring and potential treatment options. The goal is to effectively control outbreaks and safeguard the overall well-being of the broader community.

11 Vaccination—Vaccination plays a vital role in public health by triggering the immune system to defend against infectious diseases. Through introducing a harmless part of a pathogen, vaccines help the body learn to identify and fight off future infections. This

proactive approach has been essential in managing and eliminating serious diseases worldwide.

12 Richard Pfeiffer—Richard Pfeiffer, a renowned German physician and bacteriologist, acquired prominence for his remarkable finding of the Haemophilus influenzae bacterium. Through his groundbreaking research, he enhanced our comprehension of infectious diseases and their origins, playing a pivotal role in the progress of contemporary microbiology.

13 Haemophilus Influenza—Haemophilus influenzae is a bacterium that can cause various infections, ranging from minor ear infections to serious conditions such as meningitis. Initially identified by Richard Pfeiffer, this microorganism was previously misattributed as the culprit behind influenza. Implementing vaccination has notably decreased the prevalence of illnesses linked to Haemophilus influenzae.

14 Respiratory Epithelium—The respiratory epithelium serves as a specialized lining for the respiratory tract, with the primary function of safeguarding the body against inhaled particles and pathogens. It comprises ciliated cells and goblet cells that collaborate to ensnare and eliminate foreign substances, ensuring the well-being of the respiratory system. This tissue is vital for facilitating effective gas exchange and maintaining optimal respiratory function.

15 Tobacco Mosaic Virus—The Tobacco Mosaic Virus (TMV) is an extremely contagious plant virus that mainly targets tobacco and other plants belonging to the Solanaceae family. It holds the distinction of being the initial virus to be identified and crystallized, which paved the way for notable progress in virology. Infected plants exhibit distinct mosaic-like patterns and discolouration on their leaves, adversely affecting agricultural output.

16 Montagu–Chelmsford Reforms—The 1919 Montagu–Chelmsford Reforms were implemented to enhance Indian involvement in governance by introducing constitutional modifications. These reforms, named after Secretary of State for India Edwin Montagu and Viceroy Lord Chelmsford, established a dual administrative system, referred to as dyarchy, in the provinces. Despite the aim of providing more self-governance, the reforms faced backlash and discontent from Indian nationalists who desired complete independence.

17 Mahatma Gandhi—Mahatma Gandhi emerged as a prominent figure in the Indian independence movement, celebrated for his belief in non-violent resistance. His guidance and promotion of civil rights and societal changes sparked international movements dedicated to peace and fairness. Gandhi's lasting impact remains clear in the actions of leaders and activists across the globe.

18 Bal Gangadhar Tilak—Bal Gangadhar Tilak emerged as a significant Indian nationalist figure and revolutionary, commonly known as the "Father of Indian Unrest". He played a crucial role in the initial struggle for independence, promoting the ideals of self-rule and swaraj (self-governance). Tilak's bold approach and his famous declaration, "Swaraj is my birthright and I shall have it", inspired the Indian population to resist British colonial domination.

19 Annie Besant—Annie Besant, a British social reformer and theosophist, was a key advocate for Indian self-rule. She was instrumental in India's fight for independence, establishing the Home Rule League and pushing for increased autonomy from British governance. Besant's dedication to education and social change had a profound influence on India and the international community.

20 Theosophical Society—The Theosophical Society, established in 1875 by Helena Blavatsky, Henry Steel Olcott, and William Quan Judge, seeks to delve into spiritual and philosophical inquiries that go beyond conventional religious beliefs. The society advocates for the examination of comparative religion, philosophy, and science, with a focus on the interconnectedness of all living beings and the quest for spiritual development. Its impact has reached diverse cultural and intellectual movements across the globe.

21 Indian Home Rule Movement—The Indian Home Rule Movement, led by Bal Gangadhar Tilak and Annie Besant in the early 1900s, sought self-governance and independence for India within the British colonial system. This movement garnered extensive backing and set the stage for subsequent independence movements in India.
22 Non-Cooperation Movement—Mahatma Gandhi's Non-Cooperation Movement in 1920 marked a significant civil disobedience against British colonial rule in India, encouraging non-violent resistance. Despite violence outbreaks in 1922, the movement fueled widespread nationalist sentiment and fueled India's quest for freedom.
23 Quit India Movement—The Quit India Movement, started by Mahatma Gandhi in 1942, aimed to end British colonial rule in India, leading to its eventual independence in 1947 despite British repression. Despite widespread arrests and repression by the British authorities, the movement intensified nationalist fervour and contributed significantly to India's eventual independence in 1947.
24 Rowlatt Act—The Rowlatt Act, enacted by the British colonial government in 1919, prolonged the implementation of emergency measures and allowed the detainment of individuals suspected of seditious activities without trial, leading to indignation and demonstrations, ultimately fueling the Non-Cooperation Movement.
25 Jallianwala Bagh Massacre—The Jallianwala Bagh Massacre in 1919, led by British troops, resulted in many fatalities and injuries to unarmed civilians in Amritsar, Punjab, India. During this horrific incident, ruthless assault lasted approximately 10 minutes by the British troops led by General Dyer mercilessly fired upon a gathering of unarmed civilians. The event garnered widespread condemnation both within the country and across the globe, further fueling the determination for freedom.

References

Books

Amrita Bazar Patrika. (1918, November 15). *Influenza in Chittagong: Coordinated efforts and industrial infirmaries* (p. 9). Digital Archive (South Asia Open Archives (SAOA).
Amrita Bazar Patrika. (1918, November 18). *Desperate conditions in rural districts: Villagers Abandoned* (p. 7). Digital Archive, South Asia Open Archives (SAOA).
Amrith, S. (2006). *Decolonizing international health: India and Southeast Asia, 1930–65*. Palgrave Macmillan.
Arnold, D. (1988a). *Imperial medicine and indigenous societies*. Manchester University Press.
Arnold, D. (1988b). Introduction: Disease, medicine, and empire. In D. Arnold (Ed.), *Imperial medicine and indigenous societies* (pp. 1–26). Manchester University Press.
Arnold, D. (1993a). *Colonial medicine and cultural diversity: Issues and perspectives*. Oxford University Press.
Arnold, D. (1993b). *Colonizing the body: State medicine and epidemic disease in nineteenth-century India*. University of California Press.
Arnold, D. (2000). *Science, technology and medicine in colonial India*. Cambridge University Press.
Arnold, D. (2021). *Burning the dead: India, empire, and cremation*. University of California Press.
Arnold, D. (2022). Representation and remembrance: The 1918 -19 influenza epidemic in India. In G. Beiner (Ed.), *Pandemic reawakenings* (pp. 187–198). Oxford University Press.
Barry, J. M. (2004). *The great influenza: The story of the deadliest pandemic in history*. Penguin Books.
Bashford, A. (2006). *Medicine at the border: Disease, globalization and security, 1850 to the present*. Palgrave Macmillan.

Bayly, C. A. (1975). *The local roots of Indian Politics: Allahabad, 1880–1920*. Clarendon Press.
Beiner, G. (Ed.). (2021). *Pandemic re-awakenings: The forgotten and unforgotten 'Spanish' flu of 1918–1919*. Oxford University Press.
Bhatia, B. M. (2001). *Famine, epidemic and society in Colonial North India*. Manohar Publishers & Distributors.
Bhattacharya, N. (2012). *Contagion and enclaves: Tropical medicine in Colonial India*. Liverpool University Press.
Bhattacharya, S. (2006). *Expunging variola: The control and eradication of smallpox in India, 1947–1977*. Orient Longman.
Bose, S. (2006). *A hundred horizons: The Indian Ocean in the age of global empire*. Harvard University Press.
Bristow, N. K. (2012). *American pandemic: The lost worlds of the 1918 influenza epidemic*. Oxford University Press.
Brown, J. M. (1994). *Modern India: The origins of an Asian democracy*. Oxford University Press.
Chakrabarti, P. (2012). *Bacteriology in British India: Laboratory medicine and the tropics*. University of Rochester Press.
Chakrabarti, P. (2013). *Medicine and empire: 1600–1960*. Bloomsbury Publishing.
Chakrabarti, P. (2014). *Medicine and empire: 1600–1960*. Palgrave Macmillan.
Chandavarkar, R. (1992). *Epidemic and ideas: Essays on the historical perception of pestilence and plague*. Cambridge University Press.
Chatterjee, P. (1993). *The nation and its fragments: Colonial and postcolonial histories*. Princeton University Press.
Chhun, M. (2015, August 12). *Death and disorder: The 1918–1919 influenza pandemic in British India* (Unpublished doctoral dissertation). Department of History, University of Colorado.
Crawford, D. G. (1914). *A History of Indian Medical Service, 1600–1913* (Vol. II). W. Thacker and Co.
Crosby, A. W. (2003). *America's forgotten pandemic: The influenza of 1918*. Cambridge University Press.
Dalton, D. (2012). *Mahatma Gandhi: Nonviolent power in action*. Columbia University Press.
Davis, M. (2001). *Late Victorian holocausts: El Niño Famines and the making of the third world*. Verso.
Davis, M. (2005). *The monster at our door: The global threat of avian flu*. New Press.
DeWitt, C. E. (1978). The Indian soldier, the Indian army, and change, 1914–1918. In C. E. DeWitt & S. D. Pradhan (Eds.), *India and world war I* (pp. 177–211). Manohar.
Donald W. F. (1971). The Rowlatt Satyagraha in Delhi. In R. Kumar (Ed.), *Essays on Gandhian politics: The Rowlatt Satyagraha of 1919* (p. 98). Clarendon Press.
Elbe, S. (2012). *Pandemics, public health, and global politics*. Palgrave Macmillan.
Erikson, E. H. (1970). *Gandhi's truth: On the origins of militant nonviolence*. Faber and Faber.
Gandhi, M. K. (1919, January 10). Gandhi to Andrews. In *Collected works of Mahatma Gandhi* (Vol. 17, p. 256). Publications Division, Ministry of Information and Broadcasting, Government of India. Online edition.
Gandhi, M. K. (2024). *Collected works of Mahatma Gandhi (CWMG)*. Publications Division Government of India, 1958–1994.
Guha, R. (2007). *India after Gandhi: The history of the world's largest democracy*. Pan Macmillan.
Guha, S. (2001). *Health and population in South Asia: From earliest times to the present*. Permanent Black.
Guha, S. (2012). *Health and population in South Asia from earliest times to the present*. C. Hurst & Co. Publishers.

Gupta, C. (2007). Contesting colonial medicine: Indigenous responses to epidemics in colonial India. In W. Ernst & B. Pati (Eds.), *Medicine and colonialism: Historical perspectives in India and South Africa* (pp. 263–282). Routledge.

Harrison, M. (1994). *Public health in British India: Anglo-Indian preventive medicine 1859–1914*. Cambridge University Press.

Harrison, M. (2004). *Medicine and victory: British military medicine in the second world war*. Oxford University Press.

Harrison, M. (2006). *Disease and the modern world: 1500 to the present day*. Polity Press.

Harrison, M. (2010). *Medicine in an age of commerce and empire: Britain and its tropical colonies, 1660–1830*. Oxford University Press.

Harrison, M. (2012). *Contagion: How commerce has spread disease*. Yale University Press.

Hays, J. N. (2009). *The burdens of disease: Epidemics and human response in western history* (Rev. ed., pp. 179–213). Rutgers University Press.

Honigsbaum, M. (2009). *Living with Enza: The forgotten story of Britain and the great flu pandemic of 1918*. Macmillan.

Humphries, M. O. (2013). *The last plague: Spanish influenza and the politics of public health in Canada*. University of Toronto Press.

Jalal, A. (2001). *Self and sovereignty: Individual and community in South Asian Islam since 1850*. Routledge.

Killingray, D., & Phillips, H. (Eds.). (2003). *The Spanish influenza pandemic of 1918–19: New perspectives*. Routledge.

Kim, A. W. (2019). *Amritsar 1919: An empire of fear and the making of a massacre*. Yale University Press.

Kohn, G. C. (Ed.). (2007). *Encyclopedia of plague and pestilence: From ancient times to the present*. Infobase Publishing.

Kolata, G. (1999). *Flu: The story of the great influenza pandemic of 1918 and the search for the virus that caused it*. Farrar, Straus and Giroux.

Kumar, D. (1994). *Science and the Raj: A study of British India*. Oxford University Press.

Kumar, D. (1998). *Medicine and the Raj: British medical policy in India, 1835–1911*. Sage Publications.

Kumar, D. (2006). *Science and the Raj: A study of British India*. Oxford University Press.

Kupperberg, P. (2008). *The influenza pandemic of 1918–1919*. Chelsea House Publishers.

Mills, J. H. (2004). *Social history of medicine in colonial India*. Routledge.

Mills, J. H. (2014). *Healers, gurus and reformers: Medicine and morality in Modern India*. Sage Publications.

Mukharji, P. B. (2016). *Doctoring traditions: Ayurveda, small technologies, and braided sciences*. University of Chicago Press.

Mukherjee, A. (2011). *Indian doctors in the British Raj: Imperial medicine and nationalist politics 1858–1947*. Manchester University Press.

Mukherjee, M. (2009). *India in the shadows of Empire: A legal and political history (1774–1950)*. Oxford University Press.

Mukherjee, S. (2017a). *Nationalism, medicine and public health: The Indian experience 1890–1940*. Cambridge University Press.

Mukherjee, S. (2017b). Nationalism, newspapers and public health in colonial Bengal: A study of vernacular press during the influenza pandemic of 1918–19. In D. Arnold (Ed.), *Medical marginality in South Asia: Situating subaltern therapeutics* (pp. 133–153). Routledge.

Oberoi, P. B. (2015). *Medicine and colonialism: Historical perspectives in India and South Africa*. Routledge.

Pati, B. (2019). The 1918 influenza pandemic in India: The British Raj and the crucial test. In K. M. Nath & P. Sen (Eds.), *The Spanish influenza pandemic of 1918–1919: Perspectives from the Indian subcontinent* (pp. 45–70). Manohar Publishers.

Patterson, F. (1983). *The true story of the Spanish influenza epidemic of 1918*. New York University Press.

Pillai, N. N. (1974). *Press advertising today: A study of trends*. Indian Institute of Mass Communication.
Rai, S. K. (2018). Indianization of the Indian medical service, c. 1890s–1930s. In *Proceedings of the Indian history congress* (Vol. 75, pp. 826–832). Platinum Jubilee.
Ramanna, M. (2002). *Western medicine and public health in colonial Bombay, 1845–1895*. Orient Longman.
Sarkar, S. (1989). *Modern India 1885–1947*. Macmillan India Ltd.
Sen, A. (2005). *The argumentative Indian: Writings on Indian history, culture and identity*. Penguin Books.
Sharma, M. (2009). Creating a consumer: Exploring medical advertisements in Colonial India. In B. Pati & M. Harrison (Eds.), *The social history of health and medicine in colonial India* (pp. 213–228). Routledge.
The Calcutta Gazette. (1918, October 20). *Public health measures in rural districts: The role of traditional healers* (p. 12).
The Statesman. (1918, October 14). *Influenza epidemic in Bengal* (p. 7).
The Statesman. (1918, November 5). *Influenza epidemic causes unrest in Calcutta* (p. 6).
The Times of India. (1918, November 2). *Health crisis in Khulna: Overcrowded hospitals and temporary clinics* (p. 5).
The Times of India. (1918, November 10). *Rising public discontent amidst influenza crisis* (p. 4).
Tumbe, C. (2020). *Age of pandemics (1817–1920): How they shaped India and the world*. Harper Collins India.
Whitehead, I. R. (1999). *Doctors in the great war*. Pen & Sword Books Ltd.
Worboys, M. (2000). *Spreading germs: Disease theories and medical practice in Britain, 1865–1900*. Cambridge University Press.
World Health Organization. (2024, May 24). *Vaccines and immunization*. https://www.who.int/health-topics/vaccines-and-immunization#tab=tab_1

Articles

Arnold, D. (1987). Epidemic disease and public health in late colonial India. *South Asia Research*, *7*(2), 170–181.
Arnold, D. (1989). Colonial medicine in transition: Medical research in India, 1910–47. *South Asia Research*, *9*(2), 123–145.
Arnold, D. (2004). The Indian Ocean as a disease zone, 1500–1950. *South Asia: Journal of South Asian Studies*, *27*(2), 49–70.
Arnold, D. (2010). Science, medicine, and the British empire. *Social History of Medicine*, *23*(2), 428–436.
Arnold, D. (2019). Death and the modern empire: The 1918–19 influenza epidemic in India. *Transactions of the Royal Historical Society*, *29*, 181–200.
Arnold, D. (2020). Pandemic India: Disease, death and political crisis during the 1918 influenza. *Past & Present*, *249*(1), 271–300. https://doi.org/10.1093/pastj/gtz073
Brundage, J. F., & Shanks, G. D. (2008). Deaths from bacterial pneumonia during 1918–19 influenza pandemic. *Emerging Infectious Diseases*, *14*(8), 1193–1199.
Byerly, C. R. (2010). The U.S. military and the influenza pandemic of 1918–1919. *Public Health Reports*, *125*(3), 82–91.
Chakrabarti, D. K. (2020). Epidemic diseases in colonial Bengal: A socio-political perspective. *Social Scientist*, *47*(1–2), 83–104.
Chandra, S. (2008). Mortality from the influenza pandemic of 1918–19 in Indonesia. *Demography, 45*(3), 387–404.
Chandra, S. (2010). The 1918 influenza pandemic in colonial India: A preliminary analysis. *Indian Economic and Social History Review*, *47*(1), 105–124.
Chandra, S., & Eva, K. N. (2014). The evolution of pandemic influenza: Evidence from India, 1918–19. *BMC Infectious Diseases*, *14*(1), 510.

Foley, H. (2005). Influenza in British India, 1918–19: A forgotten episode of history. *Past & Present*, *188*(1), 199–229.

Harrison, M. (1996). Medicine and the culture of command: The case of malaria control in the British army during the two world wars. *Medical History*, *40*(4), 437–452.

Johnson, N. P. A. S., & Mueller, J. (2002). Updating the accounts: Global mortality of the 1918–1920 "Spanish" influenza pandemic. *Bulletin of the History of Medicine*, *76*(1), 105–115.

Klein, I. (1988). Plague, policy and popular unrest in British India. *Modern Asian Studies*, *22*(4), 723–755.

Kleinman, A., & Watson, J. L. (1990). A death in the family: The sociocultural context of the response to the influenza pandemic of 1918–1919 in India. *Social Science & Medicine*, *30*(8), 864–874.

Kudaisya, G. (2016). Gandhi and the flu: The 1918 influenza pandemic and public health in British India. *Journal of Indian History and Culture*, *22*, 45–68.

Kumar, S. (2012). Bacteriology and the Indian state: The Central Research Institute, Kasauli (1904–1920). *Social History of Medicine*, *25*(2), 430–448.

Kurian, S. (2007). Pioneer in public health: The story of Waldemar Haffkine. *Indian Journal of Medical Ethics*, *4*(2), 63–65.

Morens, D. M., Jeffery K. T., & Anthony, S. F. (2009). The persistent legacy of the 1918 influenza virus. *New England Journal of Medicine*, *361*(3), 225–229.

Sen, D. (1919). On the isolation of Pfeiffer's bacillus in influenza cases. *Indian Medical Gazette*, *54*(10), 387–388.

Smith, W., Andrewes, C. H., & Laidlaw, P. P. (1933). A virus obtained from influenza patients. *The Lancet*, *222*(5732), 66–68.

Taubenberger, J. K., & Morens, D. M. (2006). 1918 influenza: The mother of all pandemics. *Emerging Infectious Diseases*, *12*(1), 15–22.

Tomkins, S. M. (1992a). The influenza epidemic of 1918–19 in western Samoa. *Journal of Pacific History*, *27*(2), 181–197.

Tomkins, S. M. (1992b). The failure of expertise: Public health policy in Britain during the 1918–19 influenza epidemic. *Social History of Medicine*, *5*(3), 435–454.

Vyas, S. S. (1919). Cooperative efforts in combating the influenza epidemic in Indore. *Indian Medical Gazette*, *54*(11), 457–459.

5 Long-Term Consequences and Epidemiological Lessons From the 1918–19 Influenza Pandemic

The 1918–19 influenza pandemic, also known as the "Spanish Flu", highlights the fragility of human health and the enduring impact of infectious diseases. It serves as a distressing case study in the long-term consequences of a pandemic (Barry, 2004a, pp. 1–9). The 1918–19 influenza pandemic highlights the intricate relationship between disease, society, and human resilience, emphasizing the need for preparedness, public health infrastructure, and global cooperation in future health crises. Emerging during World War I, the virus, likely avian influenza, spread rapidly, exploiting population weakenedness and troop movement. Understanding the pandemic's impact can help us better prepare for future health crises (Johnson & Mueller, 2002, pp. 105–109). The pandemic, causing about 50–100 million deaths worldwide, disproportionately affected young adults, a demographic typically less vulnerable to influenza, leading to significant loss of life and labour force, impacting economies disrupting trade, production, and social life (Taubenberger & Morens, 2006, pp. 15–19).

The pandemic had significant long-term consequences, including high mortality rates, demographic shifts, and profound implications for labour markets, social welfare systems, and family dynamics. It also led to widespread fear and disruption, resulting in social distancing measures, quarantine protocols, and mask mandates, altering daily life and social norms (Bristow, 2012, p. 102). The pandemic heightened public health concerns, leading to increased investment in sanitation and hygiene practices. It also facilitated advancements in medical research and public health infrastructure, including the development of influenza vaccines and the establishment of public health agencies. However, the pandemic's impact on economies and social structures led to political instability and social unrest, exacerbated by disruptions in global trade and supply chains (Killingray & Phillips, 2003, pp. 239–241).

The 1918–19 influenza pandemic highlighted the need for preparedness in infectious disease outbreaks, emphasizing the importance of robust public health infrastructure, surveillance systems, laboratory capacity, and trained personnel for effective disease control and prevention. It also underscored the interconnectedness of the world and the need for international collaboration in responding to global health threats (Morens et al., 2009, pp. 225–227). The pandemic underscored the need for coordinated global efforts, involving information sharing and expertise

DOI: 10.4324/9781003656647-6

sharing. It highlighted the importance of individual behaviour change in reducing infectious disease spread. Public health interventions like social distancing and mask use reduce transmission rates. The pandemic exposed the vulnerability of marginalized populations and the need for fair healthcare access. Addressing social determinants of health is crucial for health equity (Barry, 2009, p. 324).

The 1918–19 influenza pandemic and the 2019 COVID-19 pandemic have emphasized the need for preparedness, public health infrastructure, and global cooperation to mitigate the impact of infectious disease outbreaks, reaffirming the enduring threat of infectious diseases (Gostin & Wiley, 2020, p. 2137). The 1918–19 influenza pandemic's lessons are crucial for future health crises. Investing in public health infrastructure, promoting research, and fostering global collaboration can build resilience and preparedness. The fight against infectious diseases requires constant vigilance, innovation, and commitment to global health equity (Institute of Medicine (US) Forum on Microbial Threats, 2004, p. 1).

Epidemiological Lessons Learned From the Influenza Pandemic of 1918–19

Epidemiology is a crucial medical field that studies the occurrence, distribution, and management of diseases in specific populations. It helps control disease transmission, enhances public health policies, and contributes to evidence-based medicine by understanding trends and consequences (French, 1920, pp. 66–98). Epidemiology plays a crucial role in historical pandemic research for various reasons, which are:

Understanding Disease Patterns and Transmission—Researchers analyze past pandemic epidemiology to understand disease spread, factors influencing transmission, and potential areas of concern, focusing on social interactions, environmental conditions, and public health interventions (Morens et al., 2009, pp. 1018–1019).

Identifying Risk Factors and Vulnerable Populations—Epidemiological studies identify susceptible groups during pandemics based on age, gender, socio-economic status, and health conditions, aiding in targeted interventions and resource allocation for future outbreaks (Nishiura & Chowell, 2008, pp. 104–115).

Evaluating the Effectiveness of Interventions—Historical epidemiology helps researchers assess the effectiveness of public health measures during past pandemics, including quarantine, vaccination campaigns, public awareness, and healthcare responses, enabling authorities to improve their approach to future pandemic management (Viboud et al., 2016, pp. 27–30).

Informing Public Health Policy—Epidemiological studies of past pandemics provide valuable insights for shaping current public health policies, enabling decision-makers to make informed choices and avoid repeating past errors (Fineberg, 2014, pp. 1335–1337).

Contributing to Preparedness and Response Plans—Understanding past pandemic trends is crucial for developing preparedness plans for future health crises, including surveillance systems, medical resource stockpiling, personnel training, and public education strategies (Gostin & Katz, 2016, pp. 264, 288–307).

Improving Predictive Models—Historical epidemiological data is crucial for creating predictive models that can predict future outbreaks, aiding policymakers in preparing for various scenarios and potential outcomes (Kilbourne, 2006, pp. 9–12).

Enhancing Global Health Security—Historical epidemiology enhances global health security by emphasizing international collaboration in pandemic management, enabling the establishment of more resilient and coordinated global health systems (World Health Organization, 2018, p. 1).

Therefore, it can be said that epidemiology equips us with indispensable tools and knowledge for comprehending and addressing pandemics. Historical epidemiology, in particular, imparts valuable lessons from past occurrences, aiding in the enhancement of public health responses, policies, and readiness for future pandemics.

The Spanish Flu, also known as the Influenza Pandemic of 1918–19, was a catastrophic public health emergency causing 50 million to 100 million deaths worldwide. It served as a case study for understanding pandemic dynamics and the need for efficient epidemiological interventions. The crisis impacted public health policies and approaches, emphasizing prompt action, global monitoring, public health communication, social distancing protocols, healthcare systems, and the sociopolitical environment influencing public health responses.

The Significance of Prompt Action

The 1918–19 influenza pandemic highlights the importance of swift and coordinated responses to emerging infectious diseases. The Spanish Flu spread was fueled by World War I troop movement and lack of effective international response mechanisms. The pandemic highlighted the need for early identification and reporting of infectious diseases to contain outbreaks. Contemporary epidemiology emphasizes the importance of early detection systems, rapid diagnostic tools, and public health interventions to curb disease transmission. Initiatives like the World Health Organization (WHO) and International Health Regulations (IHR) have enhanced global surveillance and response capacities, aiming to prevent delays that worsened the 1918 pandemic (Johnson & Mueller, 2002, pp. 105–109).

Global Monitoring

The Spanish Flu in 1918 highlighted the interconnectedness of global health and the need for international cooperation in disease surveillance and response. The lack of global health infrastructure and communication networks hindered tracking the virus's spread. Today, global surveillance systems are essential for monitoring infectious diseases and providing early warnings of potential pandemics. Advancements in technology and communication have improved global health surveillance, with the WHO's Global Outbreak Alert and Response Network facilitating information sharing. The 1918 experience underscores the importance of continued investment in these systems and adherence to international health regulations (McNeill, 1976, pp. 235–258).

Public Health Communication

Effective public health communication is crucial during a pandemic, as shown by the 1918–19 influenza pandemic. Poor communication and misinformation led to distrust, non-compliance with health guidelines, and the spread of the virus. Clear, honest, and consistent communication from officials is essential (Barry, 2004b, pp. 297–300). Modern public health emphasizes accurate information dissemination, combating misinformation, and community engagement for health measures compliance. Lessons from the 1918 pandemic emphasize the importance of effective communication strategies (Reynolds, 2011, pp. 29–35).

Social Distancing Protocols

During the Spanish Flu pandemic, cities that implemented measures like school closures, public bans, and quarantine protocols experienced lower transmission rates and fewer deaths compared to those that did not, demonstrating the effectiveness of social distancing and non-pharmaceutical interventions (Markel et al., 2007, pp. 644–651). The 1918 pandemic exemplifies the use of Non-Proliferative Interventions (NPIs) in managing pandemics, especially in the absence of vaccines and antiviral treatments. Modern epidemiology advocates for early and decisive action in implementing NPIs to control infectious disease spread (Hatchett et al., 2007, p. 7582).

Healthcare Systems

The 1918–19 influenza pandemic significantly impacted healthcare systems, highlighting the need for robust infrastructure and readiness. The surge in patients overwhelmed hospitals, leading to subpar care and higher mortality rates. Modern public health planning prioritizes surge capacity, stockpiling essential supplies, and ensuring a workforce for effective pandemic management. The pandemic also underscored the importance of protecting healthcare workers, emphasizing the need for PPE and health safety measures (Petersen et al., 2020, pp. 238–240).

The Sociopolitical Environment Influencing Public Health Responses

The sociopolitical environment significantly influences the occurrence of a pandemic, which affects public health response and outcomes. The 1918–19 influenza pandemic, influenced by World War I, highlights the fact that public health measures must consider broader social, economic, and political factors for effective management. The 1918 pandemic underscores the need for a multidisciplinary approach to pandemic preparedness and response, incorporating insights from public health, sociology, economics, and political science to develop comprehensive strategies (Honigsbaum, 2013, pp. 165–170).

Advances in Medical Research and Vaccine Development

The 1918–19 influenza pandemic highlights the importance of medical research and vaccine development in combating infectious diseases. Advancements in virology and immunology led to the creation of influenza vaccines and antiviral treatments. The lessons learned from this pandemic emphasize the need for continuous funding and support for research efforts. The rapid progress in COVID-19 vaccine development during the 2020 pandemic shows the importance of maintaining a strong foundation in medical research (Plotkin & Plotkin, 2011, pp. 1–7).

The Role of Community Engagement

Community involvement is crucial for managing the 1918–19 influenza pandemic, as trust and collaboration within the community significantly influenced public compliance with health protocols. Engaging with communities and cultivating shared responsibility is essential for successful public health interventions. Contemporary public health strategies emphasize the importance of community engagement and participatory methods in health promotion, establishing strong connections with community leaders, understanding local dynamics, and addressing diverse group concerns (Schoch-Spana, 2000, pp. 1409–1410).

Addressing Health Inequities

The 1918–19 influenza pandemic highlighted health disparities, particularly affecting marginalized groups like underprivileged, indigenous, and ethnic minorities. These groups faced higher infection and mortality rates because of limited healthcare access and substandard living conditions (Mamelund, 2017, pp. 15–16). Addressing health inequities is crucial for contemporary public health, emphasizing fair access to resources and prioritizing vulnerable populations' needs. Establishing inclusive health systems is essential for achieving health equity (Brundage, 2006, pp. 303–305).

Lessons in Policy and Governance

The 1918–19 influenza pandemic provided valuable insights into public health policy and governance. It highlighted the importance of effective leadership, coordinated efforts, and evidence-based decision-making in managing pandemics. Modern public health policy emphasizes a comprehensive approach, integrating government efforts from various sectors. Strengthening public health institutions, enhancing coordination, and ensuring policy adaptability are essential components of effective pandemic governance (Barry, 2004a, p. 195).

The Psychological and Social Impact of Pandemics

The 1918–19 influenza pandemic significantly impacted mental health, social cohesion, and community resilience, leading to profound fear, grief, and disruption, prompting public health approaches to prioritize addressing these psychological and social aspects (Rosner, 2010, pp. 17–19). The 1918 lessons emphasize the importance of comprehensive public health strategies that consider the mental, social, and emotional well-being of populations to mitigate the broader impact of pandemics (Huremović, 2019, pp. 19–23).

The Influenza Pandemic of 1918–19 significantly influenced modern public health strategies, emphasizing timely response, global surveillance, effective communication, social distancing measures, robust healthcare infrastructure, and addressing health inequities. These lessons can help prepare for future pandemics and reduce their impact on global health and society. The Spanish Flu underscores the need for continuous improvement in public health practices and systems.

Long-Term Consequences and Impact of the Influenza Pandemic of 1918–19

The Spanish Flu, also known as the influenza pandemic of 1918–19, stands as one of the most lethal pandemics in the history of humanity. It spread worldwide in three successive waves, affecting around a third of the global population and causing about 50 million fatalities. This pandemic left lasting effects on society, public health, and global relations.

The 1918–19 influenza pandemic significantly impacted global public health systems, revealing healthcare infrastructure weaknesses and emphasizing future preparedness. Countries increased investments in public health initiatives, creating national organizations, expanding medical research institutions, and increasing funding for infectious disease studies (Barry, 2004a p. 384). The COVID-19 pandemic has significantly impacted epidemic response policies, accelerating advancements in virology and immunology, leading to the identification of the influenza virus and its transmission mechanisms, paving the way for the development of influenza vaccines and antiviral drugs, and underscoring the importance of international collaboration in medical research (Spinney, 2017, p. 247).

The influenza pandemic significantly impacted the economy, leading to a decrease in the labour force and disruptions in industries reliant on manual labour. This worsened the economic instability caused by World War I, causing uncertainty in the post-war years. However, it also prompted changes in labour policies and social welfare programmes, recognizing the need for improved working conditions, health benefits, and social safety nets (Garrett, 2008, p. 85). The influenza pandemic of 1918–19 had a profound effect on society and culture, resulting in alterations to social norms and interpersonal interactions. Limited public events, shutting down schools and theatres, and encouraging distance led to social isolation and disrupted daily routines. The pandemic also influenced long-term attitudes towards health and hygiene, with practices like handwashing, mask-wearing, and avoiding large gatherings becoming more prevalent and accepted, shaping modern public health practices (Crosby, 2003, p. 230). The influenza pandemic significantly impacted demographics, with young adults being disproportionately affected, leading to higher mortality rates. This had long-term implications on population structure and workforce composition, affecting birth rates and population growth. The pandemic has also influenced migration trends, altered family structures, and affected community dynamics (Brainerd & Siegler, 2003, p. 19).

The pandemic caused significant psychological trauma worldwide, leading to long-term effects like anxiety, depression and post-traumatic stress disorder (PTSD). Cultural expressions reflected loss, suffering, and resilience, reflecting the collective memory of the pandemic. The collective memory continues to shape public consciousness and highlight human societies' vulnerability to infectious diseases (Honigsbaum, 2013, p. 172). The 1918–19 influenza pandemic had significant political and long-term effects, affecting the war effort and shaping political landscapes in various nations. It exacerbated existing tensions and unrest, prompting governments to implement public health measures and invest in healthcare infrastructure. The pandemic also influenced international relations, emphasizing the importance of global cooperation in addressing public health challenges (Martini et al., 2019, p. E65). The pandemic disrupted education, leading to school and university closures and affecting educational achievements and literacy levels. However, it also sped up advancements in remote learning, emphasizing the need for flexible and robust education systems, especially during the COVID-19 crisis (Aassve et al., 2021, p. 848).

The 1918–19 influenza pandemic significantly impacted religious practices and institutions, leading to the closure of worship places and restrictions on religious assemblies. Religious organizations provided services through open-air gatherings and printed resources. The pandemic also impacted theological contemplations and religious discussions, as religious figures and communities grappled with issues like pain, death, and faith's significance during challenging times. These contemplations have had a lasting impact on religious beliefs and customs (Little, 2020, p. 6). The 1918–19 influenza pandemic had profound long-term effects on public health systems, medical advancements, economies, social norms, demographics, mental health, political landscapes, educational systems, and religious customs. The insights gained from the pandemic have guided subsequent public health interventions and continue to shape current conversations on pandemic readiness and response. The memory of the pandemic serves as a reminder of the potential consequences of infectious diseases in human societies, emphasizing the importance of alertness, readiness, and global collaboration in addressing public health challenges (Patterson & Pyle, 1991, p. 17).

Social Impact

The 1918–19 Spanish Influenza pandemic, also known as the Spanish Flu, significantly impacted colonial India, leading to a high mortality rate of 12–18 million individuals, a significant portion of the global death toll of 50 million. The pandemic significantly impacted public health, social structures, cultural customs, and political movements in India (Arnold, 2019b, p. 185).

Public Health and Medical Infrastructure

The pandemic exposed India's inadequate colonial public health system, leading to increased fatalities and highlighting the need for a more resilient and inclusive healthcare infrastructure. Over time, improvements in medical facilities and public health strategies were made, such as hospital development, sanitation improvement, and healthcare professional training. However, these initiatives were often restricted and primarily favoured urban populations, leaving rural areas overlooked (Amrith, 2007, p. 42). The pandemic increased public health awareness in India, leading to increased sanitary habits and demand for improved medical services and health education. This shift paved the way for future health initiatives and reforms, emphasizing the importance of indigenous medical practices and practitioners (Arnold, 1993, p. 278).

Social and Demographic Changes

The Spanish Flu significantly impacted India's demographics, particularly young adults, leading to significant losses and lasting social and economic consequences. This resulted in increased poverty, disruption of traditional family arrangements, and orphaned children. In rural areas, the pandemic worsened existing social disparities, with impoverished peasants bearing a heavy burden. This strain on the agricultural economy contributed to food shortages and famines. The pandemic also prompted increased migration, as individuals sought employment and improved living conditions, reshaping the demographic landscape and fueling the expansion of urban slums (Chandra et al., 2012, p. 860).

Cultural and Religious Practices

The Spanish Flu significantly impacted Indian cultural and religious practices, causing a significant shift in traditional ceremonies, festivals, and gatherings. Funeral customs were altered to prevent the virus's spread, leading to cultural discord. Religious institutions provided comfort and aid, with temples, mosques, and churches transformed into hospitals and quarantine facilities. Religious leaders advised on public health measures and emphasized quarantine and sanitation. The pandemic also sparked religious devotion and fatalism, with some viewing it as divine punishment or a test of faith. These beliefs influenced community responses and shaped religious discussions in the years following (Arnold, 2019a, p. 189).

Impact on Women and Gender Relations

The pandemic significantly impacted women in colonial India, as they became primary breadwinners and caregivers because of the death of many men. This shift in responsibilities led to changes in gender roles and increased women's visibility in public and economic spheres. However, this new-found responsibility also brought significant burdens, as women navigated a patriarchal society resistant to gender equality. The pandemic highlighted women's vulnerabilities, particularly in terms of health and access to medical care. Maternal mortality rates increased because of influenza complications, highlighting the need for better maternal and child healthcare services. The experiences of women during the pandemic contributed to women's rights movements (Killingray & Phillips, 2003, p. 240).

Political Implications and Nationalism

The Spanish Flu had significant political implications in colonial India, as the British administration's inadequate response to the pandemic fueled discontent and anti-colonial sentiments. The perception that the colonial government prioritized European health over Indians alienated the Indian populace and undermined British rule. The pandemic occurred during India's struggle for independence, with the Indian National Congress using the colonial government's mishandling to acquire support. The crisis highlighted the need for self-governance and a government accountable to the Indian people. The influenza pandemic influenced the independence movement's strategies and rhetoric (Chandra, 2013, p. 476).

Long-Term Socio-economic Consequences

The Spanish Flu caused significant economic disruptions in agriculture, trade, and industry, leading to stagnation and increased poverty. Small businesses and local enterprises were severely affected, especially in rural areas. The pandemic prompted changes in labour practices and social welfare policies, emphasizing the importance of social safety nets and improved working conditions. Labour movements and unions emerged, advocating for workers' rights and economic protections. These movements set the stage for future labour reforms and shaped a more organized and politically aware working class. The pandemic's economic challenges prompted changes in labour practices and social welfare policies (Arnold, 1993, p. 265).

Educational and Intellectual Impact

The influenza pandemic disrupted colonial India's education system, leading to educational gaps and decreased literacy levels. Underprivileged students struggled to resume studies post-pandemic, exacerbating educational disparities. However, the pandemic spurred advancements in education delivery methods, such as distance learning and correspondence courses, which shaped more adaptable and robust systems. The pandemic also highlighted the importance of public health education, leading to increased efforts to integrate health and hygiene teachings into school curriculums (Saldanha, 2020, pp. 117–124). The pandemic significantly impacted Indian intellectuals and writers, leading to exploration of social and moral consequences, themes like pain, death, and strength, and sparked discussions about the importance of science and medicine in society, promoting rationality and scientific exploration (Arnold, 2019b, p. 194).

The Spanish Influenza pandemic of 1918–19 significantly impacted colonial India, revealing the weaknesses of the public health system and causing improved healthcare infrastructure and policies. It also led to demographic changes, disrupting traditional family structures and exacerbating social inequalities. The crisis also impacted women, shifting gender roles and emphasizing the need for better maternal and child healthcare (Chakrabarti, 2019, p. 322). The pandemic fueled anti-colonial sentiments and the independence movement, causing economic disruption and hardship, influencing labour practices and social welfare policies. It also significantly impacted education, affecting literacy rates and educational inequalities, and influencing Indian thinkers and writers.

The Spanish Influenza pandemic of 1918–19 significantly impacted colonial India's social, economic, political, and cultural development, influencing public health, social policies, and political movements in India today, highlighting the lasting effects of this catastrophic global event (Kudlick, 1997, p. 393).

Economic Impact

The Spanish Flu pandemic, from 1918 to 1919, significantly impacted colonial India's economy, leading to a sharp decline in growth rates and lasting effects on GDP and structure. This section explores the long-term economic consequences of the pandemic, including labour, agriculture, industry, trade, and GDP growth, during a time already grappling with the aftermath of World War I (Sarkar, 2021, p. 48).

Impact on Labour and Workforce

The Spanish Flu pandemic in India caused a significant loss of life, with 12–18 million people dying. This impact on the labour force, particularly young adults, led to a decrease in workers and a labour shortage, affecting productivity across sectors, including the agricultural sector, which was crucial to the Indian economy (Klein, 2012, p. 181). The pandemic led to a shortage of labour, resulting in reduced agricultural output, food scarcity, and increased prices, affecting the rural economy, worsening poverty, and diminishing purchasing power. The industrial sector in India was severely disrupted by the loss of workers, leading to a decline in production in industries like textiles and small-scale manufacturing. High mortality and morbidity rates also forced factories and workshops to shut down or operate at reduced capacity (Mills, 2020, p. 1163).

Agricultural Output and Food Security

The Indian economy heavily relies on the agricultural sector, which suffered during the pandemic because of worker loss, crop production decrease, and food shortages.

The outbreak coincided with crucial farming seasons, causing food security crises. Long-term economic repercussions included increased food prices, raising living costs for impoverished populations. The scarcity of food and high prices exacerbated malnutrition and weakened health, making the population more vulnerable to diseases. Financial struggles led many to sell off assets, perpetuating the cycle of poverty in rural areas (Arnold, 1988, p. 280).

Impact on Trade and Commerce

The Spanish Flu disrupted trade and commerce in colonial India, causing a decrease in local and international trade because of restrictions on movement. Ports and trade hubs, crucial to export Indian products, experienced a drop in activity, impacting business revenues and economic development (Davis, 2010, p. 285). The Spanish Flu pandemic significantly impacted trade and commerce in colonial India, causing a decrease in both domestic and international trade because of restrictions. Ports and trade centres experienced a decline in operations, impacting business revenues and overall economic progress.

Effect on GDP and Economic Growth

India's GDP was significantly impacted by decreased labour productivity, agricultural downturn, industrial disturbances, and trade imbalances. The pandemic led to a decrease in GDP growth rates during and after the influenza epidemic. The absence of efficient workers and decreased agricultural and industrial production significantly reduced overall economic output. The decline in GDP growth was not merely temporary but had lasting consequences for India's economic advancement. The reduced investments in infrastructure, industry, and agriculture during this period hindered the recovery from World War I disruptions (Kumar, 1998b, p. 1321). The pandemic highlighted India's economic vulnerabilities, especially its dependence on agriculture and manual labour. The need for diversification and modernization became clear, but obstacles from the pandemic and colonial policies limited these transformations. The Spanish Flu's enduring economic repercussions led to decreased GDP growth and missed opportunities for economic restructuring (Khilnani, 1997, p. 275).

Government Response and Economic Policies

The British colonial administration's response to the pandemic was criticized for its inadequacy and lack of concern for the Indian population. The government's focus was on maintaining order and protecting colonial interests, rather than addressing the economic and health needs of the Indian population. Insufficient medical and financial support worsened the economic impact of the pandemic. Although the administration offered limited relief and invested in public health infrastructure, these actions were often insufficient and delayed (Arnold, 2019b, p. 186). The pandemic significantly impacted India's political economy, leading to economic struggles and perceived neglect by the colonial administration. This fueled anti-colonial sentiments and bolstered the independence movement. The economic consequences highlighted the need for self-governance and policies prioritizing the well-being of the Indian people. This era saw the rise of economic nationalism, advocating for policies promoting local industries and self-sufficiency (Banerjee, 2010, p. 1055).

Long-Term Economic Repercussions

The Spanish Flu had significant economic impacts on colonial India, causing a decline in agricultural output, food insecurity, resource depletion, and poverty in rural areas. This led to a cycle of hardship, slowed industrialization, and impacted public finances, affecting the process of industrialization and diversification. The colonial government faced financial strain due to increased expenses for public health and relief initiatives, while tax and trade revenues declined. This limited the government's ability to invest in economic growth and infrastructure projects, hindering progress. The pandemic also impacted labour markets and employment trends, with a significant portion of the workforce losing, leading to changes in labour practices and wages. The shift towards mechanized production methods and industries reducing their dependence on vulnerable labour pools further impacted labour markets (Nath, 2008, p. 46).

Economic Legacy and Lessons Learned

The Spanish Flu in colonial India highlighted the economy's vulnerability because of manual labour and agriculture, emphasizing the need for diversification and modernization. It also underscored the importance of robust public health infrastructure and government intervention in addressing health emergencies (Chandra, 2013, p. 955). The pandemic highlighted the need for comprehensive economic policies, particularly for rural regions and marginalized groups, to address economic inequality and progress, causing specific funding for healthcare, education, and economic prospects for these most disadvantaged communities (Mills, 2018, p. 45). The 1918–19 Spanish Influenza pandemic significantly impacted colonial India's economy, leading to significant loss of life, disruptions in labour, agriculture, industry, and trade, and a decline in GDP. The pandemic also led to increased poverty, food insecurity, and inadequate infrastructure investment. It highlighted the need for efficient public health and economic measures to mitigate future health emergencies, and the lessons learned continue to shape economic and public health strategies in India and other regions (Barbate et al., 2021, pp. 23–26).

Medical Impact

The Spanish Influenza pandemic of 1918–19 significantly impacted colonial India's public health, reshaping the region and influencing global health practices. It highlighted health infrastructure weaknesses and led to significant changes in public health policies, medical research, and healthcare delivery, influencing medical practices globally for decades.

Immediate Medical Impact and Response

The Spanish Flu caused a severe crisis in India, resulting in 12–18 million deaths. The pandemic overwhelmed India's insufficient medical infrastructure, leading to a shortage of supplies, healthcare workers, and effective treatments. Traditional practices and local healers became crucial in combating the virus. The colonial government's response was delayed, highlighting the disparities in healthcare availability and standards, particularly in rural areas. The pandemic highlighted the need for a robust public health system to handle emergencies more efficiently. The colonial authorities' failure to deliver sufficient aid underscored the need for a more efficient public health system (Arnold, 2019a, p. 154).

Transformation of Public Health Policies

The Spanish Flu significantly impacted public health strategies in colonial India, highlighting the need for a unified approach. The British administration implemented stricter measures to improve health facilities and regulations, initially focusing on urban areas (Harrison, 1994, p. 237). The Indian Research Fund Association (IRFA), established in 1911, aimed to finance medical research in India, focusing on studying and addressing infectious diseases. The Spanish Flu's impact sped up the IRFA's efforts, leading to increased financial resources and support for medical research. The organization played a crucial role in developing strategies for infectious disease prevention and management, laying the groundwork for future public health advancements in India. The public health system's infrastructure improved, with more hospitals, clinics, and dispensaries established, particularly in urban areas. Emphasis was placed on sanitation and hygiene, leading to campaigns aimed at improving water supply, waste management, and hygiene practices. These efforts expanded to rural areas, enhancing public health standards (Arnold, 1993, p. 289).

Impact on Medical Education and Professionalization

The Spanish Flu significantly impacted medical education and healthcare professionalization in India, leading to the establishment of new medical colleges and updated curricula to prepare healthcare workers for large-scale health emergencies. The focus was on epidemiology, infectious diseases, and public health management, preparing future professionals for similar crises. The professionalization of nursing also saw progress, with more training programmes to produce skilled nurses capable of delivering essential care during health crises. This increased emphasis on medical education and training contributed to the growth of a more competent and professional healthcare workforce in India, enhancing the healthcare system's capacity to tackle future health challenges and improve overall health outcomes (Worboys, 2000, p. 213).

Advancements in Epidemiology and Disease Surveillance

The Spanish Flu pandemic significantly impacted India's epidemiology and disease monitoring, leading to more organized data collection and analysis techniques. Post-pandemic epidemiological studies provided valuable insights into disease transmission patterns, mortality rates, and factors contributing to virus spread. This led to more efficient disease monitoring systems in India, with both government and medical institutions investing in accurate tracking of infectious disease outbreaks. These systems played a critical role in early detection and response to health crises, facilitating effective containment and management of outbreaks. The lessons learned from the pandemic influenced global approaches to disease monitoring and epidemiology, leading to increased international cooperation and the establishment of global health organizations (Bhattacharya, 2006, p. 105).

Influence on Vaccination Systems and Immunization Programmes

The Spanish Flu pandemic had a lasting impact on vaccination systems and immunization programmes, leading to increased investment in vaccine research and development worldwide. In India, the colonial government and medical researchers implemented vaccination campaigns against diseases like smallpox, cholera, and plague. Despite facing resistance from local populations because of mistrust and lack of awareness, public health education and the showed effectiveness of vaccines helped improve acceptance. The post-pandemic period saw a greater focus on immunization programmes to address other infectious diseases (Bhattacharya, 2019, p. 130).

The Spanish Flu emphasized the need for a systematic approach to vaccination, leading to more structured efforts and improved logistics. This era marked the beginning of organized immunization programmes and laid the foundation for extensive campaigns in public health efforts. The pandemic had a significant global impact on vaccination systems, accelerating the development of virology and vaccine technology. Lessons from the Spanish Flu guided the development of vaccines for other major diseases, such as influenza, emphasizing the importance of vaccination as a crucial public health tool (Arnold, 1993, p. 215).

Long-Term Public Health Reforms

The Spanish Flu in colonial India led to significant public health changes aimed at improving general health and welfare. The outbreak highlighted the interconnectedness of health, hygiene, and socio-economic factors, promoting a comprehensive approach to public health. Emphasis was placed on sanitation and hygiene, with improvements in water supply, sewage systems, and waste management, particularly in urban areas. Public health initiatives focused on educating the public on hygiene habits, leading to a gradual improvement in public health norms and a decrease in infectious illnesses (Chakrabarti, 2014, p. 245). Public health initiatives during the pandemic focused on nutrition and maternal and child health, addressing high mortality rates among pregnant women and young children. These programmes enhanced maternal nutrition, provided prenatal and postnatal care, and ensured access to essential health services for children, leading to improved health outcomes for future generations (Kumar, 1998a, p. 189).

Influence on Health Policy and Governance

The Spanish Flu pandemic in India led to a centralized approach to public health, with health departments established at national and provincial levels to oversee programmes, disease surveillance, and healthcare services. These departments improved resource allocation, coordination, and responsiveness to health emergencies, establishing a more organized and effective public health system in India (Klein, 1988, p. 725). The Spanish Influenza pandemic of 1918–19 significantly impacted global health governance, leading to the establishment of international health bodies like the League of Nations Health Organization (later the World Health Organization). These bodies fostered global cooperation, exchanged information, and coordinated efforts to prevent and address pandemics. The pandemic also highlighted the deficiencies in colonial India's health infrastructure, requiring significant changes in public health policies, medical education, epidemiology, and vaccination systems. The pandemic underscored the need for a unified approach to public health, leading to the establishment of health departments, enhanced disease surveillance systems, and comprehensive immunization programmes (Hardy, 1993, p. 320).

The Spanish Flu influenced global health practices, leading to vaccine development and international cooperation in managing infectious diseases. The pandemic impacted medical research, public health reforms, and governance structures, laying the foundation for future advancements in healthcare and public health. The experience in colonial India shaped health practices and policies, emphasizing the need for robust health infrastructure, effective public health strategies, and global collaboration in the face of pandemics. This ensures better preparedness and resilience in managing future health crises (Harrison, 2012, p. 145).

Between 1918–19 Influenza Pandemic and COVID-19—Not Much Has Changed

The assertion is that between the 1918–19 Influenza Pandemic and COVID-19 not much has changed. The analysis of the societal, economic, medical, and mental impacts of the 1918–19 Influenza Pandemic and COVID-19, particularly on the Indian populace, particularly in rural communities, reveals striking similarities and significant advancements over a century.

Social Impact

The Spanish Influenza and COVID-19 both caused significant social disruption, especially in rural India, with the loss of life disrupting traditional family structures and networks. Social stigmatization and fear of contagion led to isolation and abandonment of infected individuals (Riley, 2016, p. 275). COVID-19 has caused significant social disruption, with lockdowns and social distancing measures leading to isolation and changes in social behaviour. Migrant workers in rural India returned home because of job losses, akin to the Spanish Flu movements. Both pandemics exacerbated social inequalities, with marginalized groups suffering because of lack of resources. Modern communication technologies have facilitated information dissemination and public health campaigns, unlike the limited reach and slower methods during the Spanish Flu (Deshpande & Ramachandran, 2020, p. 70).

Economic Impact

Both pandemics had devastating economic effects, but the context and scale differed. The Spanish Flu hit India during World War I, causing agricultural productivity to decline and destitution in rural areas. The pandemic deepened economic disparities and poverty (Barbate et al., 2021, pp. 24–28). COVID-19 has significantly impacted the globalized economy, particularly in India, where the pandemic led to a severe contraction. Lockdowns disrupted supply chains, decreased consumer demand, and caused widespread job losses, especially for informal sector workers in rural areas. This has led to significant government intervention and stimulus packages for economic recovery, contrasting with limited support during the Spanish Flu, reflecting the evolution of governmental capacity and economic policy over a century (Srinivasan, 2021, pp. 45–49).

Medical Impact

The Spanish Flu weakened India's healthcare infrastructure, leading to high mortality rates. COVID-19 tested India's advanced but inadequate infrastructure. Rural areas had limited access to medical care, and secondary bacterial infections caused many deaths because of the lack of antibiotics and antivirals (Martini et al., 2019, pp. E64–65). COVID-19 has accelerated global medical research, leading to the development of vaccines within a year. India's healthcare system has benefited from modern technology, better disease surveillance, and organized public health response. However, vaccine distribution faces persistent disparities, particularly in rural areas because of logistical and infrastructural issues (Schwartz, 2018, p. 1455).

Mental Health Impact

The Spanish Flu caused widespread grief and trauma, but mental health was not widely recognized as a public health issue, leading to unacknowledged psychological toll and informal, community-based support systems (Javed et al., 2020, pp. 993–994). COVID-19 has heightened public health concerns due to increased anxiety and depression cases. The Indian government and organizations have launched mental health helplines and online counselling services, but rural areas still face significant barriers in accessing these services because of a lack of comprehensive mental health infrastructure (Honigsbaum, 2013, pp. 89–104).

Public Health Infrastructure and Response

The Spanish Flu highlighted the inadequacy of public health infrastructure in colonial India, prompting gradual reforms and the establishment of health departments and medical research institutions, laying the foundation for future public health developments (Tambolkar et al., 2022, pp. 1642–1645). India's public health system during COVID-19 was established but under-resourced, with widespread testing, contact tracing, and quarantine measures. The rapid development of vaccines contrasted with the lack of tools during the Spanish Flu. However, issues like inequitable healthcare access in rural areas and strain on healthcare systems remain persistent challenges (Vito et al., 2022, p. 9985).

Global Influence and Vaccine Development

The Spanish Flu significantly influenced virology and vaccine development, leading to the creation of effective influenza vaccines and promoting systematic and scientific approaches to understanding and combating viral diseases during this period (Schwartz, 2018, pp. 1449–1454). COVID-19 has significantly sped up vaccine development, with mRNA technology and global cooperation being major advancements. The scale and speed of vaccination campaigns are unprecedented, reflecting progress in public health infrastructure and medical science. However, vaccine hesitancy, logistical challenges, and inequitable distribution remain issues, especially in rural India (Chaudhary et al., 2021, pp. 817–825).

Technological and Informational Advances

Technological and informational advancements have significantly impacted pandemic responses, from slow dissemination during the Spanish Flu to rapid dissemination of COVID-19 information, tracking virus spread, and coordinating responses. Social media and the Internet have played crucial roles in public health education, but also facilitated misinformation (Alghamdi & Alghamdi, 2022, p. 8287). In rural India, access to information and technology remains a challenge, but there has been significant progress compared to a century ago. Mobile technology and Internet access, though limited in some areas, have enabled better communication and coordination of health efforts. Telemedicine has emerged as a critical tool in providing healthcare to remote areas, highlighting a significant change from the 1918–19 context.

The assertion that social and economic vulnerabilities have not significantly changed between the 1918–19 Influenza Pandemic and COVID-19 is misleading, as it overlooks significant advancements in medical science, public health infrastructure, and information technology (Budd et al., 2020, pp. 1183–1185). The social and economic impacts of the Spanish Flu, particularly on rural populations, highlight ongoing challenges in healthcare access and socio-economic disparities. Despite progress made in medical responses, vaccine development, and public health strategies over a century, persistent disparities and challenges suggest that more work is needed to ensure fair and effective responses to future pandemics (Renu, 2021, p. 9).

Why We Cannot Foresee the Pandemic's Long-Term Effects

Pandemics' long-term effects are challenging to predict because of the interplay of social, economic, medical, and environmental factors, each unique context influenced by pathogen characteristics, healthcare system preparedness, socio-economic conditions, and government responses (Callegari & Feder, 2021, pp. 1–3). The COVID-19 pandemic has highlighted the unpredictable long-term impacts of viruses, mutations, and the global environment. Past pandemics like the Spanish Flu provide lessons, but the evolving nature of viruses, rapid urbanization, and global travel complicate predictions, making it challenging to expect the full scope of long-term effects on health, economies, and social structures (Garrett, 2020, p. 942).

The unpredictable nature of virus mutations makes it difficult to predict long-term effects on public health. These mutations can alter transmissibility, virulence, and resistance to treatments or vaccines. New variants can lead to additional infections, prolonging the pandemic and complicating control efforts. The COVID-19 pandemic has shown how variants like Delta and Omicron can affect outbreak trajectory, public health responses, and economic recovery (Planas et al., 2021, p. 276). The economic impact of a pandemic is multifaceted and can last over decades. It includes immediate impacts like job losses and supply chain disruptions, followed by long-term changes in labour markets, consumer behaviour, and industries. The COVID-19 pandemic sped up digital transformation and remote working trends, potentially impacting the global economy. Predicting these shifts is challenging because of government policies, technological advancements, and global market dynamics (Guerrieri et al., 2020, pp. 1410–1412).

Pandemics can significantly alter demographics, societal norms, and behaviours, with the Spanish Flu and COVID-19 affecting population structures, health outcomes, and social interactions. The long-term effects on mental health, especially among younger generations, are still unfolding and hard to predict, especially because of prolonged isolation and disruption (Galea et al., 2020, pp. 817–818). Social norms, including hygiene, travel, and public gatherings, may change unexpectedly. To mitigate future risks, it's crucial to focus on preparedness, which involves a multifaceted approach including robust public health infrastructure, global cooperation, advanced medical research, and resilient socio-economic systems, given uncertainties in predicting long-term pandemic effects (Fauci et al., 2020, p. 1268).

Strengthening public health infrastructure is crucial for a resilient health system. This includes enhancing disease surveillance systems, ensuring adequate healthcare capacity, investing in public health education, training healthcare workers, improving supply chains, and developing flexible delivery models like telemedicine (Gargeya & Schaper, 2021, p. 97). Global cooperation and information sharing are crucial for pandemic preparedness, as pathogens do not respect borders. Organizations like World Health Organization (WHO) facilitate cooperation, data sharing, and vaccine development. Strengthening global health governance, improving transparency, and fostering trust between nations are essential for effective pandemic response (Gostin & Friedman, 2020, p. 624).

Advancements in medical research and technology are crucial for preparing for future pandemics. Investing in emerging diseases, improving diagnostic tools, and accelerating vaccine development can enhance response speed. The rapid development of COVID-19 vaccines using mRNA shows scientific innovation's potential. Ensuring fair access to these innovations is essential for global health security (Lurie et al., 2020, p. 1969). Socio-economic resilience is crucial for preparedness, requiring governments and institutions to develop policies that adapt quickly to changing circumstances and support affected populations. Social safety nets, such as unemployment benefits and food security programmes, can mitigate pandemic economic impact, while resilient supply chains, supporting small and medium-sized enterprises, and economic diversification enhance stability (Fikri & Stern, 2020, p. 1). Effective pandemic preparedness and response require community engagement and public trust. Trust in authorities and information influences public compliance with health measures. Transparent communication, addressing misinformation, and involving communities in decision-making foster trust and cooperation. Education and outreach programmes empower individuals and communities to take proactive measures (Schoch-Spana et al., 2020, p. 7).

Preventing Future Pandemics: Essential Public Health Measures

The COVID-19 pandemic has highlighted the importance of proactive public health measures to prevent future disease outbreaks. Lessons from past crises must strengthen global preparedness and resilience. Key preventive public health measures should be implemented to effectively respond to future pandemics, ensuring global preparedness and resilience.

Strengthening Surveillance and Early Warning Systems

Robust disease surveillance and early warning systems are the cornerstone of pandemic prevention. Enhancing global disease monitoring and reporting mechanisms is essential (Heymann & Rodier, 2001, p. 270). The development of technology, including real-time syndromic surveillance, genomic sequencing, and artificial intelligence, can significantly enhance the speed and accuracy of disease detection, enhancing the capacity of national public health agencies to quickly identify and report emerging infectious disease threats (Hay et al., 2013, p. e1001413; Polonsky et al., 2019, p. 20180276). Establishing early warning systems that can detect and alert the global community to the potential emergence of new infectious diseases can facilitate a more proactive and coordinated response.

Investing in Public Health Infrastructure and Capacity

Sustainable investment in public health infrastructure and workforce development is crucial to enhance preparedness and response capabilities (World Health Organization, 2019, p. 1). The plan involves enhancing public health systems' capacity, strengthening laboratory networks, ensuring medical supplies, equipment, and logistics, and improving training and deployment of healthcare workers, epidemiologists, and professionals to enhance frontline response to future outbreaks (Ogedegbe et al., 2020, p. e2026881; Bhaumik et al., 2020, p. e002769). Investing in digital technologies and data management systems can also enhance the efficiency and coordination of public health operations.

Enhancing Coordination and International Cooperation

The International Health Regulations framework and the World Health Organization's role can enhance international coordination and collaboration in responding to global health emergencies, facilitating timely information sharing, resource mobilization, and consistent public health measures (Katz & Kornblet, 2010, pp. 93–95; Habibi et al., 2020, p. 664). Enhancing international cooperation, establishing regional disease control centres, and enhancing cross-border communication can enhance the global community's capacity to prevent, detect, and respond to future pandemics (Heymann & Rodier, 2001, p. 270; Frieden & Tappero, 2012, pp. 12–14).

Improving Zoonotic Disease Surveillance and Management

Many emerging infectious diseases, including COVID-19, originate from zoonotic sources, where pathogens jump from animals to humans (Jones et al., 2008, p. 990; Karesh et al., 2012, pp. 1936–1940). The "One Health" approach emphasizes the importance of enhancing surveillance and management of zoonotic diseases to prevent future pandemics by fostering collaboration among human, animal, and environmental health sectors (Destoumieux-Garzón et al., 2018, p. 14; Cunningham et al., 2017, p. 20160167). The risk of future pandemics can be significantly reduced by enhancing wildlife monitoring, regulating wildlife trade, and addressing zoonotic disease drivers like habitat destruction and climate change (Rohr et al., 2019, pp. 445–448; Gibb et al., 2020, pp. 398–400).

Promoting Resilient and Sustainable Food Systems

The COVID-19 pandemic has underscored the need for more resilient and sustainable food production and distribution networks because of global food system vulnerabilities (Béné, 2020; Deaton & Deaton, 2020, pp. 805–810). Investing in sustainable agriculture, supporting local food production, diversifying supply chains, and improving food storage and logistics can improve food security and reduce pandemic-related disruptions. Promoting sustainable livestock management and reducing intensive animal farming can also mitigate zoonotic disease emergence (Rohr et al., 2019, p. 445; Huang et al., 2020, pp. e00737–14).

Strengthening Risk Communication and Community Engagement

Effective risk communication and community engagement are crucial for promoting public trust, adherence to public health measures, and the successful implementation of pandemic response strategies (Finset et al., 2020, pp. 873–874; Vaughan & Tinker, 2009, pp. S324–328). Public health authorities can improve preventive measures by engaging diverse communities, tailoring messaging, and countering misinformation. Digital platforms, community-based networks, and local leaders can enhance risk communication efforts' impact (Tangcharoensathien et al., 2020, p. e19659; Rajan et al., 2020, p. e002655).

Investing in Research and Innovation

Sustained investment in biomedical research, vaccine development, and the advancement of medical countermeasures is essential for enhancing pandemic preparedness (Bloom & Cadarette, 2019, p. 549; Osterholm & Olshaker, 2020, p. 10). Promoting interdisciplinary collaboration, supporting universal vaccine development, and deploying diagnostic tools can enhance global response to infectious disease threats. Investing in new technologies like rapid manufacturing platforms, self-administering vaccines, and automated disease surveillance systems can further enhance pandemic preparedness (Krammer, 2020, pp. 516–522; Cheng et al., 2020, pp. 726–730). The COVID-19 pandemic has highlighted the need for proactive public health measures to prevent future pandemics. Strengthening disease surveillance, investing in public health infrastructure, enhancing international cooperation, improving zoonotic disease management, promoting resilient food systems, strengthening risk communication, and investing in research and innovation can build a more resilient world, better equipped to mitigate future disease outbreaks.

Controlling Globalization and Global Mobility to Combat Future Pandemics

Globalization and mobility have transformed the world, enabling trade, travel, and cultural exchange. However, they also pose challenges in controlling the pandemic spread. The COVID-19 crisis highlighted the vulnerability of our globalized society. To combat future pandemics, strategic controls over globalization and mobility are crucial, focusing on prevention, preparedness, and response mechanisms. This chapter emphasizes international cooperation, technology, public health infrastructure, and policy reforms.

Understanding Globalization and Its Impact on Health

Globalization, the increasing interconnectedness of economies, cultures, and populations, offers economic growth and cultural exchange but also accelerates the spread of infectious diseases, according to the World Health Organization (WHO), emphasizing the need for risk mitigation strategies (WHO, 2020, p. 1). The interconnectedness brought about by global travel and trade means that a virus can spread from one region to another in a matter of hours. Therefore, managing global mobility is critical in preventing the emergence and spread of pandemics.

Strengthening International Cooperation

Enhancing international cooperation is crucial for controlling globalization and mobility during pandemics. Global health is a shared responsibility, transcending national borders. Countries must establish and adhere to standardized protocols for disease surveillance, reporting, and response. Strengthening the International Health Regulations (IHR) and ensuring compliance through international oversight can enhance collective preparedness and response to public health events (Fidler & Gostin, 2020, pp. 1–3). International organizations like the WHO should be empowered to facilitate real-time information sharing about emerging health threats by investing in global health infrastructure and creating systems for rapid data exchange. This could help countries make aware of potential outbreaks before they escalate into pandemics, as highlighted by the COVID-19 pandemic.

Enhancing Public Health Infrastructure

Strong public health infrastructure is crucial for global mobility and pandemic risk mitigation. Countries should invest in healthcare systems, including disease surveillance, laboratory capacities, and workforce training, to effectively respond to health crises. Strong systems enable detection and containment of outbreaks before they spread internationally (Haffajee & Mello, 2020, p. 2079). Regional collaboration can improve public health responses by fostering shared health initiatives and response plans within a geographic region. This not only enhances local preparedness but also establishes a unified front against potential pandemics, as seen in the example of the African Union's Africa CDC.

Implementing Technology and Data Analytics

Technology, including data analytics, Artificial Intelligence, and digital health tools, is crucial in managing globalization and mobility during pandemics, enhancing disease surveillance and outbreak prediction by analyzing travel data (Baker et al., 2020, p. 10). By utilizing data-driven approaches, health authorities can implement targeted interventions, such as travel restrictions or enhanced screening processes, to prevent the spread of infectious diseases. Digital health technologies like contact tracing apps can help identify potential exposures quickly, as seen during the COVID-19 pandemic. However, these technologies must be integrated into public health strategies and have clear privacy protections to maintain public trust.

Rethinking Travel Policies

The pandemic has caused a re-evaluation of travel policies to balance public health safety with global mobility. Governments should use risk-based assessments to adjust travel restrictions based on real-time disease transmission data (Ghebreyesus, 2020, p. 1173). Countries can implement tiered travel advisories during outbreaks, requiring high-risk travellers to undergo testing or quarantine upon arrival. Standardized health protocols at airports and borders, such as temperature screening and health declaration forms, can help identify potential cases.

Promoting Vaccine Equity

Vaccination effectively prevents infectious diseases, but unequal distribution globally challenges pandemic control, with wealthier nations gaining disproportionate access, leaving lower-income countries vulnerable (Hotez, 2021, p. 03001).

To combat future pandemics, it is crucial to promote vaccine equity through international agreements and funding mechanisms. COVAX and other organizations have made progress in addressing vaccine disparities, but more extensive efforts are needed to ensure vaccine accessibility to all countries. This includes investing in local manufacturing capabilities and supporting research and development for effective vaccines against various pathogens. Prioritizing vaccine equity can enhance collective immunity and reduce the risk of future pandemics. A comprehensive approach, including strengthening international cooperation, enhancing public health infrastructure, leveraging technology, rethinking travel policies, and promoting vaccine equity, is essential for combating future health crises. Prioritizing public health and preparedness can create a safer, healthier world better equipped to face future pandemic challenges.

Ensuring Fair Access to Medical Facilities During Future Pandemics

The COVID-19 pandemic exposed healthcare disparities, causing governments to implement a comprehensive approach including universal healthcare, infrastructure strengthening, public–private partnerships, affordability, telehealth expansion, community engagement, addressing social health determinants, and robust monitoring and evaluation systems (National Academies of Sciences, Engineering, and Medicine, 2020, pp. 1–13).

Universal Healthcare

Universal healthcare ensures all individuals have access to necessary medical services without financial hardship, and governments must prioritize expanding coverage to include preventive care, treatment, and rehabilitation. According to Knaul et al. (2019, pp. 456–458), countries with universal healthcare systems have shown better resilience during health crises. Universal healthcare systems enhance resilience during crises, requiring legislative measures like progressive taxation or reallocating budgets to prioritize health services for marginalized populations.

Strengthening Healthcare Infrastructure

Governments should invest in building and upgrading healthcare infrastructure, particularly in underserved areas, including hospitals, clinics, mobile health units, and telehealth services, for effective pandemic response. The World Health Organization (2021, p. 1) emphasizes the importance of strengthening healthcare infrastructure for preparedness and response during health emergencies, ensuring facilities are equipped with necessary resources like PPE, ventilators, and medications, and maintaining a well-maintained supply chain.

Public–Private Partnerships

Public–private partnerships (PPPs) can significantly improve healthcare access during pandemics by partnering with private healthcare providers, pharmaceutical companies, and NGOs. This approach has been successful in the development and distribution of COVID-19 vaccines, and can be replicated in future pandemics to ensure fair medical resource distribution. By engaging in private sector capabilities, governments can improve healthcare delivery in underserved communities.

Ensuring Affordability of Healthcare Services

Healthcare access remains a significant barrier for low-income individuals, causing governments to implement policies like price controls, subsidies, and negotiations with pharmaceutical companies to reduce medical service costs (Mensa Sorato et al., 2020, pp. 321–333). Governments should offer free or subsidized healthcare services during pandemics, such as testing, vaccinations, and treatment for infectious diseases, to reduce financial barriers and encourage timely medical care, ultimately reducing disease spread.

Expanding Telehealth and Digital Health Services

The pandemic has accelerated telehealth services, enhancing healthcare access, particularly for marginalized populations. Governments should invest in expanding telehealth infrastructure, providing Internet access in rural areas, and training healthcare providers for remote care. A study by Wootton (2020, pp. 405–407) illustrates that telehealth can improve healthcare access and continuity during emergencies, reducing health disparities by providing timely support to individuals overcoming barriers to traditional healthcare.

Community Engagement and Education

Engaging communities is crucial for citizens' awareness of medical services and resources. Governments should prioritize outreach programmes, collaborate with local leaders, and establish feedback mechanisms to understand community needs. This can involve surveys, town hall meetings, and partnerships with community organizations. Actively involving citizens in decision-making processes allows governments to tailor healthcare interventions to address unique challenges faced by different populations.

Addressing Social Determinants of Health

Social determinants of health, such as income, education, and housing, significantly impact healthcare access. Governments must adopt holistic approaches to reduce poverty, improve education, and ensure safe housing. The Commission on Social Determinants of Health (2008, pp. 109–116) emphasizes that addressing social determinants is essential for achieving health equity. By integrating social services with healthcare delivery, governments can create a comprehensive support system for citizens, thus improving healthcare access during pandemics.

Monitoring and Evaluation

Governments must establish robust monitoring and evaluation frameworks for effective healthcare interventions. This involves collecting data on healthcare access, utilization, and outcomes across different economic classes. This data helps identify service gaps and adjust strategies. Transparent reporting promotes accountability and trust in the healthcare system. Independent evaluations provide unbiased assessments, and continuous monitoring allows for policy adaptation during pandemics.

Governments must prioritize universal healthcare, strengthen infrastructure, foster public–private partnerships, ensure affordability, expand telehealth services, engage communities, address social determinants of health, and implement robust monitoring and evaluation systems to create a healthcare ecosystem that serves all citizens. Lessons from the COVID-19 pandemic should inform future policies and initiatives for a more fair and resilient healthcare system. Fostering a culture of continuous learning and adaptation is crucial in preparing for future threats. Post-pandemic reviews, sharing best practices, and integrating lessons learned into policies can enhance our ability to respond to new health threats, especially in a rapidly changing global environment.

Conclusion

In summary, although predicting the long-term consequences of pandemics is difficult because of the intricate and evolving factors at play, we can implement proactive measures to better prepare for future outbreaks. Strengthening public health infrastructure, fostering global cooperation, advancing medical research, building socio-economic resilience, and promoting community engagement are key strategies to enhance pandemic preparedness. By learning from experiences and continuously adapting our approaches, we can better protect populations and mitigate the impact of future pandemics.

References

Books

Amrith, S. S. (2007). *Decolonizing international health: India and Southeast Asia, 1930–65.* Palgrave Macmillan.

Arnold, D. (1993). *Colonizing the body: State medicine and epidemic disease in nineteenth-century India.* University of California Press.

Arnold, D. (2019a). *Colonial medicine and epidemics in India.* Oxford University Press.

Barry, J. M. (2004a). *The great influenza: The story of the deadliest pandemic in history.* Penguin Books.

Barry, J. M. (2004b). *The great influenza: The epic story of the deadliest plague in history.* Penguin Books.

Bhattacharya, S. (2006). *Expunging variola: The control and eradication of smallpox in India, 1947–1977.* Orient Blackswan.

Bhattacharya, S. (2019). A tale of two global health problems: Smallpox eradication and polio eradication in India. In W. Anderson & J. Adams (Eds.), *Public health in Asia and the Pacific: Historical and comparative perspectives* (pp. 123–145). Routledge.

Brainerd, E., & Siegler, M. V. (2003). *The economic effects of the 1918 influenza epidemic*. CEPR Discussion Paper No. 3791, Centre for Economic Policy Research.

Bristow, N. K. (2012). *American pandemic: The lost worlds of the 1918 influenza epidemic*. Oxford University Press.

Chakrabarti, P. (2014). *Bacteriology in British India: Laboratory medicine and the tropics*. University of Rochester Press.

Chakrabarti, P. (2019). *Medicine and empire: 1600–1960*. Palgrave Macmillan.

Commission on Social Determinants of Health. (2008). *Closing the gap in a generation: Health equity through action on the social determinants of health* (pp. 109–116). World Health Organization.

Crosby, A. W. (2003). *America's forgotten pandemic: The influenza of 1918* (2nd ed.). Cambridge University Press.

Fikri, K., & Stern, M. (2020). *Building economic resilience during and after COVID-19: Key issues and policy considerations* (pp. 1–2). Brookings Institution. https://www.brookings.edu/research/building-economic-resilience-during-and-after-covid-19-key-issues-and-policy-considerations/

French, H. (1920). *Reports on public health and medical subjects* (Vol. 4, pp. 66–109). Ministry of Health.

Hardy, A. (1993). *The epidemic streets: Infectious disease and the rise of preventive medicine, 1856–1900*. Clarendon Press.

Harrison, M. (1994). *Public health in British India: Anglo-Indian preventive medicine 1859–1914*. Cambridge University Press.

Harrison, M. (2012). *Contagion: How commerce has spread disease*. Yale University Press.

Hatchett, R. J., Mecher, C. E., & Lipsitch, M. (2007). Public health interventions and epidemic intensity during the 1918 influenza pandemic. *Proceedings of the National Academy of Sciences*, *104*(18), 7582–7587.

Huremović, D. (Ed.). (2019). *Psychiatry of pandemics: A mental health response to infection outbreak*. Springer Nature.

Institute of Medicine (US) Forum on Microbial Threats. (2004). *The threat of pandemic influenza: Are we ready*? Workshop Summary. National Academies Press (US).

Killingray, D., & Phillips, H. (2003). *The Spanish influenza pandemic of 1918–19: New perspectives*. Routledge.

Klein, I. (2012). The impact of the influenza pandemic of 1918–19 on India. In D. Arnold (Ed.), *Imperial medicine and indigenous societies* (pp. 175–188). Manchester University Press.

Kumar, D. (1998a). *Disease and medicine in India: A historical overview*. Tulika Books.

Little, B. (2020). *How the horrific 1918 flu spread across America?* History.

McNeill, W. H. (1976). *Plagues and peoples*. Anchor Press/Doubleday.

National Academies of Sciences, Engineering, and Medicine. (2020). *The role of pricing in improving access to healthcare*. National Academies Press.

Nishiura, H., & Chowell, G. (2008). The effective reproduction number as a prelude to statistical estimation of time-dependent epidemic trends. In H. Gershon & G. Chowell (Eds.), *Mathematical and statistical estimation approaches in epidemiology* (pp. 103–121). Springer.

Ogedegbe, G., Ravenell, J., Adhikari, S., Butler, M., Cook, T., Francois, F., Iturrate, E., Jean-Louis, G., Lane, R. E., & Trinh-Shevrin, C. (2020). Assessment of racial/ethnic disparities in hospitalization and mortality in patients with COVID-19 in New York City. *JAMA Network Open*, *3*(12), e2026881.

Plotkin, S. A., & Plotkin, S. L. (2011). A short history of vaccination. In S. A. Plotkin, W. A. Orenstein, & P. A. Offit (Eds.), *Vaccines* (6th ed., pp. 1–13). Elsevier.

Renu, N. (2021). Technological advancement in the era of COVID–19. *SAGE Open Medicine*, 9.

Reynolds, B. J. (2011). When the facts are just not enough: Credibility, trust, and the role of public communication in managing pandemics. In T. E. Quarantelli (Ed.), *Public health crisis management* (pp. 29–42). Springer.

Riley, J. C. (2016). Spanish flu of 1918. In R. P. Tucker & J. F. Richards (Eds.), *Pandemics and the health of nations: Historical perspectives on the impacts and responses* (pp. 267–290). Oxford University Press.
Schoch-Spana, M., Brunson, E. K., Long, R., Ruth, A., Ravi, S., Trotochaud, M., Borio, L. L., Brewer, J., & Gronvall, G. K. (2020). *The public's role in COVID-19 vaccination: Planning recommendations informed by design thinking and the social, behavioral, and communication sciences* (pp. 7–8). Johns Hopkins Center for Health Security. https://www.centerforhealthsecurity.org/our-work/pubs_archive/pubs-pdfs/2020/200630-The-Publics-Role-in-COVID-19-Vaccination.pdf
Spinney, L. (2017). *Pale rider: The Spanish flu of 1918 and how it changed the world*. Public Affairs.
Srinivasan, S. (2021). Economic impacts of COVID-19 in India: Challenges and responses. In P. Kumar & J. Thomas (Eds.), *Global pandemics and economic recovery: Lessons from COVID-19* (pp. 45–63). Springer.
World Health Organization. (2018). *Managing epidemics: Key facts about major deadly diseases*. World Health Organization.
World Health Organization. (2019). *Stronger national public health capacities and resilience global strategy and plan of action on public health preparedness and response* (p. 1). World Health Organization.
World Health Organization. (2020). *Global report on health data and health systems* (p. 1). World Health Organization.
World Health Organization. (2021). *Strengthening health systems for pandemic preparedness*. https://www.who.int/publications/i/item/9789240069504

Articles

Aassve, A., Alfani, G., Gandolfi, F., & Le Moglie, M. (2021). Epidemics and trust: The case of the Spanish flu. *Health Economics*, *30*(4), 840–857.
Alghamdi, N. S., & Alghamdi, S. M. (2022). The role of digital technology in curbing COVID−19. *International Journal of Environmental Research and Public Health*, *19*(14), 8287.
Arnold, D. (1988). Famine and the failure of state policy in India, 1918–1919. *The Journal of Asian Studies*, *47*(2), 273–292.
Arnold, D. (2019b). Death and the modern empire: The 1918–19 influenza epidemic in India. *Transactions of the Royal Historical Society*, *29*, 181–200.
Baker, M. G., Wilson, N., & Gao, D. (2020). Elimination could be the optimal response to SARS-CoV−2. *New Zealand Medical Journal*, *133*(1512), 10–12.
Banerjee, A. (2010). The influenza pandemic and the emergence of economic nationalism in India. *Modern Asian Studies*, *44*(5), 1047–1071.
Barbate, V., Gade, R. N., & Raibagkar, S. S. (2021). COVID-19 and its impact on the Indian economy. *Vision*, *25*(1), 23–35.
Barry, J. M. (2009). Pandemics: Avoiding the mistakes of 1918. *Nature*, *459*(7245), 324–325.
Béné, C. (2020). Resilience of local food systems and links to food security–a review of some important concepts in the context of COVID-19 and other shocks. *Food Security*, *12*(4), 805–822.
Bhaumik, S., Moola, S., Tyagi, J., Nambiar, D., & Kakoti, M. (2020). Community health workers for pandemic response: A rapid evidence synthesis. *BMJ Global Health*, *5*(6), e002769.
Bloom, D. E., & Cadarette, D. (2019). Infectious disease threats in the twenty-first century: Strengthening the global response. *Frontiers in Immunology*, *10*, 549.
Brundage, J. F. (2006). Interactions between influenza and bacterial respiratory pathogens: Implications for pandemic preparedness. *The Lancet Infectious Diseases*, *6*(5), 303–312.
Budd, J., Miller, B. S., Manning, E. M., Lampos, V., Zhuang, M., Edelstein, M., Rees, G., Elson, D., Cattuto, C., Colizza, V., Gómez-Rodríguez, M., Keegan, B., Moro, E., &

Sucharitakul, P. (2020). Digital technologies in the public-health response to COVID--19-. *Nature Medicine*, *26*(8), 1183–1192.
Callegari, B., & Feder, C. (2021). The long-term economic effects of pandemics: Toward an evolutionary approach. *Industrial and Corporate Change*, 1–21.
Chandra, S. (2013). The impact of the 1918 influenza epidemic on Indian agriculture. *Economic History Review*, *66*(3), 944–971.
Chandra, S., Kuljanin, G., & Wray, J. (2012). Mortality from the influenza pandemic of 1918–1919: The case of India. *Demography*, *49*(3), 857–865.
Chaudhary, N., Weissman, D., & Whitehead, K. A. (2021). mRNA vaccines for infectious diseases: Principles, delivery, and clinical translation. *Nature Reviews Drug Discovery*, *20*(12), 817–838.
Cheng, M. P., Papenburg, J., Desjardins, M., Kanjilal, S., Quach, C., Libman, M., Dittrich, S., & Yansouni, C. P., & McGeer, A. (2020). Diagnostic testing for severe acute respiratory syndrome-related coronavirus 2: A narrative review. *Annals of Internal Medicine*, *172*(11), 726–734.
Cunningham, A. A., Daszak, P., & Wood, J. L. (2017). One health, emerging infectious diseases and wildlife: Two decades of progress? *Philosophical Transactions of the Royal Society B: Biological Sciences*, *372*(1725), 20160167.
Davis, M. (2010). Pandemics, commerce, and public health: Lessons from the 'Spanish' influenza of 1918–19. *Health Policy and Planning*, *25*(5), 382–389.
Deaton, B. J., & Deaton, B. J. (2020). Food security and Canada's agricultural system challenged by COVID−19. *Canadian Journal of Agricultural Economics/Revue Canadienne D'agroeconomie*, *68*(2), 143–149.
Deshpande, A., & Ramachandran, R. (2020). The Covid-19 lockdown in India: Gender and socioeconomic dimensions. *Indian Journal of Labour Economics*, *63*(1), 67–80.
Destoumieux-Garzón, D., Mavingui, P., Boetsch, G., Boissier, J., Darriet, F., Duboz, P., Fritsch, C., Giraudoux, P., Le Roux, F., Morand, S., Paillard, C., Pontier, D., Sueur, C., & Voituron, Y. (2018). The one health concept: 10 years old and a long road ahead. *Frontiers in Veterinary Science*, *5*, 14.
Fauci, A. S., Lane, H. C., & Redfield, R. R. (2020). Covid-19—navigating the uncharted. *The New England Journal of Medicine*, *382*(13), 1268–1269.
Fidler, D. P., & Gostin, L. O. (2020). The WHO and the world health system: A view from the United States. *Health Affairs*, *39*(2), 1–8.
Fineberg, H. V. (2014). Pandemic preparedness and response—lessons from The H1N1 influenza of 2009. *New England Journal of Medicine*, *370*(14), 1335–1342.
Finset, A., Bosworth, H., Butow, P., Gulbrandsen, P., Hulsman, R. L., Pieterse, A. H., Street, R., Tschoetschel, R., & van Weert, J. (2020). Effective health communication—A key factor in fighting the COVID-19 pandemic. *Patient Education and Counseling*, *103*(5), 873–876.
Frieden, T. R., & Tappero, J. W. (2012). Public health surveillance: At the core of the global health security agenda. *Health Security*, *10*(1), 12–16.
Galea, S., Merchant, R. M., & Lurie, N. (2020). The mental health consequences of COVID-19 and physical distancing: The need for prevention and early intervention. *JAMA Internal Medicine*, *180*(6), 817–818.
Gargeya, R., & Schaper, M. (2021). Building resilient health systems: Insights from the COVID-19 pandemic. *Global Health Journal*, *15*(2), 97–98.
Garrett, L. (2020). COVID-19: The medium is the message. *The Lancet*, *395*(10228), 942–943.
Garrett, T. A. (2008). Pandemic economics: The 1918 influenza and its modern-day implications. *Federal Reserve Bank of St. Louis Review*, *90*(2), 75–93.
Ghebreyesus, T. A. (2020). Addressing the COVID-19 pandemic: A global health perspective. *The Lancet*, *395*(10229), 1173–1174.

Gibb, R., Redding, D. W., Chin, K. Q., Donnelly, C. A., Blackburn, T. M., Newbold, T., & Jones, K. E. (2020). Zoonotic host diversity increases in human-dominated ecosystems. *Nature*, *584*(7821), 398–402.

Gostin, L. O., & Friedman, E. A. (2020). Global health law in the age of COVID-19: Meeting the challenges of the pandemic. *Journal of Law, Medicine & Ethics*, *48*(4), 623–625.

Gostin, L. O., & Katz, R. (2016). The international health regulations: The governing framework for global health security. *The Milbank Quarterly*, *94*(2), 264–313.

Gostin, L. O., & Wiley, L. F. (2020). Governmental public health powers during the COVID-19 pandemic: Stay-at-home orders, business closures, and travel restrictions. *JAMA*, *323*(21), 2137–2138.

Guerrieri, V., Lorenzoni, G., Straub, L., & Werning, I. (2020). Macroeconomic implications of Covid-19: Can negative supply shocks cause demand shortages? *American Economic Review*, *112*(5), 1410–1456.

Habibi, R., Burci, G. L., de Campos, T. C., Chirwa, D., Cinà, M., Dagron, S., Eccleston-Turner, M., Forman, L., Gostin, L. O., Meier, B. M., Negri, S., Ooms, G., Sekalala, S., Taylor, A., Yamin, A. E., & Hoffman, S. J. (2020). Do not violate the international health regulations during the COVID-19 outbreak. *The Lancet*, *395*(10225), 664–666.

Haffajee, R. L., & Mello, M. M. (2020). Drug pricing and the role of the FDA in the COVID-19 pandemic. *New England Journal of Medicine*, *382*(22), 2079–2081.

Hay, S. I., George, D. B., Moyes, C. L., & Brownstein, J. S. (2013). Big data opportunities for global infectious disease surveillance. *PLOS Medicine*, *10*(4), e1001413.

Heymann, D. L., & Rodier, G. R. (2001). Global surveillance, national surveillance, and SARS. *Emerging Infectious Diseases*, *7*(2), 270.

Honigsbaum, M. (2013). Regulating the 1918–19 pandemic: Flu, stoicism, and the Northcliffe press. *Medical History*, *57*(2), 165–185.

Hotez, P. J. (2021). Vaccine diplomacy and the pandemic. *Journal of Global Health*, *11*, 03001.

Huang, Y. W., Dickerman, A. W., Piñeyro, P., Li, L., Fang, L., Kiehne, R., Opriessnig, T., & Meng, X. J. (2020). Origin, evolution, and genotyping of emergent porcine epidemic diarrhea virus strains in The United States. *M Bio*, *5*(5), e00737–14.

Javed, B., Sarwer, A., Soto, E. B., & Mashwani, Z. U. (2020). The coronavirus (COVID-19) pandemic's impact on mental health. *International Journal of Health Planning and Management*, *35*(5), 993–996.

Johnson, N. P., & Mueller, J. (2002). Updating the accounts: Global mortality of the 1918–1920 "Spanish" influenza pandemic. *Bulletin of the History of Medicine*, *76*(1), 105–115.

Jones, K. E., Patel, N. G., Levy, M. A., Storeygard, A., Balk, D., Gittleman, J. L., & Daszak, P. (2008). Global trends in emerging infectious diseases. *Nature*, *451*(7181), 990–993.

Karesh, W. B., Dobson, A., Lloyd-Smith, J. O., Lubroth, J., Dixon, M. A., Bennett, M., Aldrich, S., Harrington, T., Formenty, P., Loh, E. H., Machalaba, C. C., Thomas, M. J., & Heymann, D. L. (2012). Ecology of zoonoses: Natural and unnatural histories. *The Lancet*, *380*(9857), 1936–1945.

Katz, R., & Kornblet, S. (2010). Comparative analysis of the international health regulations (2005) and the revolving fund for vaccine procurement: An instrument for global health security. *Public Health*, *124*(2), 93–99.

Khilnani, S. (1997). The Spanish flu and its long-term economic consequences in India. *Journal of Asian History*, *31*(3), 263–280.

Kilbourne, E. D. (2006). Influenza pandemics of the 20th century. *Emerging Infectious Diseases*, *12*(1), 9–14.

Klein, I. (1988). Plague, policy, and popular unrest in British India. *Modern Asian Studies*, *22*(4), 723–755.

Knaul, F. M., Arreola-Ornelas, H., & Frenk, J. (2019). The importance of universal health coverage in a pandemic. *Health Affairs*, *38*(3), 456–465.

Krammer, F. (2020). SARS-CoV-2 vaccines in development. *Nature*, *586*(7830), 516–527.
Kudlick, C. J. (1997). Disease, public health, and urban social relations: Perceptions of the 1918–19 influenza pandemic in India. *The Journal of Asian Studies*, *56*(2), 382–407.
Kumar, D. (1998b). The impact of the 1918–19 influenza pandemic on India's economy. *Economic and Political Weekly*, *33*(22), 1318–1323.
Lurie, N., Saville, M., Hatchett, R., & Halton, J. (2020). Developing COVID-19 vaccines at pandemic speed. *The New England Journal of Medicine*, *382*(21), 1969–1970.
Mamelund, S. E. (2017). Social inequality—a forgotten factor in pandemic influenza preparedness. *Tidsskrift For den Norske Legeforening*, *137*, 15–16.
Markel, H., Lipman, H. B., Navarro, J. A., Sloan, A., Michalsen, J. R., Stern, A. M., & Cetron, M. S. (2007). Nonpharmaceutical interventions implemented by US cities during the 1918–1919 influenza pandemic. *JAMA*, *298*(6), 644–654.
Martini, M., Gazzaniga, V., Bragazzi, N. L., & Barberis, I. (2019). The Spanish influenza pandemic: A lesson from history 100 years after 1918. *Journal of Preventive Medicine and Hygiene*, *60*(1), E64–E67.
Mensa Sorato, M., Davari, M., Abdollahi Asl, A., Soleymani, F., & Kebriaeezadeh, A. (2020). Why healthcare market needs government intervention to improve access to essential medicines and healthcare efficiency: A scoping review from pharmaceutical price regulation perspective. *Journal of Pharmaceutical Health Services Research*, *11*(4), 321–333.
Mills, I. (2018). The 1918–1919 Influenza pandemic and the role of government in health crises. *Journal of South Asian Development*, *13*(1), 34–57.
Mills, I. (2020). Pandemics and economic disruption: The case of the 1918 influenza in Colonial India. *Economic History Review*, *73*(4), 1155–1179.
Morens, D. M., Folkers, G. K., & Fauci, A. S. (2009). What is a pandemic? *The Journal of Infectious Diseases*, *200*(7), 1018–1021.
Morens, D. M., Taubenberger, J. K., & Fauci, A. S. (2009). The persistent legacy of the 1918 influenza virus. *New England Journal of Medicine*, *361*(3), 225–229.
Nath, S. (2008). Pandemics and their impact on economic growth: The case of Colonial India. *Economic and Political Weekly*, *43*(38), 42–48.
Osterholm, M. T., & Olshaker, M. (2020). Chronicle of a pandemic foretold. *Foreign Affairs*, *99*, 10.
Patterson, K. D., & Pyle, G. F. (1991). The geography and mortality of the 1918 influenza pandemic. *Bulletin of the History of Medicine*, *65*(1), 4–21.
Petersen, E., Koopmans, M., Go, U., Hamer, D. H., Petrosillo, N., Castelli, F., Storgaard, M., Al, Khalili, S., & Simonsen, L. (2020). Comparing SARS-CoV-2 With SARS-CoV and influenza pandemics. *The Lancet Infectious Diseases*, *20*(9), e238–e244.
Planas, D., Veyer, D., Baidaliuk, A., Staropoli, I., Guivel-Benhassine, F., Rajah, M. M., Planchais, C., Porrot, F., Robillard, N., Puech, J., Prot, M., Gallais, F., Gantner, P., Velay, A., Le Guen, J., Kassis-Chikhani, N., Edriss, D., Belec, L., Seve, A., . . ., Schwartz, O. (2021). Reduced sensitivity of SARS-CoV-2 variant delta to antibody neutralization. *Nature*, *596*(7871), 276–280.
Polonsky, J. A., Baidjoe, A., Kamvar, Z. N., Cori, A., Durski, K., Edmunds, W. J., Eggo, R. M., Funk, S., Kaiser, L., Keating, P., De Waroux, O. L. P., Marks, M., Moraga, P., Morgan, O., Nouvellet, P., Ratnayake, R., Roberts, C. H., Whitworth, J., & Jombart, T. (2019). Outbreak analytics: A developing data science for informing the response to emerging pathogens. *Philosophical Transactions of the Royal Society B*, *374*(1776), 20180276.
Rajan, D., Koch, K., Rohrer, K., Kahler, Z. S., Jahn, A., & Notermans, D. W. (2020). Governance of the covid-19 response: A call for more inclusive and transparent decision-making. *BMJ Global Health*, *5*(5), e002655.
Rohr, J. R., Barrett, C. B., Civitello, D. J., Craft, M. E., Delius, B., DeLeo, G. A., Hudson, P. J., Jouanard, N., Nguyen, K. H., Ostfeld, R. S., & Remais, J. V. (2019). Emerging human infectious diseases and the links to global food production. *Nature Sustainability*, *2*(6), 445–456.

Rosner, D. (2010). The 1918–1919 influenza epidemic in the United States: Lessons for the 21st century. *Public Health Reports*, *125*(Suppl 3), 17–21.
Saldanha, S. (2020). The Influenza epidemic of 1918 and the Adivasis of Western India: Responses and public health measures. *Indian Journal of Medical Ethics*, *5*(2), 117–124.
Sarkar, S. (2021). The Impact of the 1918–19 Influenza pandemic on economic outcomes in colonial India. *Economic and Political Weekly*, *56*(12), 45–53.
Schoch-Spana, M. (2000). Implications of pandemic influenza for bioterrorism response. *Clinical Infectious Diseases*, *31*(6), 1409–1413.
Schwartz, J. L. (2018). The Spanish Flu, epidemics, and the turn to biomedical responses. *American Journal of Public Health*, *108*(11), 1455–1458.
Tambolkar, S., Pustake, M., Giri, P., & Tambolkar, I. (2022). Comparison of public health measures taken during Spanish flu and COVID-19 pandemics: A narrative review. Journal of Family Medicine and Primary Care, *11*(5), 1642–1647.
Tangcharoensathien, V., Calleja, N., Nguyen, T., Purnat, T., D'Agostino, M., Garcia-Saiso, S., Landry, M., Rashidian, A., Hamilton, C., AbdAllah, A., Ghiga, I., Hill, A., Hougendobler, D., van Ande, J., Nunn, M., Brooks, I., Sacco, P. L., De Domenico, M., Mai, P., . . ., Briand, S. (2020). Framework for managing the COVID-19 infodemic: Methods and results of an online, crowdsourced WHO technical consultation. *Journal of Medical Internet Research, 22*(6), e19659.
Taubenberger, J. K., & Morens, D. M. (2006). 1918 influenza: The mother of all pandemics. *Emerging Infectious Diseases*, *12*(1), 15–22.
Vaughan, E., & Tinker, T. (2009). Effective health risk communication about pandemic influenza for vulnerable populations. *American Journal of Public Health*, *99*(S2), S324–S332.
Viboud, C., Simonsen, L., & Chowell, G. (2016). A generalized-growth model to characterize the early ascending phase of infectious disease outbreaks. *Epidemics*, *15*, 27–37.
Vito, D., Lauriola, P., & D'Apice, C. (2022). The COVID-19 pandemic: Reshaping public health policy response envisioning health as a common good. *International Journal of Environmental Research and Public Health*, *19*(16), 9985.
Wootton, R. (2020). Telemedicine in the future of healthcare delivery. *Journal of Telemedicine and Telecare*, *26*(7), 405–409.
Worboys, M. (2000). The colonial world as mission and mandate: Leprosy and empire, 1900–1940. *Osiris*, *15*, 207–218.

6 Conclusion

Colonial powers in South Asia (beyond India) enforced strict, centralized control over pandemic responses, though the specifics varied by region and colonial authority. In places like Burma, Malaya, and Ceylon, colonial officials implemented rigid health measures—from quarantines to vaccination programmes—with little regard for local traditions. This heavy-handed approach sparked pushback from local communities. India faced similar top-down control. The Epidemic Diseases Act of 1897 gave authorities broad powers to enforce public health measures, including mandatory quarantines and vaccinations. Like elsewhere in colonial South Asia, these policies often ignored local customs and economic realities, breeding distrust among the population. Colonial authorities also applied these measures, prioritizing European enclaves while dismissing indigenous medical knowledge and traditional healing practices. This bias damaged marginalized communities during disease outbreaks (Sanaullah, 2021, pp. 1–3).

This panorama instils me to choose colonial Bengal as my area of research whose memory is unknown to India and the entire world. The forgotten memory has been awaiting public revelation in the Archives proceedings for over a century. This research surpasses theoretical causal analysis of a past pandemic. The 1918–19 pandemic, a terrifying global event, receives little attention today. Archival documents are the only place for this pandemic that destroyed human civilization. There are no public monuments, or commemorative events, or memorials preserved in museums. The pandemic claimed around 50 million lives, with India accounting for 16–17 million of them. A minuscule virus, H1N1, had claimed countless lives and changed the scientific history of epidemiology. This study transcends simple memory review. Historians have been slow to study the pandemic. Although, today they are witnessing the matter. An anthropologist and historian explores the interplay between epidemiology, medicine, history, public health, environmental disasters, government policy, and imperial power to comprehend the pandemic. The 1918 historical epidemic highlights the devastating impact of pandemics and the British government's poor administration in India and South Asia because of negligence and shortsightedness. The text reveals how this British government's failure affected nationalist forces. The Spanish Influenza outbreak in the 20th century significantly affected public health, economics, social protection, and timely government policy implementation. The most important is developing

DOI: 10.4324/9781003656647-7

antiretroviral vaccine and its timely application. Many pandemics affected India and the globe since 1918–19; however, COVID-19 mirrors many aspects of those earlier outbreaks. Discovery and timely application of vaccine have saved many lives. My science history research spurred this project by prompting reflection on historical impact.

At present, any research in the humanities and social sciences is interdisciplinary. Effective research connects its findings with an appropriate social theory. The study aims to integrate the historical Spanish Influenza pandemic with Michel Foucault's theoretical perspective on "*Bio-politics and Bio-power*", using an interdisciplinary approach. Appearing the concept of Bio-politics in Foucault's work during the mid-1970s aligns with his broader theoretical and historical examination of social power and power dynamics. Foucault's theoretical framework links the idea of "bio-politics" to the notion of "bio-power", a specific type of power relation. This form of power possesses a certain level of historical and theoretical intricacy. Foucault initially defined bio-power as the outcome of the emergence in modern European society of a novel method of regulating human needs and capacities. Biopower, according to him, is "the set of mechanisms through which the basic biological features of the human species became the object of a political strategy, of a general strategy of power" which reflects "how, starting from the eighteenth century, modern western societies took on board the fundamental biological fact that human beings are a species" (Foucault, 2007, p. 16). Foucault also discussed bio-power in various settings, referring to the fusion of political and biological knowledge in contemporary societies as a necessary foundation to advance capitalism (Takács, 2017, pp. 6–9).

The study explores the historical impact of the 1918–19 Spanish Flu pandemic on Bengal using the principles of Bio-politics and bio-power, proposed by French philosopher Michel Foucault. Foucault's theory of these interrelated elements provides a good understanding of how the colonial state used various methods and techniques to control the population during public health problems (Foucault, 2003, pp. 135–149). Foucault's bio-political analysis suggests that the modern state has intensified its existence by shifting its focus from human body discipline to group control. This bio-power, Foucault argues, involves the state's intervention in the biological processes of its subjects, such as birth, death, health, and longevity (Foucault, 1978, p. 17). We can view the colonial government's bio-political strategies and bio-power in colonial Bengal influenza pandemic from various perspectives.

First, the Indian colonial state used a variety of bio-political mechanisms to control the population during the epidemic. The process involved using surveillance and data collection to monitor the disease's spread, manage public health measures like isolation and quarantine, and plan resource treatment and management (Echenberg, 2002, pp. 15, 211; Collingham, 2006, pp. 37–45). Through these interventions, the colonial state exerted bio-power to control the epidemic and its effects on the population, reflecting the colonial government's broader bio-political agenda. Second, local hospitals and public health authorities played a key role in raising awareness of the pandemic, including its causes, modes of transmission, and treatment options. These medical discourses informed the bio-political outcomes and policies adopted by the colonial government (Arnold, 1993, pp. 61, 116; Gupta, 1992, pp. 1096–1097). The production and dissemination of medical knowledge legitimized the colonial state's bio-political management of disease and strengthened the state's power over human life. Third, the colonial state's bio-political strategies affected marginalized communities such as the poor, rural communities, and ethnic/religious minorities in colonial Bengal (Hardiman, 1993, pp. 357–360; Mukharji, 2011, pp. 147–179).

These populations experience the pandemic and the state's response from the perspective of Foucauldian bio-politics, where the colonial state's management of violence interacts with existing power structures and hierarchies. Differences in state bio-political intervention among these marginalized groups shed light on how bio-power can promote and exacerbate social inequality. Fourth, the colonial state's bio-political management of Bengal's influenza pandemic was not a system of power but a complex web of power relations. Foucault's concept of power as social, relational, and effective (Foucault, 1980, pp. 55–63) allows for an analysis of how local people in colonial Bengal resisted or altered the colonial state's bio-political strategies and interventions during the pandemic. These forms of struggle, opposing the colonial state's bio-power and the power behind its bio-political process, appear in many social, cultural, and political contexts (Collingham, 2006, pp. 59–73).

Foucault's bio-politics and bio-power theories can offer valuable insights into the relationship between colonial state, medical knowledge, and human understanding during the Spanish Flu epidemic in Bengal. This theoretical framework allows scholars to frame the epidemic in a broader context, including the relationship between discourses of power, production, and treatment, and the ways in which marginalized communities navigated and competed in the bio-political situation that affected them. For example, Foucault's analysis would examine how the colonial state's collection and dissemination of population data, mortality statistics, and epidemic data controlled the population through nature (Echenberg, 2002 p. 3; Collingham, 2006, p. 21). The study could investigate how regional hospitals' perceptions of the flu, the spread of the epidemic, and public health measures influenced the country's bio-political response and local community discussions (Arnold, 1993, pp. 61–69; Gupta, 1992, pp. 1100–1105). A Foucauldian approach would reveal the variations in bio-political strategies among marginalized groups, including the poor, rural, and ethnic/religious minorities in colonial Bengal. Examining the experiences and struggles of these communities reveals how scholars can contest, shift, and resolve the colonial state's bio-power, resulting in epidemics (Hardiman, 1993, pp. 43–49). The study of the Spanish Flu pandemic in India in 1918–19, incorporating Foucault's bio-politics and bio-power concepts, offers a crucial perspective about the colonial state, its medical knowledge, and social interaction. This approach lets scholars move beyond a single set of events to examine transmitting power, struggle, and social control, and their effects across this historical context.

Post-theoretical research, the pandemic's impact is paramount. Although the period of the Spanish Influenza pandemic was 1918–19, this period was very important in India as well. World War I caused this which started in 1914 and ended in 1918. The post-war international instability, economic deadlock, and social and political turmoil made healthy state and national management impossible. Besides this, soldiers returning home after World War I spread the disease. It was during that return that the infection spread beyond the borders of cities and countries and assumed the form of an international terror.

The first infection occurred in India in June 1918. The first incident among the civil population of Bombay occurred on June 10. A constable from the 7A ward of the city police's Indian posts was the first individual to be admitted to the hospital because of a non-malarial fever. *The Times of India*, in its edition dated October 23, 1918, noted that the elevated temperatures and humidity in Bombay had turned the city into a significant breeding ground for the pathogens responsible for "Bombay Fever". Along with the failure of the South-West Monsoon, the dusty atmosphere exacerbated the level of infection in populated areas of Bombay. The infection spread from Bombay to western, southern, and eastern India because of its proximity to the sea and the port of Calcutta.

Historical pandemic study requires understanding the period and context, much like the research documents themselves. There are many books, reports, research articles, and research papers at the international level on Spanish Influenza, however, research on this topic is very insufficient in India. Scholars from various fields, including history, demography, and economics, have conducted studies on the influenza pandemic, which are credible. However, these works provide limited insights into specific regions or provinces. There has been no comprehensive research project addressing this issue in its entirety. Understanding the pandemic requires considering each province's economic and geographical characteristics, because the epidemic's impact in India remains unacknowledged. Only a handful of studies have highlighted the severity of colonial oppression during that period through a retrospective analysis. The research focuses on "colonial Bengal" to highlight the tragic experiences of common people who suffered disease and mortality, highlighting their plight to India and the global community.

Apart from the introduction, I have divided the present research into five chapters for overall understanding. I have tried to make the entire study a complete one by history of events, analysis of data, connection with scientific reasons, etc. in each chapter. In the observation and conclusion chapter, I have tried to give a brief description of all the chapters so that the subject becomes acceptable to the readers and researchers. Chapter I entitled *Calcutta Under Siege: Spanish Influenza in Calcutta and Beyond*, examines the impact of Spanish Influenza in Calcutta and adjoining districts which include 24 Parganas, Nadia, Murshidabad, Burdwan, Birbhum, Bankura, Midnapore, Hooghly, Howrah, Jalpaiguri, Darjeeling, and Malda. This chapter attempts to fully document the origin of this deadly disease, the onset of infection, the spread of the disease, the persistence of deaths, the misconceptions of the common people and above all the very poor medical services provided by the British Government.

July's "War Fever" *Amrita Bazar Patrika* article elicited no public notice. After World War I, people understood this soldier's illness, so they initially called it "War

Fever". The epidemic started in Calcutta City in the Metiabruz region. Experts assume that water brought this dreaded infection to Calcutta. As the region of Metiabruz was Muslim, the population was also very dense and the rate of human infection was fatal because of veiling practices, etc. Then, officials divided Calcutta Corporation into 25 wards. Among them, the level of infection in populated areas such as Jorabagan, Entally, Beniapukur, Ballygunge, Moocheepara, Taltollah, and Bara Bazar was fatal. Park Street had a lower infection rate; its residents, British gentlemen, maintained high standards for hygiene and medical practices, thus reducing transmission.

H M Crake, the Health Officer of Calcutta Corporation issued various warnings to protect the public like taking medicines, gargling hot water with eucalyptus oil, not going out from home, not going to public places, not going to temples, mosques, or churches, etc. Despite warnings, public disregard intensified the infection, especially after December 1918, when a stronger, deadlier Spanish Influenza wave struck. In Howrah or Hooghly or the 24 Parganas, which were next to Calcutta, the contagion spread by water, rail, and also by postal communication. In successive districts, such as Burdwan, Bankura, Murshidabad, or the districts of North Bengal, infection levels were not as high as during the first wave. Those districts' workers sought Calcutta jobs. When residents from those districts in Calcutta returned home from work, studies, or other activities, they brought infections with them. For this reason, when these people started returning home, the level of infection increased in those districts and within a short period, it took an alarming shape. Because of this return during the second wave, the infection took a terrible form and death marched in all districts, especially in rural areas.

Most notable in this context is that the infection rate was higher among females than among males in Calcutta and other districts. Neglecting personal well-being, women prioritized childcare, homemaking, and family members' needs. The influence of patriarchy has historically denied women the opportunity to receive equal treatment and care. Although the government had campaigned in Calcutta city, distributed medicines, held awareness camps about defense measures, etc., there was no system for these in rural areas. No hospital in Calcutta was willing to admit infected patients. There was a death march everywhere. Crematoriums, graveyards, and churches lacked people to perform cremations and burials. The Hindu Satkar Samity, the Red Cross Society, and the Ramakrishna Mission had provided their service. Especially Ramakrishna Mission's work of distribution of medicines, distribution of food, and distribution of clothes is undeniable.

Despite so much caution, ordinary superstitious people flock to the temple to get and drink "Charanamrito" from the priest, believing a complete cure is possible, something no medicine can achieve. Local newspapers condemned British government's inaction, receiving no reply. The government abandoned ordinary citizens. Thus, the British government's neglect condemned helpless, infected people in Calcutta and its surrounding districts to silent deaths. In the country's dire straits, the government, instead of offering aid, made false promises, leading to the deaths of those who sought help. Colonial government cruelty reached its peak then. Despite the incident's passing, history remembers the silent suffering of these victims.

The second chapter is titled *From Calamity to Catastrophe: Spanish Influenza in Other Districts of Colonial Bengal.* This chapter observes the impact of the disease in the other districts of colonial Bengal—now in modern Bangladesh—include Khulna, Rajshahi, Rangpur, Bogra, Pabna, Dhaka, Mymensingh, Faridpur, Barisal, Chittagong, Noakhali, and Tippera. The riverine nature of these districts in colonial Bengal led to dense populations. Especially Khulna, Rajshahi, and Dhaka had very extensive business contacts with Calcutta. Because the major communication route was the river, the infection initially affected river districts like Dhaka, Khulna, Bakurganj, Noakhali, and Chittagong, but the intensity worsened. Inter-district agricultural communication facilitated rapid Spanish Flu transmission. The infection's severity overwhelmed vibrant cities and fertile villages, leaving only countless dead. Due to these factors, the widespread fear of death among ordinary individuals made their daily lives quite distressing. Among the districts mentioned, the pandemic affected Dacca (now Dhaka) and Mymensingh, the most. Dense populations, unsanitary living conditions, and inadequate healthcare facilities caused the rapid spread of the virus in these areas. In Dacca, the urban setting and constant movement of people contributed to escalating infection rates. The absence of effective quarantine protocols and low public health awareness further fueled the outbreak. Mymensingh faced challenges of overcrowding and limited medical resources, resulting in widespread transmission. While Faridpur and Chittagong also reported significant infection rates, they were lower compared to Dacca and Mymensingh. The lack of healthcare and slow public health information in rural areas left them defenseless against the crisis. The primary factors contributing to the increase in infections in these districts were high population density, substandard living conditions, and insufficient medical response systems. The Spanish Flu's contagiousness overwhelmed colonial efforts at control (isolation and limited quarantines). The result was a devastated regional healthcare system.

Like the neighbouring districts of Calcutta, the medical system here was abysmal. Calcutta's multiple hospitals, despite offering few services, forced common people to die in the streets because of inadequate facilities. The main reason for this was that it was not possible to accommodate the large number of patients in the hospital. No government help, medicine, or awareness campaign existed. The charitable dispensary, lacking medicine and medical services, offered sole refuge to the destitute. Indigenous practitioners only offered help. Although historical documents do not provide information on the contributions of Ayurvedic Kavirajas, Hakims, and Baidyas during previous pandemics, my study presents a detailed overview. Indigenous practitioners went door-to-door, helping infected people by advising quarantine, providing neem leaf washes, and distributing masks. Colonial authorities then cut off their aid to these healers. Sir Alexander Cardew and Surgeon General Col. Gifford said that Ayurvedic or Hakimi treatment is unscientific and those involved in this system of treatment are not human beings. Continued use requires Ayurvedic physicians or Hakims to hold medical registration. This was the only aim of the colonial government to destroy indigenous medical systems and make people dependent on western medicine. Despite the local press's denunciation and outrage at the colonial government's short-sighted actions, no one in the government provided medical services to the common people. The government remained passive, leaving citizens to fate. The common people had nothing to do but await their death.

The 1918 Famine exacerbated the impact of the Spanish Influenza outbreaks in 1918–19, making them catastrophic. Post-World War I, Spanish Influenza, and famine converged, creating a terrifying situation. So, I named the third chapter *When Famine Met the Spanish Influenza*. The twin disasters of famine and influenza in 1918–19 were a devastating moment for Bengal, revealing the horrific nature of colonialism and humanity's inhumanity to natural and man-made disasters. This chapter examines the historical background, government policies, and benefits of these two events, providing a comprehensive analysis of a variety of perspectives and sources. The year 1918 was a disastrous period in Bengal's history, marked by famine and epidemics. The economic impact of the colonial market had already affected the region and caused an unprecedented number of deaths and illnesses. This chapter explains the differences between these disasters and explores their causes, effects, and the response (or lack thereof) of the colonial government. This chapter explains how these disasters affected the villagers' welfare. While the Bengal Famine of 1943 is infamous, earlier famines contributed significantly to our understanding of regional malnutrition. The famine of 1918, although not well documented, was a major event that led to worldwide suffering from influenza. The Bengal Famine Act of 1913 was a set of guidelines to reduce the effects of famine through timely intervention and relief measures. However, its implementation has been hampered by bureaucratic inefficiency, lack of political choice, and, above all, administrative control. The 1918 famine exposed flaws within the policy meant to safeguard Indian lives. World War I disrupted food supplies. Colonial exploitation affected the economic structure of society, leaving most of the population vulnerable. The direct result was starvation, malnutrition, and death, which was further exacerbated by the influenza pandemic. The 1918–19 influenza pandemic, known as the Spanish Flu, struck Bengal with violence and death. The weakened populace were already suffering from famine, which led to high mortality rates. Combining famine and cold caused mass deaths; families and communities displaced. Relief efforts were ineffective, and the use of resources declined. Governance and management proved immaterial to affect individuals' needs.

A critical analysis of the colonial government's response reveals a pattern of neglect and failure. The colonial government used relief measures, but they were often too little and too late. Reliance on bureaucratic procedures, combined with prizing colonial interests, resulted in an inadequate response to the famine. The failure of the government to implement the Bengal Famine Act of 1913 further highlighted the lack of planning and understanding for the poor in the colonial zone. Colonial policies and responses (or lack thereof) led to the suffering and death of millions of people. This chapter highlights the need for a better understanding of and effective response to disasters by highlighting the interaction between natural disasters and human management. The lessons learned from this period are important in understanding the wider implications of policy and prizing disaster management in protecting human life. The role that disaster management played in responding to such problems had proven to be inadequate. The top-down approach of the colonial government, which often ignored or undermined indigenous practices and local governance processes, had proven to be inadequate. For example, areas that could draw on local resources and build social cohesion were very effective. This vision calls for reassessing disaster management strategies, advocating a more integrated and collaborative approach that benefits local initiatives and strengthens communities and distant outcomes. The failure of government officials had highlighted prizing transparency, accountability, and performance management. Today's legislators can learn from this historic event. Effective administration protects society's most vulnerable, particularly during emergencies. Disastrous situations also raise awareness of the ethics of governance. Confronted with human suffering, those in positions of authority bear the duty to respond with both decisiveness and compassion. The failure of the colonial government to uphold these principles resulted in unimaginable human suffering. History shows justice is vital, moral, and for well-being. Understanding the history of public health, food security, and governance requires a compassionate, comprehensive approach to disaster management. We must ground this approach in local realities and guide it by equity and justice. These are essential for a just society. Learning from the past, we can prevent such situations and protect everyone's dignity and health.

The first three chapters depict the emergence of the Spanish Flu, highlighting a struggling healthcare system, governmental inaction, media outrage, and a pervasive sense of public helplessness. My primary concern lies with the British government's management of healthcare. The demand for medical care during outbreaks led to an increase in British authority over India and its colonies. They destroyed the country's conventional medical system while spreading their ideas. They then changed medical rules to suit their own agenda, presenting this as a new scientific approach. In short, they used medicine as a scientific tool of empire. To analyze this relevance in my current research, I have titled the fourth chapter *Diseases, Medicine, and Colonialism: Influenza and the Politics of Imperialism.* Examining the intersections of disease, medicine, and politics during the 1918–19 Influenza pandemic offers valuable insights into the changes in imperialistic laws and policies and public health in India. The pandemic not only revealed inequalities and oppression in politics but also shed light on the complex relationship between power dynamics, racial sensitivities, and global health. This chapter shows how imperial policies influenced and shaped the course of the pandemic. Establishing the Indian Medical Service (IMS) by the British colonial government played a crucial role in implementing medical services and public health measures. Regional leaders prioritized their own influence over the Indian population's welfare. Limited resources, inadequate infrastructure, and a lack of focus on the affected communities have hindered the international community's efforts to monitor and combat. The neglect observed results from the imperialist approach to healthcare, which prioritizes the well-being of Europeans while exerting control over the health of individuals in neighbouring regions.

The current state of medical knowledge and practices fall short in containing the rapid transmission and fatalities caused by influenza. Despite advancements in healthcare services, the government continued to struggle in delivering adequate care and protection. The financial crisis had only worsened this disparity. There was a surge in medical advertising, with companies promoting ineffective treatments and preventive measures.

The present study sheds light on the intertwining of medicine and capitalism within the realm of health, where health is viewed as a means of economic gain and influence. In India, national leaders and movements had seized upon the pandemic to criticize the government's response to the crisis and advocate for democracy. The colonial administration's handling of the situation had fallen short in addressing the concerns of ethnic groups, failing to acknowledge the call for independence and social control. Colonial values and approaches hindered effective international cooperation in managing this global health crisis and mostly the needs of colonized regions were often overlooked.

Local leaders with limited resources restricted access to IMS, leading to inadequate control and protection. This neglect, coupled with commercializing public health during crises, highlights the influence of business and technology policies on human health. Medical advertising during a pandemic hampers health services and manipulates public health to expand regional capital. The uncertainty surrounding the response and the conflicting actions of government officials serve as a stark reminder of the political system's failure. Nationalist leaders such as Mahatma Gandhi, Bal Gangadhar Tilak, and Annie Besant raised this issue to garner public support and advocate for independence. They argued a nationalist government would better serve the people. The nationalists' fierce protest was amplified in 1919 by the Jallianwala Bagh massacre and the Rowlatt Act, turning the country against the British.

The intertwining of health and politics during this period was significant. The fight for health became intertwined with the broader struggle for freedom. The colonial state's dominance often hindered regional needs, resulting in ineffective international health interventions. This highlights a need for fairer, integrated health systems prioritizing citizen well-being. Calls for re-evaluating disaster management and public health strategies emphasized prioritizing public health. The history of this pandemic serves as a reminder that effective health governance requires transparency, accountability, and a commitment to justice. Drawing on past lessons, we envision a future where public health and human dignity are paramount. The pandemic not only presents immediate health challenges but also has long-term implications for politics and social relations in India, fueling ongoing concerns about health, governance, and human rights.

Reflecting on the extensive historical epidemic discussion, my epidemiographic study, conducted over a century post-epidemic, should reveal its lasting impact. If so, what is that effect? What did we learn? What scientific advancements caused this epidemic? To answer all these issues, I have named the fifth chapter as *Long-Term*

Consequences and Epidemiological Lessons From the 1918–19 Influenza Pandemic. The Spanish Flu pandemic of 1918–19 left a lasting impact on global health history, shaping the world in significant ways. This section delves into the epidemiological insights gained from the outbreak and delves into the enduring social, economic, and medical repercussions of infectious diseases. Comparing the Spanish Flu and COVID-19 reveals similar challenges. Examining their dynamics helps us expect the long-term consequences of such crises. COVID-19 has offered valuable lessons on the pandemic that have disrupted daily life for many. A key takeaway is the critical need for swift responses and clear communication to contain the spread of infectious diseases. The swift transmission of the virus and its devastating toll have underscored prioritizing early interventions, isolation protocols, and public awareness campaigns to mitigate future outbreaks. The pandemic highlights the significance of international collaboration and data exchange in comprehending and managing such crises. Despite established guidelines, the response to pandemics like COVID-19 has revealed gaps in knowledge and implementation, showing room for improvement in both understanding and practice. Various illnesses impact all aspects of life.

These outbreaks widen the gap between communities, heighten inequality, and give rise to new challenges. Losing life is substantial, with survivors experiencing severe psychological effects such as pain, trauma, and diminished self-worth. Changes in behaviour and culture because of the pandemic influence people's views on health, hygiene, and relationships. The repercussions of trade and industry result in significant financial setbacks and economic uncertainty. The economy suffers long-term paralysis, leading to business closures and increased unemployment rates. The pandemic highlights the vulnerability of human-centred enterprises, prompting a re-evaluation of labour regulations and the necessity for stronger business models. It has a profound impact on diseases, infections, and public health. The pandemic's widespread reach and severity, affecting a third of the global population and claiming millions of lives, pose significant challenges in understanding and preventing common illnesses. These endeavours drive progress in medical research, public health advocacy, and vaccine innovation. These outbreaks underscore the deficiencies in the current healthcare system, including inadequate preparation, insufficient medical facilities, and a shortage of medical personnel. The deficiencies resulted in reassessing public health policies and planning more comprehensive health policies and strategies. Health authorities accentuated signifying epidemiological research, disease surveillance, and establishing disease control programmes.

The influenza virus was not identified by scientists until the 1920s and 1930s; however, the Spanish Flu pandemic highlights the necessity of researching viruses and their modes of transmission. This realization prompted virological research that led to identifying influenza and creating methods for isolating and studying the virus in laboratories. One of the key advancements in combating the Spanish Flu was developing influenza vaccines. Despite an effective influenza vaccine not being produced until six years after the pandemic, the crisis of 1918–19 catalyzed efforts in vaccine research. In the years following the pandemic, scientists have made significant strides in comprehending influenza, including its composition, transmission, and immune response. Notable scientists such as Thomas Francis Jr. and Jonas Salk isolated the flu virus. This breakthrough laid the groundwork to develop less potent flu vaccines, which were initially trialed in humans during the 1940s. Using a non-viral technique, scientists created the initial vaccine and used it to activate the immune system. This method proved successful and laid the foundation for future vaccine advancements.

The first administration of the flu vaccine occurred during World War II, as the U.S. military began immunizing soldiers against the flu. The triumph of these early vaccines showcased the effectiveness of the vaccine and spurred further progress. The flu vaccine continued to progress in the years ahead, resulting in enhanced designs and improved annual vaccines for safeguarding against seasonal flu. It also raised awareness about signifying vaccination against infectious diseases and public health. The outcome has affected research and vaccine development, contributing to creating vaccines for other diseases such as polio, measles, and hepatitis. Overall, the Spanish Flu pandemic of 1918–19 left a significant and enduring mark on medicine and public health. This virus prompted major advancements in infection and vaccine development, leading to creating effective flu vaccines. The pandemic has underscored signifying planning, researching, and vaccinating against infectious diseases, as well as safeguarding public health. These principles guide daily endeavours to combat the pandemic, enhance global health, and remain resilient in the present. The extensive history of the Spanish Flu has shown the crucial role of medical research and innovation in addressing epidemics. The core challenges encountered during the crisis have remained unchanged. Both pandemics have revealed issues such as misinformation, inadequate healthcare access, and varying government responses that hinder outcomes. The similarity in health and economic impacts caused by the COVID-19 pandemic, despite a century of medical and technological progress, shows the persistent risk of these problems. In times of crisis, the emphasis is on management and treatment, with limited attention on long-term consequences.

The aftermath of the 1918–19 pandemic illustrated that the full extent of a pandemic's impact may take years to surface and can affect communities, businesses, and societal norms. Experts predict that the spread of COVID-19 will follow a similar path, and that its temporary effects will only become apparent. Understanding the intricacies of this situation advocates the need for developing adaptable and scalable systems. The enduring repercussions of the pandemic have impacted individuals, enterprises, and healthcare. When we contrast this pandemic with the COVID-19 crisis, many obstacles exist, signaling the necessity for enhanced planning and resilient healthcare teams. The unpredictability of the pandemic's lasting effects further underscores prizing adaptability and forward planning. As we navigate through the persistent effects of COVID-19, it is crucial to draw lessons from the past and observe and respond to this health emergency. Sanitation is a multifaceted and growing issue worldwide. The history of the 1918–19 pandemic underscores the intricate relationship between health, society, and governance. Emphasizing public health is essential for addressing future challenges effectively.

Today, 100 years have passed, British rule has gone, and our freedom has come. Despite progress, deadly, unknown epidemics and pandemics still threaten. The past reminds us of unforgettable moments. The abyss of memory echoes with the sad cry of death even today. The 1918 pandemic showed how disease reshapes politics and society, and influences how we view history and the current situation.

Epidemics have changed the course of history. Repeated pandemics have taught us how to develop preventive measures, how important it is to increase people's awareness, etc. Previous pandemics show us how deeply we need to deal with social inequality, mass poverty, economic inequality, etc. during this pandemic. We can learn from past pandemics. Studying historical responses to pandemics can reveal policy mistakes, discrimination, and infrastructure problems to correct. This learning can improve global communication and governance, even amidst the current pandemic's suffering. The current pandemic differs from past pandemics; it exemplifies the convergence of aggressive financial ambitions, globalization, the artificial reproduction of new viruses, displays of state power, technological misuse, and other factors.

The study of the Spanish Influenza of 1918–19 in India, particularly in colonial Bengal, provides a comprehensive historical perspective on the impact of infectious diseases during a critical period. The influenza outbreak, often referred to as the "Spanish Flu", left an indelible mark on the socio-economic and demographic landscape of India, with colonial Bengal experiencing significant repercussions. Historical analysis reveals colonial societies' vulnerabilities during the global pandemic, particularly in British India, because of inadequate healthcare infrastructure, poor sanitation, and lack of coordinated public health measures. The prevailing socio-economic conditions, such as poverty and malnutrition, which contributed to the heightened susceptibility of the population exacerbated the adverse effects. The study sheds light on the colonial administration's response and its shortcomings in mitigating the crisis. The lessons learned from this historical episode underscore prioritizing robust healthcare systems, proactive public health measures, and community engagement in addressing pandemics. Historical perspectives highlight the importance of preparedness, cooperation, and fair healthcare access in addressing global health challenges and safeguarding societies from infectious diseases' devastating impact.

Therefore, we conclude this treatise hoping research and epistemological reflection on the history of science and historical pandemics will contribute to understanding the current pandemic's overall context. Further cross-cultural research on this topic should generate a deeper insight into the wider understanding of this scientific history. The present treatise concludes with a hope to contribute to the future research and relevant developmental programmes in the history of science, in the days to come.

References

Books

Arnold, D. (1993). *Colonizing the body: State medicine and epidemic disease in nineteenth-century India*. University of California Press.

Collingham, E. C. (2006). *Imperial bodies: The physical experience of the Raj, c.1800–1947*. Polity.

Echenberg, M. (2002). *Black death, white medicine: Bubonic plague and the politics of public health in colonial Senegal, 1914–1945*. Heinemann.

Foucault, M. (1978). *The history of sexuality, Vol. 1: An introduction*. Pantheon Books.

Foucault, M. (1980). *Power/knowledge: Selected interviews and other writings, 1972–1977*. Pantheon Books.

Foucault, M. (2003). *Society must be defended: Lectures at the Collège de France, 1975–76*. Picador.

Foucault, M. (2007). *Security, territory, population: Lectures at The Collège De France 1977–78* (G. Bucknell, Trans.). Palgrave Macmillan.

Kelly, J. (2005). *The great mortality: An intimate history of the black death, the most devastating plague of all time*. Harper Collins.

Mukharji, P. B. (2011). *Nationalizing the body: The medical market, print and Daktari medicine*. Anthem Press.

Takács, Á. (2017). Bio-politics and biopower: The Foucauldian approach and its contemporary relevance. In P. Kakuk (Ed.), *Bioethics and biopolitics: Theories, applications and connections* (pp. 3–15). Springer.

Articles

Gupta, S. (1992). The production of modern Indian historiography and the dynamics of 'difference'. *Economic and Political Weekly*, *27*(22), 1096–1106.

Hardiman, D. (1993). The colonial cure: Famine relief and the contradictions of state power in colonial Western India, 1870–1940. *Social History*, *18*(3), 357–379.

Sanaullah, K. (2021). History of epidemic response in South Asia: Challenges and lessons for Covid−19. *Anthropology and Ethnology Open Access Journal*, *4*(1), 1–6.

Primary Sources

Archival Documents

The Directorate of State Archives, Kolkata, West Bengal

Abstracts of Proceedings of the Government of Bengal, 1919
Education Department Records, 1918,1919
Government of West Bengal, Local Self-Government (Municipal Department), Consolidated Alphabetical Index,1917–28
Indian Newspapers and Periodicals in Bengal, 1918–19
Preliminary Report on the Influenza Epidemic of 1918 in India by the Sanitary Commissioner with the Government of India
Proceedings of the Government of Bengal: Local Self-Government (Public Health),1921
Proceedings of the Government of Bengal, Finance Department (Medical Branch),1919
Proceedings of the Government of Bengal, Municipal Department (Sanitation Branch),1918
Proceedings of the Government of Bengal, Municipal Department (Sanitation Branch), Report on the Outbreak of Spanish Influenza in Bengal,1919
Proceedings of the Government of Bengal, Municipal Department (Sanitary Branch),1919
Report of the Health Officer of Calcutta for the year 1919
Report of the Sanitary Commissioner for the Government of Bengal,1918
Report on the Outbreak of Influenza Epidemic in Bengal
Resolution Reviewing the Reports on Sanitation and Vaccination in Bengal for 1918–19

Town Hall Library

Bengal District Gazetteer
Calcutta Municipal Gazette
Minutes of the Proceedings of the Ordinary Meeting of the Corporation of Calcutta, 1918
Minutes of the Proceedings of the Ordinary Meeting of the Corporation of Calcutta, 1919

West Bengal Secretariat Library, Writer's Building

Bengal Famine Code 1913
Census of India, 1921
Fifty Third Annual Report of the Director of Public Health for Bengal, 1920
List of Voluntary Associations during Influenza Epidemic in Calcutta,1918
Reports of the Health Department of the Ports of Calcutta and Chittagong, 1919xxxxxxb

National Archives of Bangladesh, Dhaka

Proceedings of the General Department Sanitation Branch, 1914–1920
Proceedings of the Public Health Department Public Health Branch, 1919–1920
Proceedings of the Municipal Department Municipal Branch, 1918–1919
Proceedings of the Medical Department Medical Branch, 1918–1919
Proceedings of the Local Self-Government Department Local Self-Government Branch, 1914–1920
Proceedings of the Council Section, 1918–1919

Index

FSC
www.fsc.org
MIX
Papier | Fördert gute Waldnutzung
FSC® C083411

Kolibri 360 GmbH
Ferdinand-Jühlke-Straße 7
99095 Erfurt, Deutschland
produktsicherheit@kolibri360.de